The human brain

The human brain

PAUL GLEES

*Emeritus Professor of Neuroanatomy and Histology
University of Göttingen*

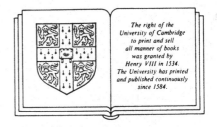

The right of the
University of Cambridge
to print and sell
all manner of books
was granted by
Henry VIII in 1534.
The University has printed
and published continuously
since 1584.

CAMBRIDGE
UNIVERSITY PRESS
Cambridge
New York   *Port Chester*
Melborne   *Sydney*

CAMBRIDGE UNIVERSITY PRESS
Cambridge, New York, Melbourne, Madrid, Cape Town, Singapore, São Paulo

Cambridge University Press
The Edinburgh Building, Cambridge CB2 2RU, UK

Published in the United States of America by Cambridge University Press, New York

www.cambridge.org
Information on this title: www.cambridge.org/9780521249744

First published 1988
Reprinted 1990
This digitally printed first paperback version 2005

A catalogue record for this publication is available from the British Library

Library of Congress Cataloguing in Publication data

Glees, Paul
The human brain.
Bibliography
Includes index.
1. Brain. 2. Neurophysiology. 3. Neuroanatomy.
I. Title. [DNLM: 1. Brain. WL 300 G555h]
QP376.G53   1988   612'.82   87-24248

ISBN-13 978-0-521-24974-4 hardback
ISBN-10 0-521-24974-0 hardback

ISBN-13 978-0-521-01781-7 paperback
ISBN-10 0-521-01781-5 paperback

CONTENTS

PREFACE

Teaching in Cambridge proved to be refreshing and stimulated my wish to write a new version of my earlier book, *Das menschliche Gehirn* (Hippokrates Verlag Stuttgart, 1968), drawing upon my experience and accumulated teaching material. This new book attempts, as did an earlier one (*Experimental Neurology*, Clarendon Press, Oxford, 1961), a combination of morphological data with physiological and neurological studies.

Being primarily a morphologist rooted in the concept of the evolution of structure I have placed the emphasis on structural organisation, but functional aspects, experimental research and clinical findings have been incorporated, broadening the interest for clinical students and for students of neurobiology.

I wish to thank Professor R. J. Harrison, FRS for his offer of a base in his department from which I could take part in departmental teaching and continue my research, supported by the Deutsche Forschungsgemeinschaft; and Dr J. Herbert, Fellow of Gonville and Caius College, and Professor W. J. Macpherson, President of the College, for making me an Associate Member of the College, enabling me to teach some of their medical students. I also wish to thank students from Gonville and Caius College, in particular Pak-Lee Chau, David Evans, Diane Hopper, John Williams and Kwong-Wai Man for their help in various ways. My thanks to Petra Schuba for her great illustrative skill, to Mrs F. Glees for her secretarial help, to Tim Crane and Dennis McBrearty for their expert technical assistance and to Herr G. Koch, Gesellschaft für wissenschaftliche Datenverarbeitung, Göttingen, for help with the index. I am indebted to the staff of Cambridge University Press, for their patience and linguistic support during the preparation of this book.

Cambridge, 1987   *Paul Glees**

* Zentrum Anatomie, Abteilung Klinische Anatomie und Entwicklungsgeschichte, Universität Göttingen.

1
Introduction to brain research

For the last twenty years considerable interest has been directed towards brain research. One of the main reasons for this is the concentration by medical researchers on particular organs with the aims of understanding the total functioning of such organs and of investigating the possibility of their replacement by younger and more efficient units. Kidney and heart transplantation are now practised widely and there has been some success in overcoming initial difficulties caused by organ rejection. One problem is whether the experience gained with these organs could be applied to the central organ, the brain. Let us first consider the technical aspects. The multiple nervous connections that carry sensory input to the brain and outgoing commands to the periphery, the cranial nerves, mean that neural reconnection is biologically and technically impossible (for reasons discussed later). A second problem would be the rejoining of blood vessels. Microsurgery would make this technically feasible, but the brain's continuous need for oxygen would hardly allow sufficient time for transplantation, even if the replacement brain were cooled. But the real problem lies elsewhere. The brain represents the signature of a genetically unique person: the individual fate and memories of that particular person, his or her character. In short, the existence of individual life history makes the idea of a cerebral replacement a foolish and worthless concept.

The idea of brain transplants apart, research on brain structure and function has made great leaps forward since the development of methods for analysing morphological and functional aspects of the brain. Comparative biology and evolutionary principles soon showed that the human brain shared common features with the brains of all vertebrates. Ludwig Edinger (1904), C. U. Ariens-Kappers, G. C. Huber and Elisabeth Crosby (1936) explored and analysed these common neurological features and it became clear that while the human brain had a larger cerebral cortex, it contained no specifically human features. The macroscopic constructional principles of the vertebrate brain, especially those of primates, have a common organisational layout and differ only in the relative proportions of certain regions. The microscopic features – the wiring up of the components – appear to obey the same rules of microcircuitry in all vertebrates. The similarity in basic connections and in ultrastructure, especially among the primates, allows the full transfer and application of comparative morphological, neurophysiological and neurobiochemical studies to the human brain. This comparative approach is endorsed by evolutionary principles, which show common vertebrate features repeated in individual embryogenesis. With these advances, human neurological diseases have become better understood, and neurosurgery has gained new tools and insight, using extensively the microtechniques of animal experimentation. Psychiatry in particular has benefited from advances in neurobiochemistry and neuropharmacology.

Psychiatry needed these advances most, having been tied down for centuries by religious and philosophical concepts. A prime mover in this field was Paul Flechsig (1847–1929), best known for his studies on myelogenesis in the brain (Flechsig, 1927) and the first medical man appointed to the Chair in Psychiatry at the University of Leipzig. His predecessor, Heinroth, was a philosopher by training and maintained that mental events were independent of bodily processes, being a manifestation of the soul! Flechsig, however, was trained by the eminent physiologist Ludwig, whose pupils included the Russian experimental physiologist Pavlov. Flechsig was determined to break away from his contemporaries' belief in the mystical cause of mental diseases, and concentrated his researches on the maturation of the brain tracts and on neuropathological aspects. He was working during a period of vigorous morphological research, when the Spanish school of neurohistology of Ramón y Cajal and the Italian Golgi were both making rapid advances in the structural analysis of the nervous system. In Germany, scientists such as Edinger, Held,

Weigert, Nissl and Vogt devoted their whole lives to unravelling some of the basic components of the nervous system, some workers using the comparative approach, others the clinical. In England, in a similar endeavour, physiological and clinical methods were used by Ferrier, Sherrington and Horsley, and were later refined and developed by Adrian. The era which started around 1870 with Fritsch, Hitzig and Ferrier and ended in the 1950s with Adrian and Penfield can now be seen as the classical period of brain research. Its results and techniques have been summarised by Glees (1961a,b,c). After this period, methodology advanced rapidly, with the application of highly refined neurophysiological methods such as microelectrode recordings and tracer studies of brain metabolism using radioactively labelled substances such as glucose. The scope of morphology gained considerably from electron microscopy and studies of the transport of labelled substances or compounds of low molecular weight along the axon, towards the periphery (downstream) or towards the cell body (upstream).

2
Evolution of the nervous system

Vertebrate evolution
General considerations

Organic evolution on Earth began in the border zone between the Earth's crust and its atmosphere. The interaction of solar energy with the Earth's surface, largely covered by the oceanic basins, resulted in mainly salt solutions. These would become an essential component of life and, eventually, of nervous systems. If we accept the view that the oceans and their rocky surroundings became the fertile grounds for organic evolution, then rock formations and marine sediments become important witnesses for evolution. The remains of early life in rocks and sediments had been known for a long time but it was only in the second half of the nineteenth century that their significance was recognised by science as documentary evidence of the evolution of life on Earth. Up to that time it was the teaching of the Church that the Earth and its inhabitants were created by a single act of God about 4000 years ago. This view was also accepted by scientists, although later modified by the French anatomist Cuvier (1769–1832) who assumed several creative acts in order to explain the different fossil findings in different geological periods. By the fifteenth century the study of mineralogy had attracted Bauer, a German doctor, who studied closely excavations made for the mining industry and who laid the foundation for a close relation between evolution and geology. Berry (1968) has given an excellent account of the interrelation between the exploration of the Earth's crust and the understanding of evolution. Figure 2.1 shows the evolution of animal groups in relation to the geological history of the Earth. It shows that the beginning of vertebrate life was in the Cambrian period. Little evidence of life in the Precambrian period is available.

Considering evolution in general, it can be said that animal life started in a simple form and that early animals and plants shared common features. Animals and plants are constructed for survival and propagation. The need for adaptation to survive in varying environmental conditions shows the advantage of simple construction. A high degree of specialisation, which can arise from refinements of simple forms, may be disadvantageous in that such specialised organisms are less capable of adaptation to changing environmental conditions; this might explain the extinction of some highly specialised animal species.

The diversity of animal and plant life demands an explanation, which appears to be supplied by the concept of evolution. The variety of life as we see it today is not the product of one act of Creation but is the outcome of continuous change of modifiable species. This continuous remodelling of life, happening slowly or intermittently during geological periods, is generally accepted, but the factors which cause these evolutionary processes are still debated. Since Darwin proposed his theories, two factors appear to be the major ones:

1. Natural selection: survival of the fittest and the propagation of certain advantages – anatomical, physiological or biochemical – in the offspring.
2. Genetic mutations affecting germ cells, caused by exposure to cosmic radiation or other high-energy particles.

These genetic effects were shown to be present by Müller (see Butler, 1954) in his experiments with the fruit fly (*Drosophila*), using X-rays to affect the germ cells. The significance of germ mutation for evolution has been put forward convincingly by the Swiss zoologist Portmann, and his book *Introduction into Comparative Morphology of Vertebrates* should be consulted.

The concept of the origin of life from non-living matter and its development to more and more complicated forms was perceived by the Ancient Greeks. The term evolution usually includes a successive constructional improvement; this is in itself a justifiable assumption but does not need to be the case.

During the eighteenth and nineteenth centuries the study of fossil remains recovered from different sedimentation layers of the Earth's crust became popular. These studies led to the concept of evolution in the animal world. This was, however, rejected by Baron Cuvier (1769–1832), who postulated a series of creative acts. A comprehensive view of evolution, in particular by selective pressure, is due to Darwin (1809–1882) (Darwin, 1859), Huxley (1825–1895) and Haeckel (1834–1919) (Haeckel, 1874). Darwin's work and writings are well known, have been amply illustrated by excellent television series, and need only a brief comment here. Darwinian evolution is a slow modelling process of animals and plants and is closely related to geological history. The interconnection of great land masses favours an exchange of life forms, while separation from land masses, on islands such as Australia and the Galapagos Islands (Darwin, 1836), leads to survival of species and specialised forms not seen on the larger land masses. The fossil record and the survival of such 'primitive' forms as marsupials are important evidence for evolution.

The concept of evolution is not without its critics, however. Among them was the late Arthur Koestler, who found the principle of natural selection and survival of the fittest unsatisfactory and believed that Lamarck's view on the inheritance of acquired characteristics still had some justification. Koestler stressed most emphatically his conviction that evolution does not act blindly but follows definite biological and constructive principles. Koestler's (1967) book, *The Ghost in the Machine*, should be consulted for its stimulating and thoughtful approach to evolution and Man's creativity. Koestler's arguments against Darwin's views are, however, often the products of philosophical humanitarian motives rather than critical scientific reasoning.

An important introduction to the history of evolutionary thinking can be found in the biographies of Darwin and Huxley by Irvine (1955) and *Early Man* by Clark Howell (1966). A comprehensive review of evolution, based on an extensive bibliography, was published by Julian Huxley in 1964.

Fig. 2.1. Evolution of the vertebrates related to the geological history of the earth (from Glees, 1971).

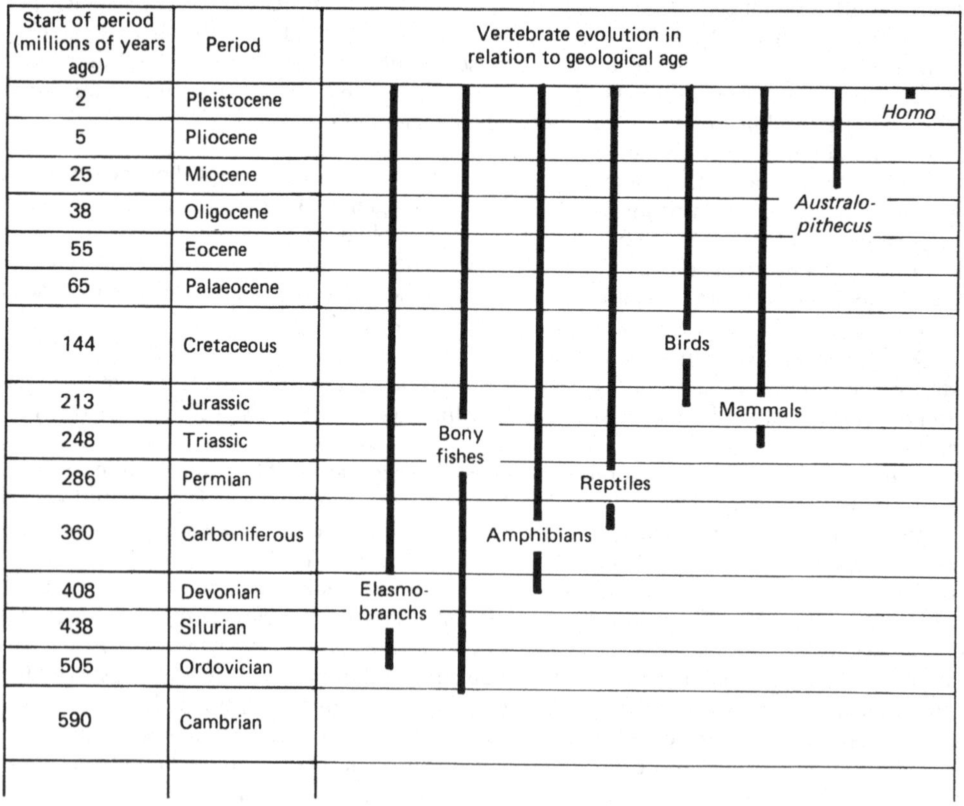

Start of period (millions of years ago)	Period	Vertebrate evolution in relation to geological age
2	Pleistocene	Homo
5	Pliocene	
25	Miocene	
38	Oligocene	Australopithecus
55	Eocene	
65	Palaeocene	
144	Cretaceous	Birds
213	Jurassic	Mammals
248	Triassic	Bony fishes
286	Permian	Reptiles
360	Carboniferous	Amphibians
408	Devonian	Elasmobranchs
438	Silurian	
505	Ordovician	
590	Cambrian	

Brief overview

A biological model of primitive vertebrates is the lamprey *Petromyzon* (see Fig. 2.2). These cyclostomes appeared 400 million years ago. They and the hagfish are the sole survivors of Palaeozoic agnathans (jawless fish) and are important witnesses for vertebrate evolution. Hardisty (1979) and Brodal & Fänge (1963) produced extensive reviews of the biology of lampreys, which live in rivers or in the sea and which may follow parasitic or free-living modes of life. Related to the cyclostomes are the jawed fishes (gnathostomes), bearing paired fins. In the Palaeozoic era, a bifurcation into cartilaginous and bony fishes occurred. Cartilaginous fishes still exist (e.g. sharks and rays), while the bony fishes (teleosts) are the dominant fishes today in both fresh and sea water. From the early types of bony fishes, lungfishes developed; usually found in the estuaries of rivers, they breathe air, rising to the surface of the water to gulp, and are capable of survival in dry periods by burrowing in the mud. It is reasonable to assume that a similar fish, capable of breathing on land, might have used its fins to crawl about and might have led to the evolution of new forms of vertebrates, the amphibians (eventually frogs, newts and others; Fig. 2.3), capable of living on land but needing to return to the water to breed. Reptiles evolved at the end of the Carboniferous period. It seems certain that the main groups of vertebrates – fishes and tetrapods – reached a high degree of specialisation very early in the Earth's history and that only minor modifications occurred later. Thus, it appears that evolutionary progress happened at a faster rate in the past than at present.

Important for progress in the evolution of reptiles was the relatively enormous size of their eggs, providing sufficient nourishment for the development of an animal capable, on hatching, of coping with the environmental factors of life on land. One basic deficiency in present-day reptiles is the lack of the ability to control body temperature in response to climatic changes or seasonal variations. When cooled, reptiles are forced to a reduction in metabolism; they are slowed down and become defenceless. Warm-blooded animals are able to live in the temperate or cold zones of the Earth, while the reptiles are today restricted to hot climates. Two animal groups became independent of temperature variations in the Mesozoic era: the birds, which developed from flying reptiles; and reptiles possessing some mammalian features. The latter group would finally give rise to the mammals.

Birds (Figs 2.4 and 2.5) are highly specialised animals which, apart from being able to regulate body temperature, are further independent of the prevailing climate, since most can fly and thus migrate to suitable geographical regions. This enables birds to escape harsh climates by choosing the most suitable surroundings and to occupy areas of rich feeding

Fig. 2.2. The lamprey (a jawless fish) is an ancient vertebrate (from Glees, 1971). Transverse and sagittal sections through the brain of this animal may be found in Fig. 2.15.

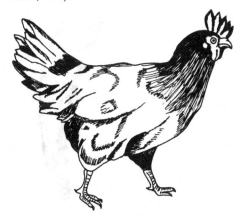

Fig. 2.4. The chicken is an example of a flying land animal whose prosencephalon, devoid of sulci, is a specialised form of the telencephalon and is thus distinguished from the brain of mammals (from Glees, 1971).

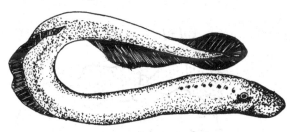

Fig. 2.3. The toad and its brain (from Glees, 1971). c = cerebellum; ms. = mesencephalon; mt. = metencephalon; p. = prosencephalon.

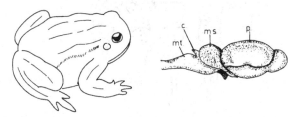

grounds. Birds and mammals have one inherent disadvantage in common. When invading new territories, they are both forced to spend much of their time in feeding their young, despite the fact that birds have a relatively short breeding time. These periods of lengthy or intensive caring for offspring impose a limit on the rate of population expansion.

The first mammals to evolve were small, mole-like creatures (Fig. 2.6) similar to present-day insectivores, which lived in burrows. The development of a placenta inside the uterus provided nourishment in a safe environment for the foetal stages. Thus, a smaller percentage of offspring died in the early stages. When compared with the highly specialised birds, however, mammals are relatively primitive animals. Mammals, with their simple limbs, cannot be compared favourably with the long-distance air travellers such as the albatross (Fig. 2.5). The bird's high body temperature (40–43 °C) is the sign of a fast metabolism, but forces them to search for food most of

Fig. 2.5. The albatross (*Diomedea*), largest of seabirds covering vast areas of the Pacific and Southern Oceans, has a great opportunity for choosing the most suitable habitat.

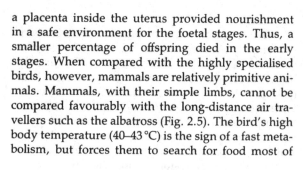

Fig. 2.6. The mole (*Talpa europaea*) is a simple mammal but has its forefeet specialised for digging (forefoot skeleton below).

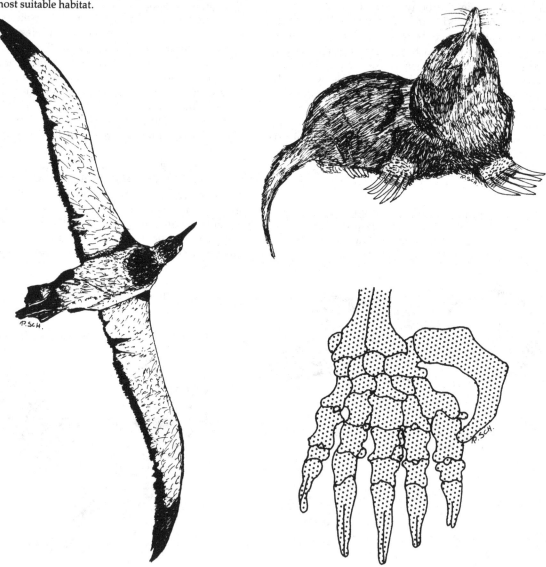

the time. Birds usually do not carry stored energy such as fat deposits, as this would hinder their flight capability (birds kept in captivity and 'fattened up' lose their ability to fly). The lack of fat for emergency nourishment has a further disadvantage: when the sudden onset of a cold period prevents access to food, birds die of starvation while mammals can utilise their fat stores. The highly effective and specialised enzymes of the bird's liver are vulnerable to the toxic insecticides used in agriculture; the less specialised small mammals survive better in a toxic environment.

The essence of mammalian basic construction is the provision for high adaptability in changing environmental conditions (Figs 2.7 and 2.8). This adaptation is shown especially in the shape of the limbs. In the mole (Fig. 2.6), short legs and large feet allow the animal to burrow deep into the ground to make tunnels. Limbs may be extremely long, even different lengths at the front and rear, as in the rabbit and kangaroo, to make for a quick getaway by jumping. The limbs need only slight changes to be suitable for swimming or for climbing and arboreal life.

The mammalian brain is similarly suited for adaptation, in contrast to the bird's nervous system. The bird is preprogrammed by genetics much more than is the mammal. The bird behaves after hatching in an automatic pattern in response to a particular trigger situation such as hunger or sex drive. We know from the works of Lorenz (1963, 1965) and Tinbergen (1951) and their pupils how greatly the bird's behaviour pattern is ritualised, predictable and stereotyped

(see Chapter 15). The difference between bird and mammal is also clearly demonstrated by the fact that the bird can hardly change its basic pattern of behaviour by experience. Mammals, however (especially

Fig. 2.8. The thick-tailed bushbaby (*Galago crassicaudatus*) and its brain, viewed from the right side. The encephalon is relatively devoid of sulci, showing only the principal sulci of the primate brain (from Glees, 1971). c. = cerebellum; f. = flocculus of the cerebellum; l.h. = left hemisphere; l.s. = lunar sulcus; m = mesencephalon; o.b. = olfactory bulb; p = pons; p.c. = palaeocortex; r.s. = rhinoid sulcus (palaeoneo-cortical sulcus); sp.c. = spinal cord; S.s. = Sylvian sulcus.

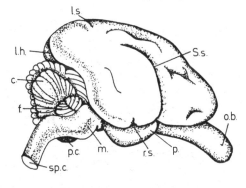

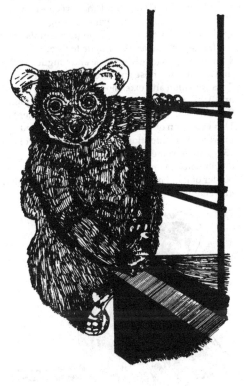

Fig. 2.7. The common tree shrew (*Tupaia glis*). A primitive mammal from southeast Asia, as regards brain development it occupies a position between the Insectivora and the prosimian primates (from Glees, 1971).

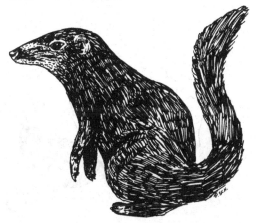

the 'higher' mammals), have the ability to use individual experience for modifying instinctive behaviour. We see that a bird, when caught in a cage, will press its head against the wires to get out, driven by the panic urge to free itself. A monkey (Figs 2.9–2.11), however, can be seen to reflect, planning its escape, or to wait for the cage door to be opened. Brain organisation in the primate allows for an intelligent assessment of the situation and the monkey is not harassed by urges and instinct like the bird. In the further chapters of this book, it will be our task to trace what factors of brain evolution and neural construction enabled mammals, and in particular Man, to achieve dominance in the animal kingdom (Figs 2.12 and 2.13). Man has conquered the Earth and pushed his close

Fig. 2.9. The baboon (*Papio*) and its brain. Baboons are intelligent and live in social groups dominated by older males. The brain of the baboon has a larger frontal lobe than that of the macaque monkey (*Macaca mulatta*) and the central sulcus takes a tortuous course (Glees, 1971). c.s. = central sulcus; f.p. = frontal pole; o.p. = occipital pole; S.s. = Sylvian sulcus; t.p. = temporal pole. The numbers refer to results of stimulation experiments and show vector points (Glees *et al.*, 1950). 1 = retraction of tongue ipsilaterally; 2 = retraction of tongue contralaterally; 3 = transitional area from tongue to face; 4 = movements involving nose and tongue; 5 = lip movements; 6 = nose and tongue movements; 7 = supination and extension of thumb and digits 2 and 3; 8 = supination and extension of wrist joint; 9 = extension of wrist; 10 = shoulder movements; 11 = extension of whole arm and hand pushed forward; 12 = extention first, then retraction of arm; 13 = arm movements combined with finger movements; 14 = extension of fingers; 15 = anterior border of hand movements and forearm extension movements.

Fig. 2.10. The gorilla and its brain. This example of a higher primate brain shows the similarity to the human brain (from Glees, 1971). c. = cerebellum; c.s. = central sulcus; f.p. = frontal pole; o.p. = occipital pole; S.s. = Sylvian sulcus (fissure); t.p. = temporal pole.

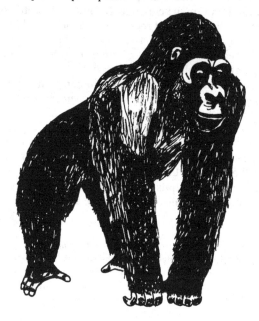

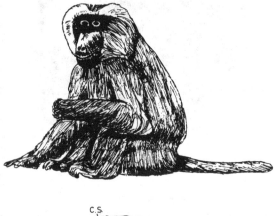

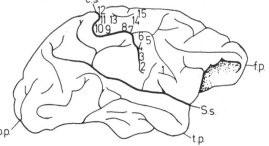

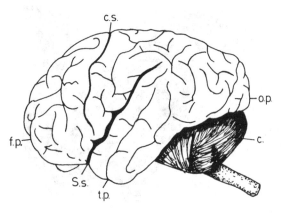

relatives among the primates into the remnants of the primeval forests. It is obvious that the greater brain volume and the brain organisation of Man must give an answer to his superiority. It appears then that a 'primitive' body construction, including a versatile digestive system, and the enormous enlargement of the forebrain were the pillars of human superiority. As we have seen, the forebrain enlargement offered a neural organisation for 'liberating' mammals, in particular primates, from the lower centres of reflex activity and instinctive behaviour. It is the elaboration of the cerebral cortex (see Figs 2.26 and 2.27) – the grey matter – which makes Man the tool-maker and inventor. (For a wide-ranging and detailed overview of the vertebrate brain and intelligence, consult Macphail (1982).)

Nervous system evolution

The primary task of a sense organ is to detect and pass on environmental information. When the

Fig. 2.11. The chimpanzee (*Pan*) is a representative of the higher apes and is found in most zoos. The body hair varies from reddish brown to black. Because of their cooperative intelligence they have been popular circus animals in the past (from Glees, 1971).

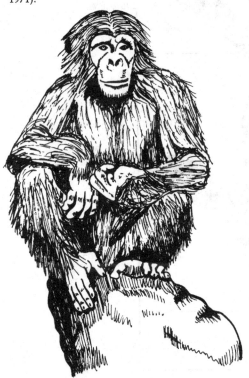

sensory information signals danger, an *escape* is initiated; should the signal indicate food, an *approach* results. In each case, innervation of appropriate muscle reaction occurs. It is a fundamental neural arrangement that sensory signals lead to well-ordered muscle contractions. The neural switchboard, the speed of sensory data processing, has been studied in great detail by classical neurophysiology and the principles of reflex action have been established. If we follow the evolutionary history of the nervous system, we find full support for the concepts of reflex actions. An animal seemingly controlled by reflex action alone is the lancelet, *Amphioxus* – a knife-blade-like silvery creature, usually buried in the sand (see Figs 2.14 and 2.15). It can be considered solely as a spinal cord creature, which either has 'given up' as useless a brain during its evolution or may never have developed one.

It is the norm in evolution, however, that the anterior end of the spinal cord enlarges to form primary brain vesicles (Fig. 2.16), which can be best studied in a vertebrate embryo. To start with, we can distinguish three vesicles. Each of these vesicles contains the neural building material for well-defined functional tasks. These vesicles, named from the anterior end of the spinal cord, are the hindbrain, midbrain and forebrain (Fig. 2.17).

These primary brain vesicles (Figs 2.18–2.20) reach different sizes in different animal species and one of the vesicles may be much larger than the two others. Casts of very early fossil skulls of seacows and elephants show these very brain divisions, as demonstrated in 1950 by Tilly Edinger (the daughter of the famous pioneer of brain research, Ludwig Edinger) (see Glees, 1952a,b). The three-vesicle brain pattern is valid for the human brain as well, as it applies in all vertebrates, but in mammals this developmental stage is surpassed early on by five vesicles. The general functional significance of these brain divisions will be discussed below. These divisions contain the imprints of the genetic programmes which emerge in birds after hatching.

Nervous system development

Phylogenetically, the nervous system develops from the outer germ layer, the ectoderm. This mode of development is also present in the ontogeny of the individual (see Fig. 2.21). The ectoderm, being the outer embryonic layer, is in contact with the surroundings. It seems common sense that this layer is destined for contact information and for the elaboration of the external stimuli. To protect the more refined nervous constructions, the data-processing part is moved

Fig. 2.12. The evolution of primates over the last 35 million years (after De Beer, 1964).

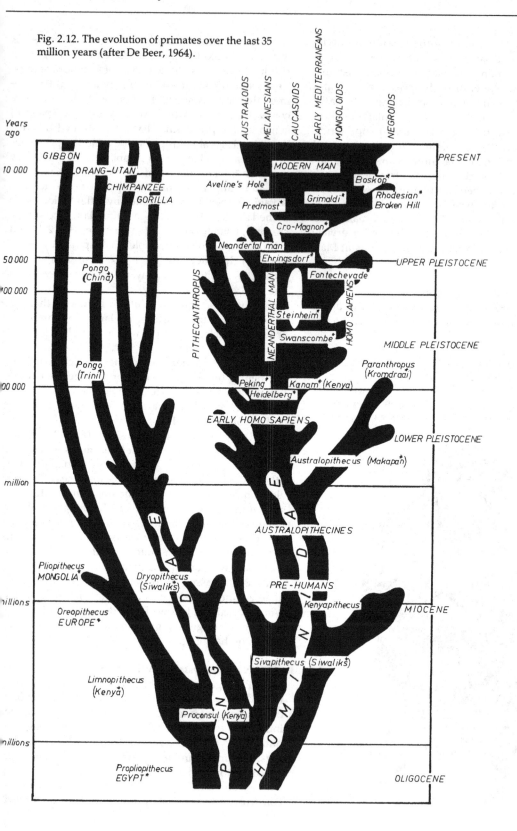

Fig. 2.13. The geographical distribution of primates
(from Glees, 1971).

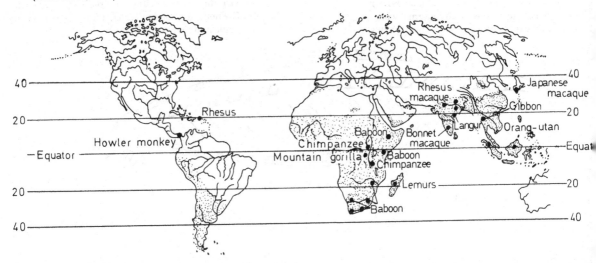

Fig. 2.14. The topography of the nervous systems of
various animals (modified from Truex, 1959).
(*a*) Detail of the nervous system of *Hydra* (*b*).
e.c. = ectodermal cell; end.c. = endodermal cell;
n.c. = nerve cell; n.c.n. = nerve cell net;
nem. = nematocyst; n.f. = nerve fibres; o.op. =
oral opening; ph.v. = phagocytic vesicle; s.c. = sensory
cell; sec.c. = secretory cell; t. = tentacle. (*c*) A
planarian worm. c.g. = cerebral ganglion; the paired
ventral nerve cords (v.n.c.) are joined by
commissures. (*d*) The earthworm (*Lumbricus*).
c.g. = cerebral ganglion; ph.g. = pharyngeal
ganglion; v.n.c. = ventral nerve cord. (*e*) *Amphioxus*.
a.o. = anal opening; b. = branchial, basket;
d.n.c. = dorsal nerve cord; m. = segm.
n. = segmental muscles and nerves; n. = notochord;
o.op. = oral opening; r.g. = rudimentary ganglion.
(*f*) The honey bee (*Apis*). a.g. = abdominal ganglia;
c.g. = cerebral ganglion; i.f. = interganglionic fibres;
th.g. = thoracic ganglia; v.n.c. = ventral nerve cord
(paired commissures linking ganglia). These
diagrams illustrate a net system (*a*), (*b*), chain-like
systems (*c*), (*d*), a continuous system (*e*) and a
nodular nervous system (*f*).

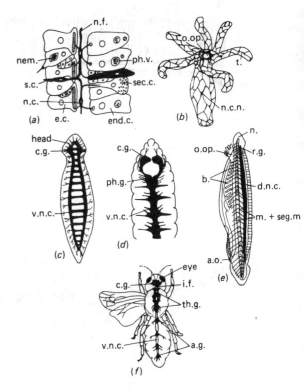

Fig. 2.15. *Amphioxus*, the lancet. (*a*) external
appearance. (*b*) Sagittal section of the anterior portion
(from Glees, 1971). bl.v. = blood vessels;
e. = ectoderm; e.w. = endodermal wall;
g.c. = ganglionic cells; h.c. = head canals;
i.o. = infundibular organ; m. = muscles;
n. = notochord; n.c. = nerve cord; n.r. = ventral
nerve rami; s.c. = subcutaneous tissue; v. = ventricle.
(*c*) The nervous system dissected free; the nerve cord
is simple and there is no brain.

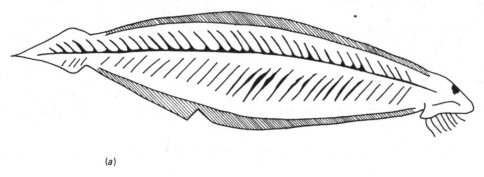

(*a*)

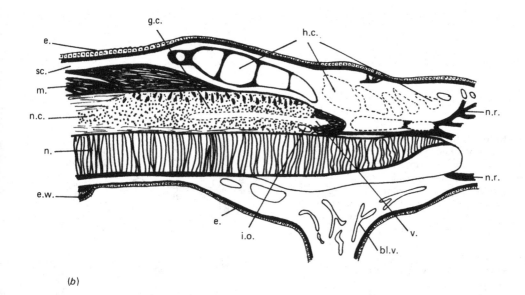

(*b*)

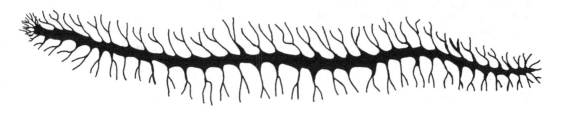

(*c*)

deeper by a process of infolding. The ensuing fold joins up, forming a tube, the precursor of the spinal cord and the cranial portions of the future brain. These sheltered parts, highly organised and interconnected, represent the central nervous system. The CNS is connected to the peripheral nerves, such as those in the skin, by way of nodes of nerve cells – the spinal and cranial ganglia (Figs 2.22–2.27). The peripheral processes of these spinal ganglia form a receptive 'information service' in the skin and internal parts of the body, while their central processes carry the information into the spinal cord and brain (Figs 2.28–2.32). This portion – the nerve cells of the spinal ganglia and their central and peripheral processes – constitutes the main sensory or receptive part of the CNS. The peripheral terminal branches of the spinal ganglia are capable of receiving information directly or are connected with special sense organs distributed in selective areas of the skin.

Fig. 2.16. A section through the elasmobranch fish *Mustelus*, a primitive vertebrate. The fundamental divisions of the brain are clearly shown. The gill clefts and nerves are important forerunners of human neck organs.

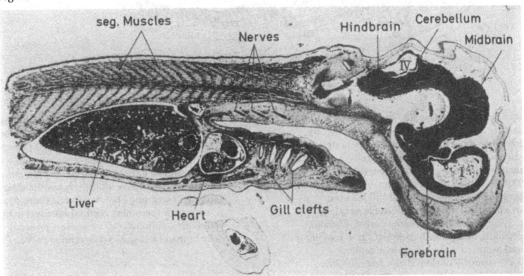

Fig. 2.17. The basic units of the vertebrate brain are the forebrain (prosencephalon), the midbrain (mesencephalon) and the hindbrain (metencephalon). They are formed at the early developmental stages of the human embryo (from Glees, 1971).

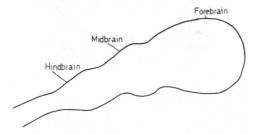

Fig. 2.18. Sagittal section through the brain of a lamprey (from Glees, 1971). al. = alisphenoid; c. = cerebellum; c.s. = corpus striatum; d.v. = diencephalic ventricle; e. = ephysis; l.v. = lateral ventricle; M = Muller cells; m.c. = mitral cells; m.v. = midbrain ventricle; n. = notochord; n.V + VII = trigeminal and facial nerve nuclei;

n.IX + X = glossopharyngeal and vagal nerve nuclei; o.l. = olfactory lobe; o.n. = olfactory nerve; op.l. = optic lobe; o.t. = optic tectum; o.tr. = optic tract; p = paraphysis; p.g. = parapineal ganglion; r.v. = rhomboid (IV) ventricle; sp.t.tr. = spino-thalamic tract; st.t. = strio-thalamic tract; t.c. = tela choroidea (choroid plexus; III = roots of third cranial nerve.

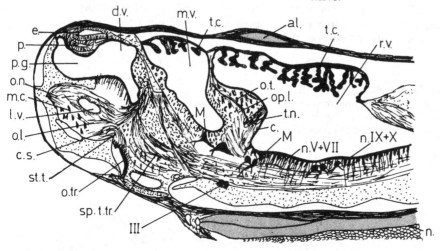

Fig. 2.19. Transverse section through the medula of a lamprey. Note the giant Müller cells which are larger than those found in higher vertebrates; they may be the precursors of the large cells in the medial reticular nucleus seen in mammals (from Glees, 1971). a.c. = part of inner ear capsule; a.f. = arcuate fibres; d.r.n.a. = dorsal root of VIII nucleus; e. = ependyma; f.n.g. = facial nerve ganglion; l.c. = lateral crest and terminal nucleus of cranial nerve VIII; M.c. = Muller cells; r.f.f.n. = root fibres of facial nerve; r.f.n. = root of facial nerve; sp.V. = spinal V nucleus; t.c. = tela choroidea; t.n.a.n. = tegmental nucleus of auditory nerve; v. = IV ventricle; v.r.n.a. = ventral root of VIII nucleus.

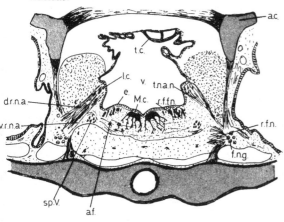

Fig. 2.20. Transverse section through the midbrain of a lamprey, showing all the typical features of the vertebrate midbrain (from Glees, 1971). M.c. = Muller cells; opt. f. = ascending optic fibres; opt. str. = optic straum; opt.t. = optic tectum; p.l.f. = posterior longitudinal fasciculus; s.th.t. = spino-thalamic tract and other ascending fibres; t.c. = tela choroidea; v. = ventricle (becoming cerebral aqueduct in higher vertebrates, although this ventricle is present in the early human foetus); III = oculomotor nerve.

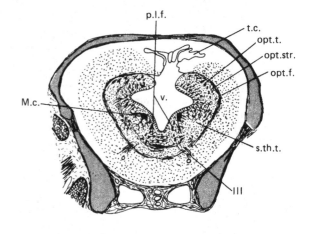

Fig. 2.21. The four important stages in the development of the vertebrate nervous system (from Glees, 1971). (*a*) The neural plate (n.p.) develops by a thickening of the ectoderm. ec. = ectoderm; en. = endoderm; m. = mesoderm; n. = notochord. (*b*) Formation of the neural groove (n.gr.). n.cr. = neural crest. (*c*) Formation of the neural tube (n.t.). (*d*) Out growths of the posterior and ventral roots of the spinal cord from neural tube connections. c.c. = central canal; s.g. = spinal ganglion; sk. = developing skin; v. = vertebra.

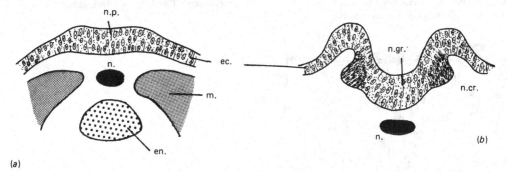

Fig. 2.22. Development of neuro-ectodermal matrix cells (from Glees, 1971).

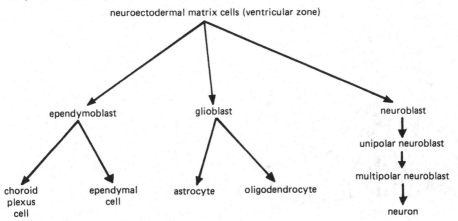

Fig. 2.23. Drawing of a transverse section through the wall of the neural tube immediately after closure. The germinal layer, consisting of the neuro-epithelial cells, has greatly increased in thickness. The nuclei of the cells behave according to the same migratory pattern as in the neural groove stage. Occasionally, however, a cell becomes detached from the lumen and moves through the germinal layer to become a primitive neuroblast. Most of the mitotic figures have their spindle fibres arranged parallel to the lumen, some are oblique and an occasional fibre is perpendicular (after Langman *et al.*, 1966). Lu = lumen; GL = germinal layer; ML = mantle layer; 1 = differentiating neuroblast; 2 = external limiting membrane (PAS$^+$v); 3 = terminal bar.

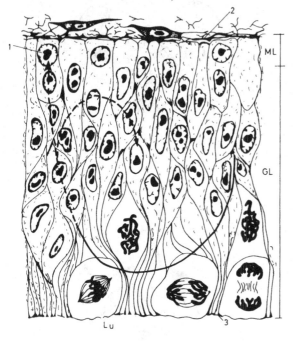

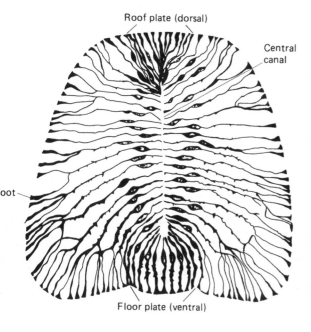

Fig. 2.24. Cross-section through the embryonic spinal cord. Giant ependymal cells extend from the central canal to the spinal cord surface and guide the migration of the neurons (Golgi silver stain) (from Glees, 1971).

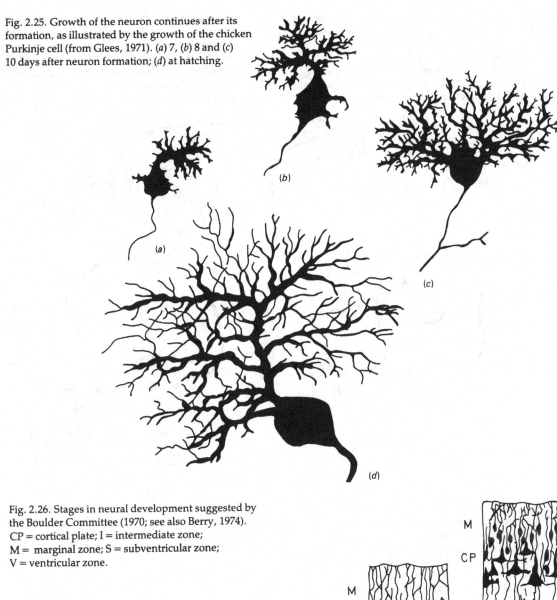

Fig. 2.25. Growth of the neuron continues after its formation, as illustrated by the growth of the chicken Purkinje cell (from Glees, 1971). (*a*) 7, (*b*) 8 and (*c*) 10 days after neuron formation; (*d*) at hatching.

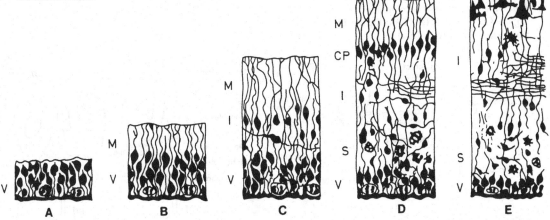

Fig. 2.26. Stages in neural development suggested by the Boulder Committee (1970; see also Berry, 1974). CP = cortical plate; I = intermediate zone; M = marginal zone; S = subventricular zone; V = ventricular zone.

Fig. 2.27. Cranial development of the neural tube. The tube undergoes dilatation and bending, resulting in the formation of cerebral vesicles. The cranial nerves are marked (from Glees, 1971).
cereb. = cerebellum; dienc. = diencephalon; inf. coll. = inferior colliculus; max.b. = maxillary branch of cranial nerve V; mand.b. = mandibular branch of cranial nerve V; mes. = mesencephalon; ol.bulb = olfactory bulb; op.b. = ophthalmic branch of cranial nerve V; opt.n. = optic nerve; opt.v. = optic vesicle; ot.v. = otic vesicle; pros. = prosencephalon; rhomb. = rhombencephalon; sp.c. = spinal cord; sup.coll. = superior colliculus; telenc. = telencephalon.

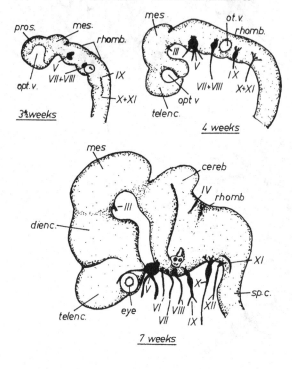

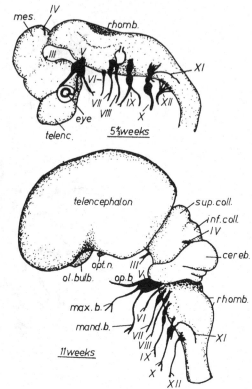

Fig. 2.28. Development of the ventricular system illustrated in stages (*a*), (*b*), (*c*), (*d*) in relation to the neural tube (*a*). The cavities contain cerebrospinal fluid and considerably enlarge in the telencephalon region producing the large lateral ventricles, following the course of hemispheral development (*b*), (*c*), (*d*). Consult Chapter 6 for finite location of ventricles (from Glees, 1971).

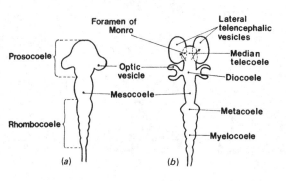

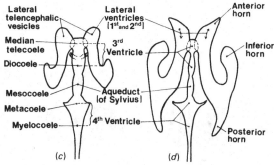

Principles of neural construction

The basic functions of nerve cells are the reception of stimuli, and the evaluation and propagation of information. Stimulus reception is carried out by polar-oriented neuroectodermal cells or by specialised neurons present in the retina (see Fig. 13.8) or the olfactory mucosa (see Fig. 11.1). These specialised cells are capable, because of their cell membrane properties, of depolarising the resting potential, producing propagated action potentials. Receptor cells and nerve cells are, in principle, of similar morphological and biochemical construction in vertebrates and invertebrates. This means that the principles for uptake of stimuli and their utilisation were realised very early on in the evolution of animal life and that future improvements were in the direction of quantity and the complexity of wiring up. Once a multicellular organisation was established, all basic requirements for improvement were present and no inherent constructional changes were necessary. This principle is not apparent in human technology, where completely new devices are frequently found, for example the change from radio valves to transistors in electronics. Life was created on the basis of miniaturisation, a principle lately realised by technical progress in 'microchips'. Regarding the animal nervous system, communication efficiency is expressed by the smallest possible size of contacts or synapses between nerve cells, their locations on the cell, their numbers, the receptivity of cell membrane portions, and the grouping and layering of nerve cells for particular functional tasks. This means, too, that these basic neural properties can be explored in invertebrates and in various species of vertebrates. The knowledge gained is valid, to some extent, for Man.

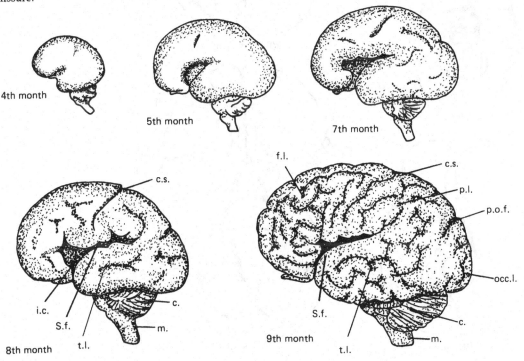

Fig. 2.29. Developmental stages of the human foetal brain, lateral view (from Glees, 1971).
c. = cerebellum; c.s. = central sulcus; f.l. = frontal lobe; i.c. = insular cortex; m. = medulla; occ.l. = occipital lobe; p.l. = parietal lobe; p.o.f. = parieto-occipital fissure; S.f. = Sylvian fissure.

The relatively simple animal (see Fig. 2.14(*b*)) *Aplysia californica*, a marine snail, has proved a fruitful model for studying the molecular mechanisms of short-term synaptic plasticity with the aim of explaining long-term memory and conditioning (Kandel & Schwartz, 1982a,b; Kandel, 1983). The respiratory chamber (gill cavity) of these animals is guarded by a protective mantle which terminates in a spout, the siphon. The siphon and the mantle are richly supplied with sensory endings which responding to light touch. This results in a withdrawal into the mantle cavity by the siphon, mantle shelf and gill. These withdrawal responses can be modified by experience, and this has been utilised by Kandel and co-workers to study the neurophysiological pathway of the reflexes involved and the biochemical mechanism of simple learning and memory habituation (see p. 106). These investigations were possible because relatively few,

Fig. 2.30. Ventral (basal) view of the foetal brain in various stages of pregnancy (from Glees, 1971).
1 = cerebral peduncle; 2 = inferior temporal sulcus; 3 = olfactory bulb; 4 = optic chiasma; 5 = hypophyseal stalk; 6 = mamillary body; 7 = pons; 8 = cortico-spinal tract; 9 = lower medula; 10 = vermis of cerebellum; 11 = frontal lobe; 12 = uncinate gyrus; 13 = a basal gyrus of temporal lobe; 14 = cerebellar hemisphere; 15 = collateral sulcus; 16 = occipital pole; 17 = rhinal fissure; 18 = occipito-temporal gyrus.

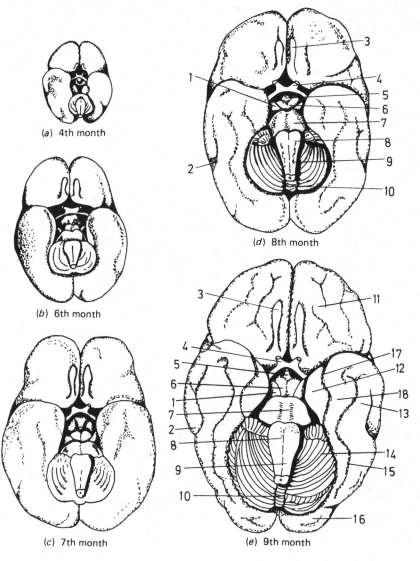

(a) 4th month

(b) 6th month

(c) 7th month

(d) 8th month

(e) 9th month

Fig. 2.31. The development of the human face and brain can be understood on a phylogenetic basis. Note the wide open face clefts, the laterally situated eyes and the remaining yolk sac in the fourth week of gestation. The human head with the dominant cranial cavity is clearly visible by week 8 (modified from Patten, 1947). 1 = opthalmic fissure; 2 = nasal cleft and process; 3 = oral cleft; 4 = ear primordium; 5 = upper extremity; 6 = heart; 7 = lung; 8 = umbilical cord; 9 = lower extremity; 10 = genital tubercle.

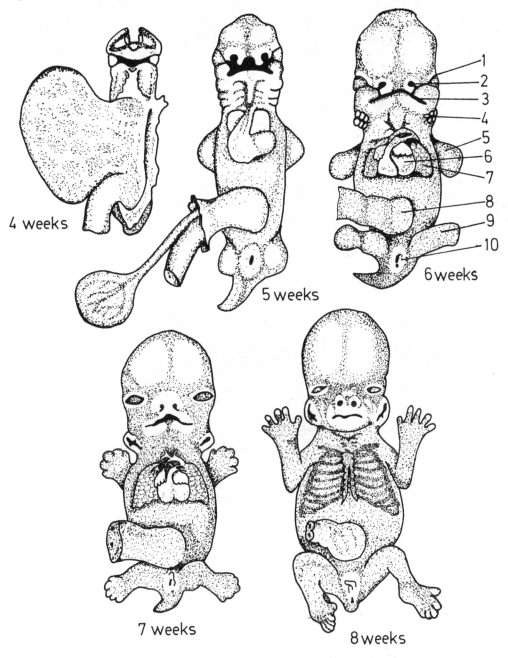

Fig. 2.32. A slightly oblique sagittal section through
the developing human brain in a foetus of about 11
weeks. B.G. = basal ganglia; m.b. = mamillary body;
F.M. = Foramen of Munro.

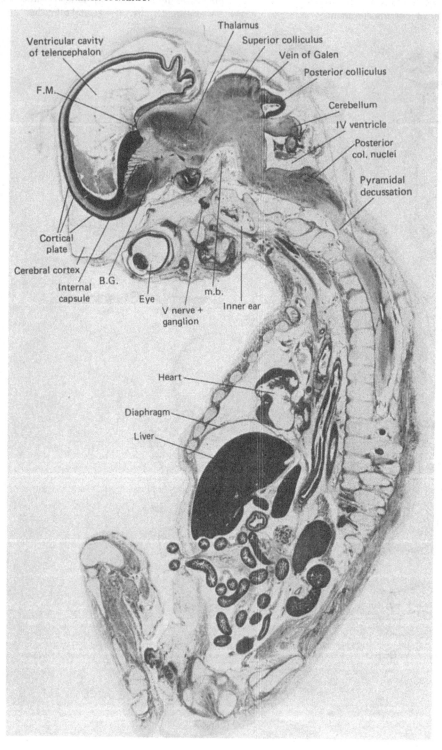

large neurons are involved and Kandel states that fewer than 50 cells have to be investigated; the vertebrate nervous system may use up to 100 000 small nerve cells for a simple behaviour pattern.

General properties of receptors

Receptors must be 'constructed' on two main principles: extreme sensitivity and the ability to localise environmental changes. The first condition, high sensitivity, has been achieved for olfaction and taste. A few molecules only of a given substance can be detected and classified with accuracy. The chemical sense has, however, one grave disadvantage in not fulfilling the second condition, for the propagation of smell or taste depends on the direction of the air or water current and no definite relation to the stimulus source is established. Smell informs efficiently that something is smelling, but additional parameters are necessary for location. Olfaction, being a diffuse alerting system, is also a powerful activator for memory processes (see p. 156).

The forebrain's original connection with olfaction proved eventually to be an evolutionary disadvantage, but the arrival of tactile and visual connections led to further evolutionary steps and to a *complete reconstruction of forebrain morphology* to form the layered cerebral cortex. For the accurate recording of sensory stimuli as reliable and verifiable projections of the outside world, it appears necessary that the pattern of a neuronal assemblage is layered and well interconnected. Layered neuronal arrangements already existed at midbrain level, receiving visual and auditory information of high quality regarding sensitivity and precise topography. As soon as the forebrain offered an even better basis by being multi-layered and precisely wired up, auditory stimuli, tactile and visual signals were also received at forebrain level, reducing the reception area for olfaction. These new information channels were relayed and filtered at a new neuronal assembly, the dorsal thalamus, a subdivision of the diencephalon. The diencephalon appears in evolution as a subdivision of the forebrain and can be divided into a ventral, evolutionarily older part, the hypothalamus, and a newer part, the dorsal thalamus, usually referred to as the thalamus. As a consequence of neocortical development, the thalamus is subdivided into condensations of neurons referred to as nuclei, which project or send their axonal processes to well-defined cortical regions (see Figs 7.10 and 9.25). The critical reactions of an animal towards environmental changes are determined by the neocortex via the thalamus. This cortical dominance is based on the function of the cerebral (layered) cortex

and an independently searching and exploring forelimb, which in primates is the hand. A further factor is the creation of a body surface capable of sensory recognition. This is achieved by a smooth, relatively hairless skin in Man; the scales of fishes, the cutaneous ossification of reptiles and the feathers of birds would be unsuitable. The projections of numerous skin receptors, particularly in the hand, onto the cerebral cortex, and the wiring up of the forebrain with auditory and visual impulses, brings the forebrain into command of sensory input and decision-making. The 'liberation' of the forebrain from being dependent solely on olfactory input, coupled with the connections of a sensory input offering precise topographical coordinates (visual input) for aimful movement, enabled the cerebral cortex to become the 'tool-maker' for Man. Provided with the neuronal resources of the cerebral cortex, Man can make changes in decades where evolution takes millions of years. We can use flight as an example. Evolution can equip various animals to fly; for example, there are flying insects, birds, fishes and mammals. Other mammals can swim underwater, such as the whale. Man does not need the help of evolution; he can create ancillary aids enabling flying, underwater swimming and even space exploration. Man alters his environment beyond recognition, for better or worse. Whole animal species are annihilated or subjected to domestication and reduced to production machinery. While Man is not necessarily the crown of 'Creation', he is the master of his destiny, even capable of his own total destruction.

General functional significance of brain vesicular divisions

The spinal cord portion of the nervous system (Fig. 2.33) receives, from the neurons of the spinal ganglia, information from outside sources, referred to as exteroceptive, and from the inside of the body, interoceptive information. This information can reach the motor neurons of the spinal cord directly or via internuncial cells. Suitable muscle contractions are caused when the signals are conveyed to motor neurons, often referred to as the motor neuron pool to stress the common purpose of an anatomical grouping of the big motor cells. The incoming signals, also referred to as afferent, can be branched off to the posterior column and ascend via two relay stations to an evolutionarily new part, the thalamus, and on to the cerebral cortex. The medulla, a part of the hindbrain, contains specialised sensory relay stations, such as the reticular system, with important ascending connections to the forebrain and descending ones to the spinal cord. The ascending connections to the fore-brain are essential for our general state of awareness. The motor tasks of the medulla are the control of respiration, of the foregut, and of the heart. The mid-brain is a coordination centre for acoustic and visual input. In mammals the forebrain is subdivided into the telencephalon (the cerebral cortex) and the thalamus and hypothalamus, called collectively the di-encephalon.

In primates, the evolutionarily older portion of the forebrain, the olfactory region, is separated from the newer cerebral cortex by the rhinal fissure and occupies a much smaller area than in 'lower' mammals. Similarly, the pyramidal or cortico-spinal projection reaches its largest in primates; the integrative

capacity of the nervous system is centred in the cerebral cortex.

Functional significance of the cerebral subdivisions

The *hindbrain*, situated at the level of neck and head (see Figs 2.33 and 2.34), has the task of regulating cardiac and respiratory activity. The heart of all vertebrates is originally situated in the neck region, close to the gills or lungs, which take up oxygen into the blood which the heart then distributes around the body. Gills are but everted lungs, to harvest the oxygen dissolved in water. The hindbrain is also responsible for the innervation of the oral opening and the skin receptors surrounding it. The receptors for taste are innervated by cranial ganglia and their nerves,

Fig. 2.33. Diagrammatic representation of fundamental neural circuits in the higher vertebrate brain (from Glees, 1971). a.c. = anterior colliculus; MoEp = motor endplate; Msp = muscle spindle; p.c. = posterior colliculus; PC = palaeocortex. 1 = olfactory tract; 2 = optic nerve; 2a = relay of optic impulses in the lateral geniculate body into the visual cortex; 2b = evolutionarily older connection to the anterior colliculus; 3 = neurons of gill clefts VII, IX and X; 4a = somato-sensory nerve; 4b = somato-motor nerve; 5 = cochlear nerve VIIIa; 6 = vestibular nerve VIIIb; 7 = posterior columns of medial lemnisci; 8 = tecto-spinal tract; 9 = cortico-spinal tract; 10 = spinal ganglion.

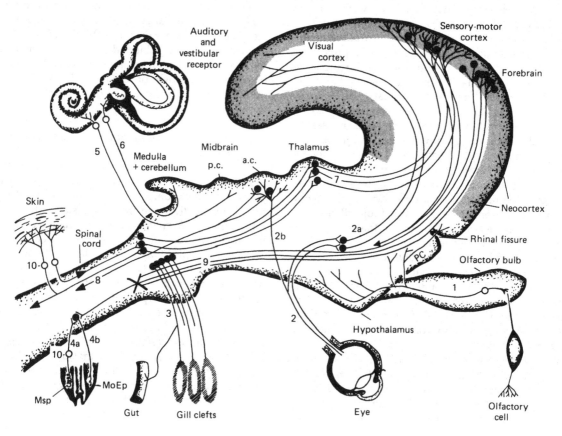

whose central terminations reach other cell bodies situated in the hindbrain. The peripheral sensory endings in the oral cavity are important in marine vertebrates for recognising sources of food immersed in sea water.

The *midbrain* is superimposed on the hindbrain (both are together referred to as the brainstem) and can be considered as an integration centre for neural information from hindbrain levels and for visual and auditory signals. The part played by the brainstem

in maintaining the state of consciousness, vital for the meaningful activity of the cerebral hemispheres (Pallis, 1984a,b) will be discussed on pp. 137–8. The integrative capacity is clearly expressed in its morphological construction, with a roof portion, the tectum, containing a multi-layered neuronal arrangement. This allows for a precise and orderly wiring up for the incoming sensory channels from the spinal cord and cranial nerves.

In contrast to this arrangement, the prime sense

Fig. 2.34. Comparative brain research has shown that the various divisions of the brain are very different in 'lower' and 'higher' vertebrates. (*a*) Cod. (*b*) Frog. (*c*) Reptile. (*d*) Bird. (*e*) Cat (after Truex, 1959). Note the enormous increase in the size of the forebrain. c = cerebellum; d = diencephalon (hindbrain); e = epiphysis (pineal body); m. = mesencephalon (midbrain); o.b. = olfactory bulb; o.t. = olfactory tract; p = prosencephalon (forebrain). Cranial nerves; I = olfactory; II = opic; III = oculomotor; IV = trochlear; V = trigeminal; VI = abducens; VII = facial; VIII = acoustic; IX = glosso-pharyngeal; X = vagus; XI = accessory; XII = hypoglossal nerve.

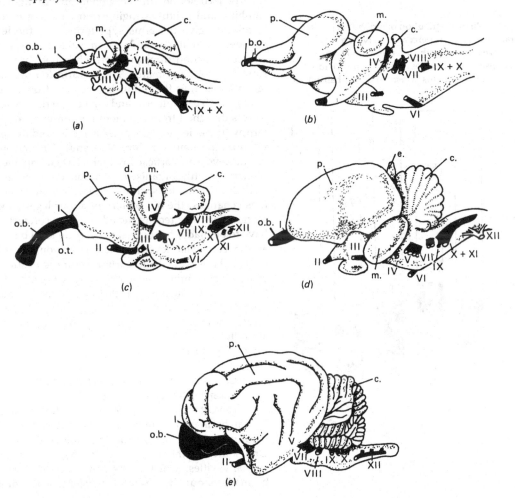

for the *forebrain*, evolutionarily speaking, is the sense of smell or olfaction. This sense and the sense of taste are chemically related and both can be classified as neurochemical transducers. Edinger referred to both senses as 'oral sense', taking the mucous membranes of the mouth and nose as a unit responsible for contact information with the external world. This was originally the sea world, where all life had started; substances that could be tasted when dissolved in sea water could be smelt in the air when on land. At first, taste and smell seem to be separate senses on land, but the salty moisture in the oral and nasal cavities restores the sea water-like environment of ancestral times.

Integration of the brain's subunits and the emergence of leading centres

The concept of neural integration, in which one cerebral vesicle takes a leading role, has also been

Fig. 2.35. Volume distribution of individual parts of the brain expressed as percentages. Note a progressive increase of the telencephalon from 'higher' insectivores (moles and hedgehogs), to Tupaiidae, to prosimians (lorises and bushbabies), to simians.

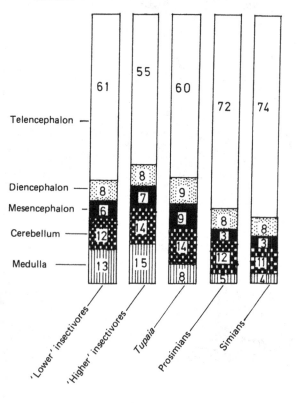

expressed as a continuous process of encephalisation and corticalisation. This evolutionary process is furthered in the individual by the processes of education and socio-cultural assimilation. Neurophysiologically and neuroanatomically this means that the input to the cerebral cortex increases, 'older' centres such as the midbrain have their main input reduced, and new channels to the thalamus and cortex are created. The functions of the old wiring schema reappear, however, when the cortex is put out of action by an anaesthetic, mishaps or injury.

To illustrate this point further we can state in general terms that mammals use all limbs for movement. To synchronise fore- and hindlimbs an integrative mechanism is located at spinal cord level. Further integration of movements occurs at midbrain level to utilise inputs from the sense of balance and from auditory and visual stimuli. The coordination mechanism of the mammal is basically constructed for a four-limb type of locomotion. In the gibbon and orang-utan, climbing and skilful swinging from one tree branch to another give the arms superiority over the legs. We see then that the hands become different in agility and construction from the feet, while both are very similar in lower primates. The forearm too becomes reconstructed, as the radius is taken out from a rigid linkage with the humerus and can be flexed. The hand is thus detached from the more rigid movement pattern with the leg and becomes an independent tool. In turn, the neuronal control is shifted from lower neural levels to cortical forebrain levels, capable of directing highly organised intentional sequences of skilled movements, such as writing in Man. Due to these changes, the old pattern of a four-legged locomotion has to be reconstructed and new connections have to be made, not only at neocortical level but also at the cerebellar levels, including a pontine relay station. However, if the cortical centre is destroyed by accident or injury caused by a stroke the older pattern emerges, causing conflicts in motor management (see p. 94). The development from the four-legged creature to an upright standing person using one hand aimfully can be studied easily in the human baby and infant (Fig. 15.1).

Comparative brain research and its value for the understanding of the human brain

Important evidence for the evolution of the human brain from primitive origins derives from comparative morphological and physiological studies. One source of this information is the casts of fossil cranial cavities, which allow general conclusions to be made about the size and divisions of the brain.

These scientific studies, referred to as palaeo-neurology, are devoted to the understanding of the nervous system of extinct species.

To further the understanding of the human brain, primitive living primates deserve the same research interest shown to living primitive Man, such as the Australian Aborigines. Comparative neurology has found rewarding objects for study in Australia and Madagascar, both islands having lost land connections to greater land masses. These islands possess primitive animal and human populations, in particular marsupials and monotremes in Australia and lemurs in Madagascar. Much of this work has been carried out at the Max Planck Institute of Brain Research in Frankfurt by Stephan & Andy (Stephan & Andy, 1964; Andy, 1964), studying the insectivores and different species of primates by relating body weight to brain weight. These two weights have definite relations and permit certain conclusions to be drawn concerning the tendency of brain evolution, taking into account that there is a minimum brain weight necessary for the control and workings of the body machinery, reflex activity and metabolism. Beyond these requirements, one brain division, such as the forebrain, can be enlarged by evolutionary pressures, giving these species greater neural resources. Equally important measurements are the relative proportions by weight of the individual parts of the brain classified by their embryological origins. Figures 2.35 and 2.36 demonstrate clearly how the telencephalon of the forebrain, and in particular the neocortex, reaches the greatest elaboration in the evolutionary scale.

Fig. 2.36. Volume distribution expressed in percentages of the divisions of the forebrain in insectivores, prosimians and simians. Note that the olfactory components decrease rapidly while the neocortex increases (from Andy, 1964).

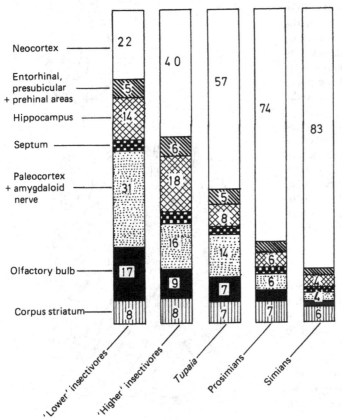

3

Fine structure of the nervous system

The macroscopic structures of the brain were described by the anatomists of Ancient Greece and Rome and were given names taken from the world of plants and animals, such as *arbor vitae* (tree of life), *hippocampus* (seahorse) and *cornus amonis* (Amon's horn). The finer structural details, however, became known only with the invention of the microscope and the histological techniques of fixation and staining. This exploratory work started in the eighteenth and nineteenth centuries and the names of Ledermüller (1758), Fontana (1782), Remark (1843) and Newport (1834) have to be mentioned. The main difficulties facing histologists were the gel-like semi-solid consistency of the brain substance and the poor power of resolution of early microscopes. Ledermüller was of the opinion that nerve fibres were hollow tubes in which a special energy circulated to convey willpower to muscles or from sense organs to the 'sensorium' of the brain. Fontana, however, proved that the nerve tubes were not empty but were filled with a colloidal substance.

Helmholtz (1821–1894), a famous physiologist of his time, who would nowadays be described as a biophysicist and who wrote his thesis on the composition of nerves (Helmholtz, 1842) under Johannes Müller (1800–1858), a physiologist and embryologist, found that the droplet-like structure of nerves postulated by van Leeuwenhoek in the seventeenth century was wrong and was caused when nerves were observed in hypotonic media.

Cellular construction

The thesis which Helmholtz wrote was of great significance for future studies, for he showed the primary importance of proper fixation for studies of preserved neural tissue. Helmholtz used alcohol to fix the brain and added acetic acid to emphasise cell borders and nuclei. Even more important was his finding that the nerve fibres stemmed from nerve cells and were not independent tubes. Ehrenberg (1834) had already proved that nerve cells were very small

independent bodies, ball-like in shape. However, the first clear description of neurons originates from Purkinje (1787–1869). While working as a physiologist at

Fig. 3.1. Purkinje (1848) had already recognized the basic structure of the cerebellum (from Glees, 1971). f.l. = fibre layer (white matter); g.s. = layer of small neurons; P = Purkinje cells.

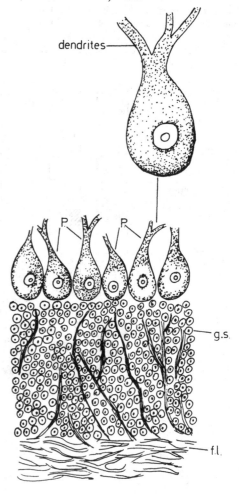

the University of Breslau, he demonstrated his findings for the first time at the meeting of German naturalists and physicians in Prague in 1837. These cerebellar cells (Fig. 3.1) are still referred to as Purkinje cells (similar important histological observations were made by Valentin and Remark). Purkinje discovered the cellular nature of the animal body before Schwann (1810–1882) had recognised the cellular nature of plants. Hannover, a Danish researcher working with Johannes Müller in Berlin, found by chance in 1840 that the nervous system revealed its structure more clearly when fixed in chromium solutions than when other fixatives of the time were used. Progress in neurohistology was due to two factors: penetrating fixation and improvement of microscopes by using achromatic lenses. This progress is well illustrated by the textbook of histology written by R. A. Kölliker in 1852 (English translation, 1853), another co-worker of Johannes Müller. This early textbook spread the recent knowledge of the structure of the brain, pointing out that the grey matter is made of nucleated cells and the white matter of myelinated fibres. Kölliker too proved the necessity for good fixation and for microtomes to cut thin sections. The knowledge of how the nerve cells were interconnected was still missing, however. Around 1850 it was assumed that nerve cells were interconnected in a net-like way; Kölliker believed that there was no substance to this assumption but technical progress brought the solution nearer. Microtome-cut thin sections could be made transparent by terpentine oil and Canada balsam. Furthermore, staining with a carmine dye introduced by Gerlach (1872a,b) revealed many surprising details. In fact many of the old dyes used remain unsurpassed. By around 1860 the basic tools of neurohistology, such as simple microtomes, fixation in acid chromium or osmium solutions, and staining in iodine and carmine, were assembled. Figure 3.2 shows the results of such technical progress: a large multipolar anterior horn cell containing the age pigment lipofucsin. Deiters proved that one special process of a nerve cell could be followed for some distance and he termed this the main process. This main process started from the cell as a thin, unmyelinated extension; it was much later that neurophysiologists realised the significance of this initial segment of the axon in the elicitation of action potentials. Deiters and Kölliker opposed the view of a syncytially organised nervous system. Further progress resulted from the work of the neurologist Stilling (1859) who used frozen sections to study thin slices of the spinal cord. A freezing microtome was constructed in Edinburgh by Shirling, who used paraffin for embedding tissue; embedding

in celloidin (Duval, 1872) proved to be still better for brain tissue. These technical advances provided considerable help for the understanding of brain cells, as can be seen in illustrations from the textbook by Schwalbe (1881).

Contact versus continuity between nerve cells

Major advances were obtained with the introduction of methods using silver and of methylene blue staining by Nissl (1894). The greatest insight, however, brought the Golgi methods (1886) (Figs 3.3 and 3.4). Golgi, an Italian psychiatrist, spent most of his time in the laboratory studying the structure of the cerebral cortex. The silver techniques reached technical perfection in the hands of the Spanish histologist

Fig. 3.2. Deiters (1865) gave the first clear description of the large anterior horn cell (motor neuron of the spinal cord) (from Glees, 1971). ax. = axon; ax.h. = axon hillock; d. = dendrites; n. = nucleus; p.g. = pigment granules (lipofucsin).

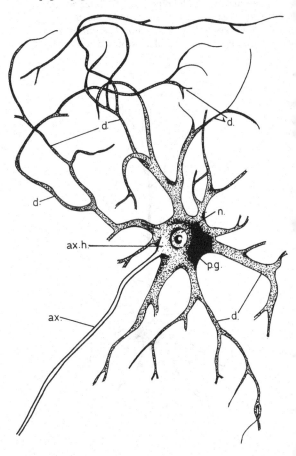

Ramon y Cajal during the years 1909 to 1906. Ramon y Cajal and Golgi were each awarded a Nobel prize in 1906 for their neurohistological discoveries. The Golgi impregnation, using potassium chromate and osmium, produced pictures of great clarity of individual neurons, in particular from embryological materials. Although this method showed neurons and their supporting cells, the neuroglia, completely isolated from each other, Golgi himself was convinced of the syncytial nature of nervous tissue and accepted the views of Gerlach (1872a,b), a famous histologist who used the gold chloride method for staining. The year 1880 was characterised by two violently opposed groups of scientists. One group, represented by Ramon y Cajal, Forel (1887), von Waldeyer (1891) and Kölliker, were referred to as 'neuronists'; the other group, represented by Golgi, Dogiel (1893a,b) and Gerlach, were the 'reticulists'. The latter view was upheld until recently by Boeke (1935), Stöhr (1951)

and K. Bauer (1948). The neuronal concept proved to be the more fruitful one and in 1906 Sherrington firmly established the physiological properties of the junctions between nerve cells, termed by him *synapses*. Sherrington, a leading English physiologist of his time, was himself a keen histologist and a friend of Ramon y Cajal, who had shown him the sections of the nervous system made with his techniques. Ramon y Cajal's silver preparations demonstrated clearly very fine, loop-like terminations (Fig. 3.5) often compared to buttons (*boutons terminaux*). Severance of nerve tracts caused recognisable degenerative structural changes in these terminal boutons, proving their identity as terminal contacts of a particular fibre connection.

The discovery that neurons are interconnected by specialised tight contacts but are not continuous also brought clarity to the nature of Golgi's *thorns* (Fig. 9.40), which are also parts of specialised contacts. The synapses were also seen and reported by the Leipzig neurohistologist Held (1906) and by Auerbach

Fig. 3.3. Pyramidal cells of the cerebral cortex, referred to as Golgi type I, are characterised by multiple branching of apical and basal dendrites (from Glees, 1971). a.d. = apical dendrites; ax. = axon; b.d. = basal dendrites; c.b. = cell body.

Fig. 3.4. Golgi type II neurons are characterised by a relatively short axon with diffuse local branches. These cells are also referred to as small stellate or small granular cells. Larger stellate cells have longer axons for spreading impulses. Type II neurons are said to make up about one third of all cortical neurons are can be divided into several types related to the mode of branching (from Glees, 1971). ax. = axon; c.b. = cell body; d = dendrites; tr.ax. = terminal branches of axon.

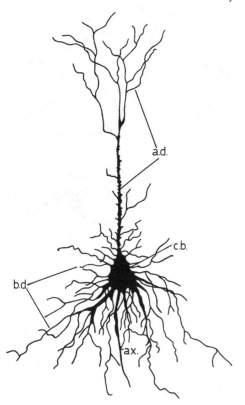

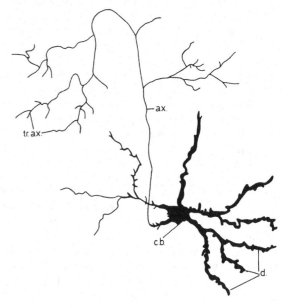

(1898a,b). Held changed his views in 1927 after seeing a very fine interconnecting fibrous matrix between the terminal bouton and the cell in his preparations. He may well have seen the amorphous substance between the pre- and post-synaptic portion of the contact. Degeneration experiments and electron microscope studies by de Robertis (1964), Gray (1959) and Vogel (1962) proved the contact theory (Fig. 3.6).

The neuron

With the light microscope and a cresyl violet stain (Nissl stain), the nerve cell shows its characteristic appearance (Fig. 3.7), with large round nucleus, filled with chromatin, and a nucleolus staining deeply blue. The cytoplasm contains similar blue-staining bodies which extend into the cell's processes except for the axon. This characteristic Nissl picture of the neuron also portrays the physiological state of nerve cells. Nissl recognised that injury to the neuron, such as severing it from its long axonal process, caused a dissolution of the organised Nissl substance into free ribosomes, a picture termed by him *'primäre Reizung'* (primary irritation (Fig. 3.7(b)). This could be accompanied by a peripheral displacement of the nucleus or by its expulsion from the cell. This cellular reaction reverts the neurons to an embryonic state and can lead to reforming of organised Nissl substance and recovery of function as far as spinal motor neurons are concerned. Such recovery of function produces a regrowth of axons which can occur after

peripheral nerve lesions or occasionally in patients after poliomyelitis, a virus disease. Nissl, a professor of psychiatry, was greatly interested in neuronal changes which might occur in mental diseases and devoted a great deal of his scientific work towards this aim. The Nissl picture of neurons is still a useful and valid criterion of the functional state of nerve cells and has *not* been superceded by electron microscopy, although this gives a much more detailed and refined picture.

An electron micrograph is shown in Figs 3.7(c) and 3.8. The nucleus is enveloped by a double membrane and filled with fine granules and a denser mass, the nucleolus. The nuclear membranes have pores through which fine granules are extruded into the cytoplasm. The cytoplasm contains complexes of tubules whose walls have protein granules attached (rough endoplasmic reticulum); each of these complexes represents the Nissl body seen in light microscopy. Close to these complexes are found numerous mitochondria, smooth endoplasmic reticulum, neurofilaments and neurotubules. The neurotubules are probably responsible for transport of substances of low molecular weight such as horseradish peroxidase (HRP) and the transport ability in *both* directions (Fig. 3.7(c)) is used for marking and mapping pathways (Figs 3.7(b),(c) and 3.9). Depending on the age of the neurons, numerous osmiophilic bodies or lipofuscin are present.

Mitochondria keep the cell metabolism going during both the resting and active states of the cell. This is the reason why nerve cells are especially vulnerable when stressed in anoxic periods such as occur in birth, anaesthesia, vascular spasms and ageing. Transplantation of organs, such as the kidney, liver and heart, has shown that these organs can survive an anoxic period of up to 10 hours under cooled condi-

Fig. 3.5. The classic picture of a silver-impregnated motor neuron of the spinal cord, showing the neurofibril content of the neuroplasm and indicating the positions of contact points referred to as terminal boutons (from Glees, 1971). A = axon; B = boutons; D = dendrites; N = nucleus.

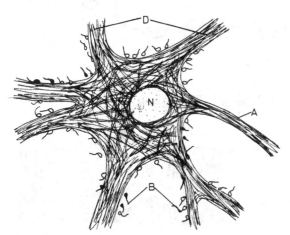

Fig. 3.6. In general terms synapses exhibit three types of pre-synaptic bag. The S-type contains round vesicles, the F-type has flat or oval-shaped vesicles and the C-type has vesicles with dense cores. The round clear vesicles are thought to be excitatory, the flat vesicles contain inhibitory substances, and the dense-cored vesicles probably contain noradrenaline (from Glees, 1971).

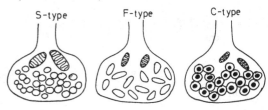

Fig. 3.7. (*a*) The classic picture of a Nissl-stained neuron, depicted diagrammatically. This is an important staining method in light microscopy and is much used for human post-mortem material (from Glees, 1971).

(*b*) The classical method for tracing connections in the CNS and peripheral nervous system used the degeneration consequent upon the severing of nerve fibres. i. represents an incision. Peripherally, there is disintegration of the axon and myelin sheath (deg.m.s.), and of the terminations, both finer branches (p.t. = preterminals) and *boutons terminaux* (b.t.). Laterally, the stem cells in A and B react by a reorganisation of their Nissl substances; the endoplasmic reticulum disperses to form free

ribosomes and the neuron reverts to a growing phase. The nucleus moves to a peripheral position. This stage is called chromotolysis (from Glees, 1961a). ax. = axon; chr.n.c. = chromotolytic nerve cell; d. = dendrite; nn. = neuroglia nucleus; n.s. = nuclei of the soleplate; R = node of Ranvier.

(*c*) Modern methods of tracing interconnections are based on the ability of neurons to transport substances. Horseradish peroxidase (HRP) is used as a marker substance. When injected intracellularly, HRP is transported towards the terminals. When injected extracellularly and close to the terminals, HRP is carried towards the cell body, probably by the action of microtubules. M = mitochondrion; mf = microfilament; mt = microtubule.

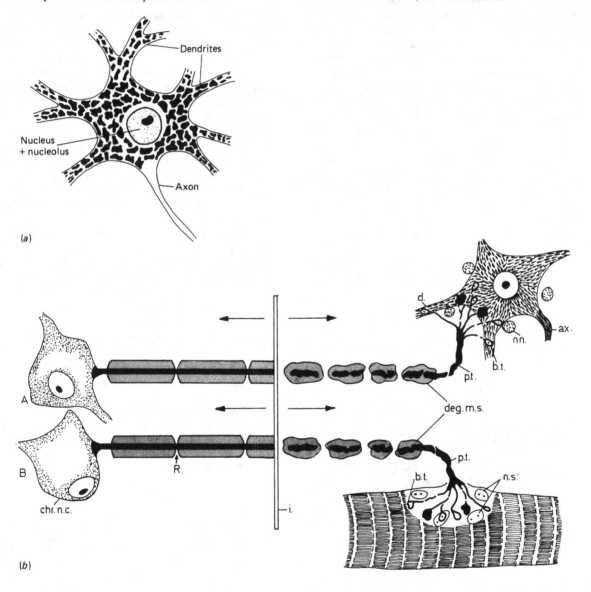

(a)

(b)

Fig. 3.7 (contd.)

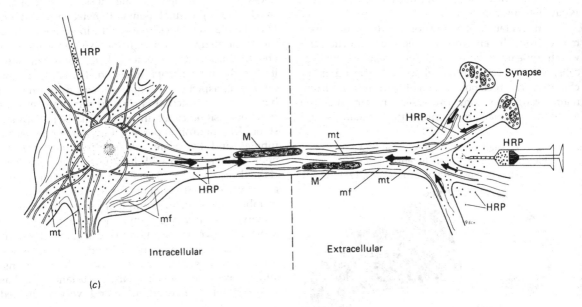

(c)

Fig. 3.8. Drawing from an electron microscope picture of a neuron (from the lateral geniculate nucleus). The finer structures such as mitochondria, microtubules and neurofilaments are shown. The great number of mitochondria testify to a state of constant activity (from Glees, 1971a). a. = axon; a.-d.s. = axo-dendritic synapse; a.-s.s. = axo-somatic synapse; d. = dendrite; e.r. = endoplasmic reticulum; f.r. = free ribosomes; m. = mitochondrion; n. = nucleus; n.f. = neurofibril; n.p. = nuclear pore; o.b. = osmiophilic body; s. = synapse; sh. = sheath.

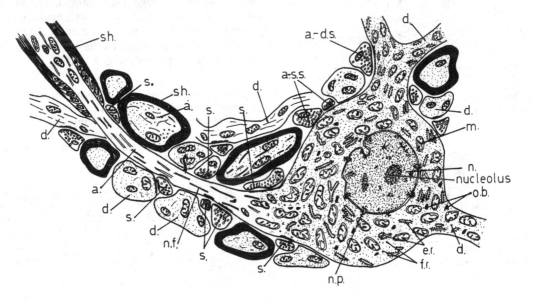

tions. This astonishingly long survival is not valid for brain cells, which last only for minutes when oxygen is cut off completely.

The metabolic demands on neurons can be estimated from the enormous density of mitochondria which appears to be even greater than that in liver cells, which each contain about a thousand mitochondria. The metabolic needs of neurons arise from: maintaining their long processes, in particular the axon; the manufacture of transmitter substances; and

Fig. 3.9. Diagrammatic representations of a mitochondrion. (*a*) Three-dimensional view. c. = cristae; (*b*) cross-section (from Glees, 1971).

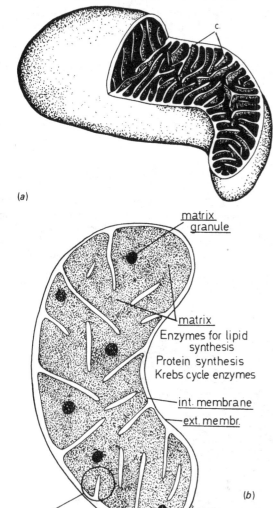

(*a*)

matrix granule

matrix
Enzymes for lipid synthesis
Protein synthesis
Krebs cycle enzymes

int. membrane

ext. membr.

(*b*)

invagination of inner membrane
Enzymes of oxidative phosphorylation
ATPase

the supply of energy for action and resting potentials necessary for the state of alertness. These changes in electrical potential demand metabolically maintained ionic exchanges between the interior and exterior of the neuron, although the axon appears to be able to conduct action potentials for some time after its cytoplasmic content is removed. The Golgi apparatus is a conspicuous tubular element of the neuron but, while its function is clear in secreting cells, its functional significance in nerve cells is not understood. The neuron is pervaded by numerous neurotubules and by protein filaments which are the neurofilaments seen with light microscopy in silver-stained sections (Fig. 3.5). The neuron is thus a conglomerate of a variety of organelles which are mainly membranous structures and it appears that neuronal activity is essentially a membrane phenomenon. The dendritic processes of the nerve cells have the same cytological structure as the cell body and are essentially receptive expansions of the cell, while the transmitting axon contains no Nissl substance but has neurofilaments, neurotubules and very elongated mitochondria.

The axon and its functional significance

The axon which conducts the discharge frequency of the cell body (the action potential) is a continuous conductor surrounded, in most cases, by a myelin sheath. The myelin sheath is composed of bilayers of phospholipids plus protein, cholesterol, glycolipids and sphingomyelin. The glycolipids contain gangliosides and cerebroside sulphates. The myelin protein contains a positively charged basic myelin, while the lipids are negatively charged. The myelin sheath is not secreted by the axon but is manufactured by non-neuronal cells, those of the neuroglia. These cells are the oligodendroglia cells in the CNS and Schwann cells peripherally (Fig. 3.10).

Fig. 3.10. Formation of the myelin sheath and enveloping action of the Schwann cell cytoplasm (from Glees, 1971). Beginning of myelinisation. a. = axon; ccSchw = cell cytoplasm. (*b*) The enveloping process. (*c*) The final result. m = myelin lamellae.

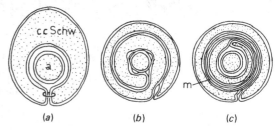

(*a*)   (*b*)   (*c*)

Fig. 3.11. Section through a peripheral nerve stained to show myelinated nerve fibres (myel.n.f.) (from Glees, 1971). b.v. = blood vessels; e. = epineurium; en. = endoneurium; f.c. = fat cells; p. = perineurium.

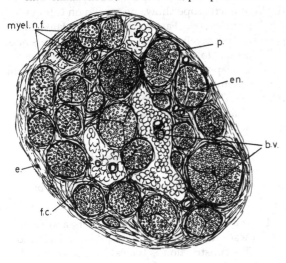

The peripheral nerves, in contrast to the central nerve fibres, possess an additional coat, the endoneural sheath of connective tissue. Peripheral nerves are axonal processes of motor neurons inside the brain and spinal cord, processes of spinal ganglion cells and processes of sympathetic and parasympathetic neurons outside the CNS. All these processes form the structure of a mixed nerve cable (Figs 3.11 and 3.12). Many of these fibres are motor in nature, conducting spinal impulses to extremities where muscles innervated by these nerves perform simple lever actions or execute finely differentiated skilled movements which have to be learned and are supervised by the cerebral and cerebellar cortex. Nerve fibres which carry impulses from the skin towards the nervous system are referred to as sensory fibres; those fibres from sympathetic or parasympathetic ganglia (Fig. 3.13) which terminate in glands or blood vessels are called autonomic fibres, being independent of volition (see p. 90). Fibres terminating in skeletal muscle are fast-conducting fibres, thickly myelinated, while those from the skin are of varying diameters. Reflex fibres reporting the degree of muscle tension needed for posture are fast-conducting fibres, since the recordings from muscle spindles and tendons have to be evaluated quickly.

Measurements of conduction speeds by Gasser & Erlanger (1927) led to the division of the mixed peripheral nerves into three main groups. The A fibres conduct most quickly (up to 120 m/s) and have a high amplitude. These are followed by B fibres (15 m/s)

Fig. 3.12. Diagrammatic representation of peripheral nerve fibres in longitudinal section (from Glees, 1971). a. = axon; e. = endoneurium; my.S. = myelin sheath; n.R. = node of Ranvier; p. = perineurium; Schw. = Schwann cell sheath enveloping an unmyelinated nerve fibre (unmy.f.); Schw.n. = Schwann cell nucleus.

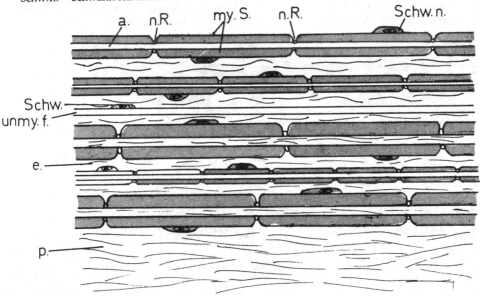

Fig. 3.13. Autonomic multipolar nerve cells stained with silver solution. This stain shows up the neurofibrils, comprised of neurofilaments and neurotubules. Neurofilaments have a diameter of about 10 nm, while neurotubules have a diameter of 20–26 nm (from Glees, 1971).

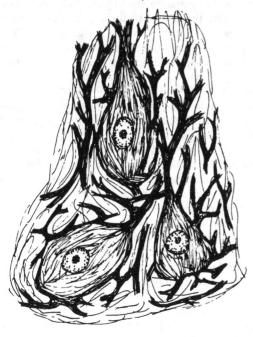

and by the very slow C fibres (0.7–2.3 m/s). The A fibres have been subdivided further into α, β and γ fibres. (Aδ fibres correspond to the original B group.) Fibres of the A and B groups are all myelinated, while the light microscope shows no myelin on C fibres but a Schwann sheath. Fast conduction is related to the presence of a myelin sheath, to axonal thickness and, in particular, to the presence of gaps in the myelin. At these gaps – nodes of Ranvier (Fig. 3.14) – the axonal membrane is open to the exterior. Action potentials (Fig. 3.15) appear to jump from node to node while non-myelinated fibre conduction is continuous.

Fundamental organisation of the nervous system

Two modes of organisation appear to be preferred:

1. Neurons are combined in clusters and each of these clusters designed for a separate function. This construction is typical for the grey matter or cell body arrangement throughout the CNS.
2. A layered structure, as in the neurons of the mammalian cerebral cortex.

The neurons of the cerebral cortex are arranged in horizontal cell bands of equal size and polar orientation (see Fig. 7.13), while the afferent and efferent fibres are grouped in vertical bundles which originate

Fig. 3.14. A node of Ranvier (n.R.) represents the joining of two Schwann cell territories (from Glees, 1971). a.c. = axon cytoplasm; e.r. = ergastoplasm; l.myel. = laminae of myelin; m. = mitochondrion; m.a. = membrane of axon; nf. = neurofilaments; nt. = neurotubules; o.m.Schw. = outer membrane of Schwann cell; Schw.c. = Schwann cell cytoplasm; Schw.n. = Schwann cell nucleus.

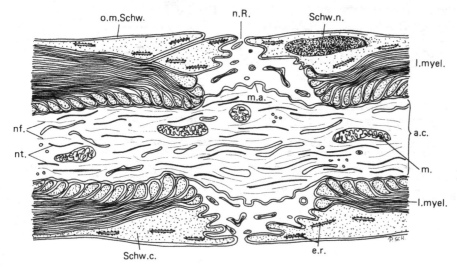

from the underlying white matter, the ascending fibres, or descend into the white matter. This arrangement provides for an orderly and precise 'wiring up' and ascending afferent fibres contact columns of cortical neurons in all layers (see Fig. 7.15). In addition, the side branches of cortical neurons allow interaction with neighbouring receptive columns of neurons.

The number of synaptic contacts of an individual neuron is very high. Sholl (1956) calculated from Golgi preparations that one cortical neuron may have as many as 4000 contacts with other neurons and one afferent cortical fibre may have contacts with 5000 neurons. The number of cortical layers increases up the evolutionary scale: evolutionarily older cortical areas have only three layers, while more recently acquired areas have six or seven layers. However, neuronal cell size decreased while the number of cell processes increased with evolution, indicating that

interconnectivity is the more important issue. This may also imply that the cell body surface is kept free from too many synaptic contacts to allow for metabolic exchanges with neighbouring capillaries and glial contacts (see Fig. 5.7). The dendrites are predominantly receptive and the excitability is modulated continuously.

Research into the functional state and structure of the cerebral cortex is progressing at great pace and has been summarised recently in a monograph by O. Creutzfeldt (1983). But the complex structure makes combined studies of morphology and function a slow task. Taking into account the regularity of the distribution of cells and their interconnections, a comparison with modern computers is obvious. While a computer can and has replaced cerebral cortex function, it is unlikely to replace the human brain as such. The human brain is preprogrammed by genetics, programmed by family and environmental influences, and continuously biased by metabolic and sociosexual demands which cannot be input into a machine. The erratic demands of the 'personality in depth', stimulated by sense organs, are normally blended with the logical and orderly resources of the cerebral cortex. But the cerebral cortex is only a part of the human brain, tied down to subcortical levels and never completely free from evolutionary instincts and ancestral tendencies.

Regeneration of neural tissue

Problems of neural repair become obvious and urgent during times of war. However, the modern way of life, with motor car accidents and terrorist activities, produces great numbers of head and spinal injuries, making the search for methods of repair a daily and distressing need.

True repair cannot realistically be expected. The very nature of neural organisation and interconnectivity precludes a positive solution. The most that can be expected are 'roundabout' interventions by rerouting muscles and their tendons or by direct electrical stimulation of efferent peripheral pathways, separated from their controlling centres. The central nervous tissue, once having reached its final steps of organisation in the foetus and very densely packed, shows no tendency for replacement apart from some subcortical areas discussed later. A spastic child with injuries suffered at birth will not regrow its corticospinal connections. Similarly, a child deprived of oxygen at birth will not develop its full brain power and will remain mentally retarded or demented. The anterior horn cells and the ganglion cells are, however, capable of regeneration assuring that a cut peripheral

Fig. 3.15. Action potentials are recorded along the nerve from the place of electrical stimulation. The action potentials arrive in a time related to the thickness of the fibre, which is in turn related to the outer nodal distance. (*a*) The $\alpha\,\beta\,\gamma$ and δ fibres arrive in sequence; (*b*) the thin c fibres propagate their potentials slowly (from Glees, 1961a).

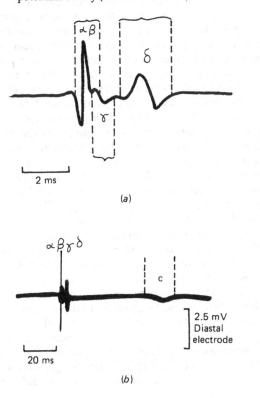

nerve will regrow and establish new connections in the periphery. This regeneration is a regrowth, not a joining up of the central and peripheral stumps. Regeneration in the peripheral nervous system has been studied in great and admirable detail by Cajal

Fig. 3.16. Diagram illustrating peripheral nerve fibre regeneration (from Ramòn y Cajal (1928)). A = central stump, containing regenerating fibres with growth cones aiming in the wrong direction a,b. C = middle region or gap showing numerous regeneration fibres 'exploring' the area. B = peripheral stump regenerating fibres entering the peripheral degenerated stump e,f. and g; d = axonal spirals.

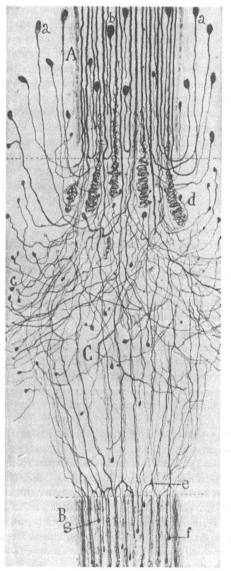

(1928), these studies, comprehensive and beautifully illustrated, are still a source for enlightenment and one basic drawing from this great work is reproduced in Fig. 3.16. Since Cajal's painstaking work based on silverstains, modern methods have been employed to investigate nerve regeneration with special reference to the neurons whose axons have been cut. The neurons were studied by using monoclonal antibodies which mark the neurofilamentous protein. These reactions show differences with the changes seen in the Nissl stained preparations of the neurons and illustrate protein synthesis needed for transport to the distant sites of regenerating axons (Moss & Lewkowicz, 1983).

After severance the peripheral stump degenerates quickly and a proliferation of Schwann cells occurs, filling the empty endoneuronal connective sheaths with the new axonal sprouts. The central stump axons, still in continuity with the cells of origin, produce at their cut ends growth cones filled with mitochondria, and sprouting of axonal filaments begins. These axonal protrusions tend to enter the peripheral stump and, depending on the interval between injury and regeneration, may enter empty endoneuronal tubes or may push their way through the débris of the injured stump. Vigorous macrophage activity indicates the removal of the old degenerating nerve fibres. Much experimental work has been done to bridge the gap with material facilitating the ingrowth of regenerating axonal sprouts, ranging from tubular plastic aids to freeze-dried, specially prepared nerve grafts from cadavers. The literature of regeneration aids is vast and the following reference should be consulted for details (Sunderland, 1968).

All attempts to achieve tract regeneration, e.g. of corticospinal fibres restoring voluntary movements after a spinal injury, have failed so far, although initial regeneration seems to occur. I believe one of the reasons for failure is the slow removal of degenerating myelin and axon material. When studying de- and regeneration one interesting fact emerges. The myelin sheath degenerates very rapidly, although the myelin-manufacturing cells – oligoglia and Schwann cells – are local features unaffected by the cuts. Axonal degeneration is easily understood, as the cut peripheral fibre is deprived of its metabolic pumping station (see Figs 3.7(*b*),(*c*), the neuron. Centrally, and in contrast to the periphery, the fragmented portions of myelin are slow to be broken up and transported to the vessels by phagocytes. In Man it may take more than one year for clearing a degenerated pathway for the possibility of regeneration. Furthermore, the gaps caused in a spinal cord by gun shots or knife wounds are large and eventually bridged by a glial scar, preventing the penetration of any axonal sprouts in their descent or ascent. Wheelchair-bound patients suffering from penetrating central injury are a permanent and lasting unhappy sign of the failure of central regeneration.

Regeneration in the central nervous system does occur in 'lower' vertebrates such as amphibians and fishes (Kirsche, 1964) but appears to be produced by a residual layer of matrix cells not present in higher vertebrates. In Man it seems inconceivable that a highly integrated nervous system, densely packed, with a cortex as an enormous storage of past events would be subject to regeneration which would be without value to Man, since memory of the past would be lost.

Swedish workers (Bjorklund, Segal & Steneri, 1979) are at present attempting to overcome the lack of regeneration in the adult rat brain by implanting replacement embryonic tissue. Embryonic locus coeruleus tissue has been implanted into adult rats in which the hippocampal connections had been severed. After 3 to 6 months, a new growth of adrenergic fibres from the implant into the hippocampus was found to have re-established the connection. The authors believe that this animal model shows promise for the replacement of lost neural tissue.

A further interesting line of research with the aim of promoting nerve regeneration has been followed up by Levi-Montalcini* and her co-workers (Levi-Montalcini, 1966). These workers discovered a nerve growth factor (NGF) present in snake venom and in mouse salivary glands. The NGF for experimental studies has been extracted from mouse salivary glands. It is a heat-labile protein. The biological activity is destroyed by a specific antiserum to this protein and has a molecular weight of 44 000. The NGF promotes vigorous growth of sensory and sympathetic ganglia, but NGF affects the sensory nerve cell only during a restricted life cycle. Tissue culture studies indicated that the growth factor stimulates the production of an essential component of the cell synthetic system (RNA).

The failure of regeneration does not exclude improvements in the condition of a patient suffering from a cerebral stroke. A stroke is caused by the occlusion of a cerebral vessel blocked by an embolus or a thrombosis, often on the basis of arteriosclerotic vascular changes. Usually the damaged vessel and its ischaemic brain area are unilateral and they may involve either the dominant or the non-dominant hemisphere (see p. 102). In the case of the dominant

* Nobel Prize 1986.

(leading) hemisphere, major impairments in speech and dexterity result. Depending on the patient's age and willpower and determination to get better, the intact hemisphere can be trained to take over or compensate to a varying degree for deficiencies associated with the stroke. A brain-injured person presents a complex problem for the neurologist, psychologist and physiotherapist. Particularly frustrating is the inability to speak or to use the right words for a particular wish. Furthermore, the brain-damaged patient is very dependent on his environment and can be at the same time moody, depressed and aggressive. The care of the brain-injured is very demanding on their family and nursing staff. This is one of the reasons why, in many countries, special rehabilitation centres have been created, caring for early nursing and therapy, where the patient can be instructed in the use of artificial devices to give some mobility. The increase in spinal injuries and the progressing number of ageing people with cardiovascular diseases leading to strokes require that these specialist centres be enlarged and equipped more fully. (In this connection, one may compare the early and now classical papers on war injuries by the late Sir Ludwig Guttmann (Guttmann, 1953).

Ageing – an important social problem of our time

Ageing is the fate of multicellular organisms whose reproductive ability and thus biological value have been lost. In taking this view, one assumes that all genetic programming has only one goal – to produce offspring; ageing is the slow decay and running down of the individual. An alternative view of the ageing process is that waste products accumulate in the cells of the body, condemning them to death.

The first view, that ageing causes the running down of the 'biological clock' towards the end of life, is generally accepted in most societies. One reason for wishing to prolong the active life of an individual, i.e. to try to postpone the running down and cessation of the 'biological clock', is that the brain is the only organ which becomes more valuable throughout life, not only for the individual concerned but also in many cases for society, as a result of its accumulated knowledge.

Signs of ageing

A sure sign of 'getting old', in the biological sense, is the loss of reproductive ability, which occurs earlier in women than in men. This loss is usually combined with ageing of other organs – the skin loses its elasticity, muscle fibres lose their contractability, and bones get brittle. Society places pressure on men and, particularly, on women to keep looking young despite advancing years; this is greatly in the interests of the cosmetic industry and plastic surgeons. The cessation of gonadal function and of the production of associated hormones at the menopause illustrates that different organs have different lifespans: the 'biological clock' is organ-specific.

Ageing of the nervous system

In relation to the early cessation of gonadal function, one might suggest that the hypothalamus, and in particular its neurosecretory neurons, is exhausted before the great majority of neurons concerned solely with impulse generation. If this were so, the hypothalamus would be the neuronal 'biological clock', setting the time span for general neural ageing. This is likely to be so, since hypothalamic disease can speed up puberty or delay maturation and also affect the rates of body growth and other functions. The consequence of this would be that neuronal ageing, particularly when combined with a lack of neurosecretion, would make ageing unavoidable and part of the general running-down process.

The running down of our neuronal machinery is even more catastrophic, in fact, since practically no new neurons appear after birth. The neuron, like the muscle cell, is a post-mitotic cell and therefore unable to divide. In view of the intense branching of neurons and their interconnectivity – already present in the foetus – a cell division would be senseless and impossible. However, Altmann (1969a,b) concluded from his autoradiographic studies in rats, guinea-pigs and cats that a great number of immature cells are present after birth. These cells are said to be capable of forming Golgi type II neurons (see Fig. 3.4) interconnecting different brain areas. Altmann and his co-workers believe that these cells, maturing relatively late, are important for learning in early infancy.

The real problem in our account of ageing is to discover the morphology of the neuronal ageing which is so obvious to us all when approaching middle age. We all note a reduction in learning ability, we become forgetful, we have difficulty in remembering the names of people we meet only occasionally. We need more rest periods, feeling more exhausted after a heavy working day than we did ten years earlier. At the same time our eyesight and hearing become less acute; this sense organ impairment may result in apparent brain deterioration which is not in fact the case.

We must also take into account the effects of nutritional damage and of drugs, including alcohol and nicotine, which may speed up the ageing process. X-rays and atomic or cosmic radiation cause marked premature ageing of the whole body.

Problems of retirement

Motor skill slows with advancing age. Although increasing automation of manufacturing should benefit the older worker, a system allowing more frequent holidays for older workers would be more advantageous. Early retirement is not necessarily a good thing, however, since the mental and physical activity of modern Man is bound up with his work. An abrupt cut-off may lead to rapid mental deterioration, enhanced by separation from colleagues and the work programme. It would improve the morale of retired workers if they could fill in for their younger colleagues on leave. Although expensive intellectual training does not bear fruit for maybe thirty years, there is now a tendency towards earlier retirement. An alternative work strategy would be to retrain older workers during their lives so that they could switch to less physically demanding jobs when getting older, rather than ceasing to work altogether. An easy transition to a relaxed time as a pensioner can be difficult.

Morphological signs of neuronal ageing

Examination of normal brains of different ages with both light and electron microscopy has demonstrated a lipid-containing pigment, lipofuchsin, in the brain cells. This pigment has a brownish-yellow colour and stains intensely black with osmic acid (Fig. 3.17). The literature on neuronal lipofuchsin is extensive; the review of Glees & Hasan (1976a) should be consulted for further information.

Diseases associated with brain ageing

Diseases closely related to ageing of the brain are senile dementia, a demented state on the basis of arteriosclerotic vascular changes, and pre-senile dementia. As discussed earlier, Flechsig was hopeful that mental diseases would have morphologically visible underlying causes. This hope proved to be true in only a few clinical pictures, while major mental disorders such as schizophrenia and the manic depressive states are biochemical disorders without a defineable structural substratum. Although not related directly to ageing, these disorders are influenced by age.

Senile dementia. Senile dementia is a disease process of advanced age, beginning around the seventies, and is observed more frequently in women than in men. Its onset is difficult to recognise but the disease progresses steadily. The family of the patient eventually

Fig. 3.17. The ageing of neurons by accumulating
granules of age pigment (lipofuscin).
(*a*) Hippocampal pyramidal cells of CA4 segment (see
Fig. 7.15), the cell bodies are filled with lipofuscin.
(*b*) A large motor neuron of lumbar spinal cord
containing a mass of lipofuscin (P). D = dendrite free
from pigment; MC = microglia cells filled with
pigment.

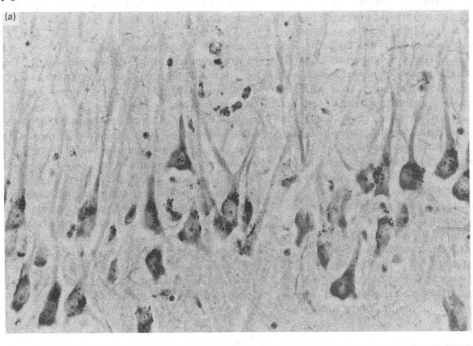

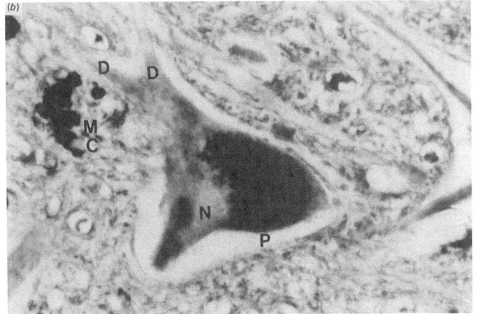

becomes aware of his/her diminishing interest in the surroundings and a flattening of emotions. At the beginning, the emotional tone of the patient is depressed or full of paranoid ideas, or he/she is occupied with feelings of being ill. Feelings of guilt, too, are freely expressed. The loss of emotions may make the old person tactless and apparently uncaring, making social integration difficult. The reduction of the relationship with the outside world forces the patient steadily to withdraw and there is a loss of interest in events previously dear to him/her, and a neglect of daily routine. Another sign is an aimless type of existence, shown by continuous perambulation about the house. Progressive loss of memory is characteristic and involves recent events most acutely – events in the distant past may still be recalled clearly. Relatives may not be recognised or may be mixed up with others who are dead. All these symptoms lead to a state of confusion. The patient is able to join in light, joking conversation but is unable to take part in serious discussion. At the same time his/her writing changes and words are omitted or used out of context. Eventually, the elderly patient is forced to remain at home, perhaps in a single room, fulfilling the classic conception of a senescent relative – wheelchair-bound and staring out of the window. If the disease worsens rapidly it may be necessary for the patient to enter an old people's home, where care and rigid routine are the rule. Such an institution may be a better solution than keeping the patient at home, since the burden of nursing is so demanding that many families are unable to cope with the problems involved.

Post-mortem examination of a patient dead from senile dementia shows marked atrophy of the brain and greatly increased ventricular cavities, the certain signs of greatly diminished brain substance; histological study shows a widespread disappearance of neurons.

Cerebral vascular sclerosis. Similar symptoms to those of senile dementia arise when arteriosclerotic changes occur, usually with progressing age after long periods of heavy smoking and high alcohol consumption. The changes involve the integrity of the personality, with reduced emotional control and marked mood swings, often ending in excessive weeping. Confusional states fluctuate with depressed phases; small strokes, causing minor impairments, are the expressions of reduced blood supply to the brain. While senile dementia shows a continuous mental deterioration, the patient suffering from cerebral vascular sclerosis can show periods of intellectual improvement, particularly when treated with vasodilatory agents which allow sufficient blood flow to reach dormant areas of the brain. In senile dementia the nerve cells themselves are affected first, although lack of blood supply does eventually cause neuronal death.

4

The nature and transmission of the nervous impulse

The bioelectric current – basis for signal transmission

As living cells are unable to utilise a metallic conductor for communication, they have chosen other means: (1) extracellular for fluid metabolic products; (2) vascular transport for hormones; and (3) ionic generation of propagated membrane potentials. Cells can accumulate negatively charged molecules inside as a result of having a selectively permeable outer membrane. Thus, a potential difference exists between the cell's interior and the outside medium, and can be used for processes of de- and repolarisation. Electrical transmission of signals by the nervous system was investigated in the first half of the nineteenth century by eminent physiologists such as Dubois-Reymond (1843) and later by Hermann (1883) and Bernstein (1902). Galvani and Volta in Italy had already recognised the presence of electric currents in frog muscle, although Volta believed that the muscle only produced a current when metals were in contact with the moisture and salt of the muscle, rather like a battery. Galvani's work was carried on by Valli and eventually it was commonly agreed that the resting muscle had an electrical potential difference across it, with a negative charge within the muscle and a positive charge on its outside. The presence of a potential difference across an inactive muscle (the resting potential) was well demonstrated by the actual flow of current which was released when the muscle was injured. Nobili (1825) for instance, recorded a marked flow of current in a frog muscle preparation, which he, not unnaturally, called the 'frog current'. (The similarity between nerves and muscles in this respect was recognised, and the discoveries made were related to nerves as well as to muscles.) The polarity recorded on the cut surface of the muscle was negative and that on the intact exterior positive. The resting potential was thus the source of electromotive power which could be released by injury; in the same way, the presence of water under pressure in a mains pipe can be demonstrated by making a hole in that pipe. It was then a logical step to assume that the wave of excitation, or action current, was also the release of the resting potential, and that the active region of the nerve fibre resembled an injured region. Such a view was expressed in a modified form by Hermann (1883), but Bernstein (1902) pointed out an important difference: the current caused by injury is monophasic (i.e. of one polarity only) while the current in the intact contracting muscle or active nerve is diphasic (of both positive and negative polarity). The first actual recording of the diphasic wave was not made until some years later by Sanderson (1895) with a much more sensitive capillary electrometer.

What then was the relation, if any, between resting potential and action current and, more important, what was the physical basis of the electromotive force provided by the resting potential? One of Hermann's original objections to the prevalent idea that nervous conduction was based on electrical activity was the slow speed at which impulses moved along the nerve fibre, compared with the speed of electricity in metal conductors. It is true that the electrons responsible for high-speed conduction were absent from living tissue, but was it not possible for an electrical charge to be available from some other source? Electrically charged ions of salt solutions are present throughout all animal tissue. On this fact Bernstein (1902) based his membrane theory of conduction. The concentrations of salts (particularly those of sodium and potassium) in a nerve fibre, and therefore its osmotic and electrical properties, differ in every respect from those of its surroundings. Whereas the sodium ion is the cation of the extracellular fluid, the intracellular fluid of the nerve fibre contains a large concentration of a different cation, the potassium ion. The difference in polarity between the resting potential within the fibre and on its surface is reflected in a difference in ionic distribution. The crux of Bernstein's whole theory lay in the presence of a non-conducting, selectively permeable membrane separating the negatively charged ions from those with a positive charge. The membrane is only a few molecules thick but possesses great electrical capacitance and resistance. Bernstein's theory stated that the arrival of a wave of excitation would then break down this membrane and in so doing would allow both anions and cations free access to any part of the fibre. This would automatically depolarise the fibre and destroy the resting potential. In essence Bernstein's theory was correct, though he erred in regarding the action current as nothing but the depolarised resting potential with negative and positive charges both reduced to zero. Hodgkin & Huxley (1939), in re-examining the theory, found that the polarity of the active region of a nerve overshoots the zero mark and is actually the reverse of the resting potential (Fig. 4.1).

The differentially permeable membrane (this physiological membrane must not be confused with the anatomical membranes round the nerve fibre – the endoneural sheath, the neurolemma and the myelin sheath), then, maintains the internal potassium level and prevents the sodium ions in the extracellular fluid from entering the nerve fibres; any which do enter are promptly 'pumped out' by the cells or by the fibres, so that the resting potential is maintained (Donnan ionic equilibrium), and thus an electrical field is established between the interior and exterior of the nerve fibre. Hodgkin & Huxley (1945) made an accurate measurement of the potential gradient of this electric field by placing a fine microelectrode inside a

particularly thick nerve fibre of the cuttlefish *Sepia*; they found that the interior of the fibre was charged to about 100 mV negative to the exterior.

The stages in the process of nervous excitation are as follows. The strength of the electrical stimulus required to initiate a propagated wave of excitation is 15–20 mV. Weaker stimuli cause only local disturbances which, as Hodgkin (1951, 1958) pointed out, remain local because of the gradual and reversible balance existing between the resting potential of the fibre and the influx of sodium ions, the permeability of the membrane being controlled by the electrical field.

As soon as the strength and duration of the electrical stimulus have reached the threshold for a nerve fibre, however, the insulating membrane suddenly 'breaks down' and the nerve fibre is immediately depolarised by a rapid influx of sodium ions, indicated electrically by the spike potential, followed after a brief interval by an outward flux of potassium ions. During the period of the spike potential the interior of the fibre ceases to be negative and reaches the charge of +40 mV. The permeability of the membrane to sodium ions continues to increase until the concentration of these ions inside and outside is almost equally balanced. Shortly before this, however, there is a considerable outward movement of potassium ions which restores the original polarity (negative within the fibre) and the resting potential, and puts an end to the influx of sodium ions.

In a squid nerve fibre studied by Hodgkin & Huxley (1945) the resting potential was −45 mV, which made a total voltage change within the fibre of 85 mV, the charge during the action potential being +40 mV. According to Hodgkin & Huxley, the rising

Fig. 4.1. The local exchanges of sodium ions and potassium ions between the interior and exterior of a myelinated nerve fibre leads to action potentials at the nodes. These are illustrated by the traces.

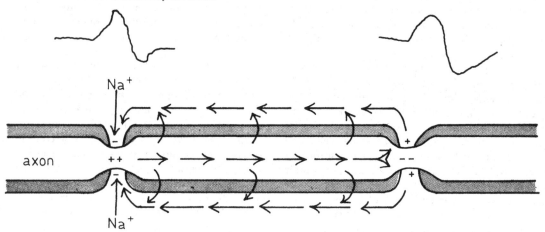

phase of the action or spike potential was produced solely by the influx of sodium ions, the outward movement of potassium ions eventually restoring the resting potential. But the fibre would thereby lose the means of generating electromotive force; sooner or later the internal potassium level must be restored by replacing the superfluous sodium with more potassium ions.

Nerve cell metabolism

It will be seen that the nerve fibre has two distinct metabolic tasks: first, the maintenance of the resting potential and, secondly, the restoration of the potential after excitation. In the inactive nerve fibre the metabolic processes are concerned with supplying the energy for the sodium pump, the mechanism which expels sodium ions from the inside of the fibre to maintain the resting potential. When the nerve becomes active and the ionic condition is changed, renewed metabolic energy is then required to restore the resting potential and the sodium pump has to 'work overtime'. The sodium pump demands at least 10% of the total metabolism of the fibre (Hodgkin & Keynes, 1954); as far as is known the potassium pump's requirements are less, but no accurate information is available about the exact amount. The metabolic activity concerned in the ionic exchange is too specialised a subject to be dealt with in detail here, and the following is little more than a pointer to further reading. The metabolic processes are normally assessed by studying oxygen consumption or carbon dioxide production and, indirectly, by measuring the heat produced by these processes. The level of oxygen required in the conduction of impulses can be studied by poisoning the pumps with dinitrophenol or cyanide. The emigration of sodium ions is studied using radioactively labelled sodium.

An inactive nerve – like other tissues – uses oxygen at a constant rate; oxygen consumption rises only when the level of excitation has lasted a considerable time, which suggests that the amount of oxygen stored is high or that not much more energy is required to generate impulses. For instance, a frog nerve will remain excitable for 2 hours at 20 °C, even when the supply of oxygen is excluded. A. V. Hill (1932) explained this by the presence of an oxygen reserve which would keep up nervous activity until exhausted. Muscle activity will, however, persist without oxygen for several days, provided that lactic acid can diffuse out. Hill has also measured the production of heat in the active and inactive nerve. In the active nerve he described, first, the initial heat which is produced during the passage of the impulse

or soon after; this he related to the partial discharge of an electrical double membrane layer on the surface of the fibre. This is followed by the 'recovery heat'. Von Muralt (1958) has calculated that the total heat produced by an active nerve is 30% higher than that found in an inactive nerve.

Other physical effects which can be observed during ionic exchange are changes in volume and in ability to reflect white light. These were investigated by D. K. Hill (1950) in the crustacean nerve trunk and in a single nerve fibre preparation of the cuttlefish, to discover if these changes had any connection with the metabolism of the fibre; the opacity was found to be due to the change in volume, itself due to an increase in osmotic pressure, and although this must be related to metabolism the exact connection is not clear.

Saltatory conduction

Katz (1952) has called the electrical excitation of a nerve an explosive and self-amplifying reaction, and it is true that the nerve impulse, once elicited, is no longer dependent on the energy of the initiating stimulus but is maintained by the energy produced by the nerve fibre and propagated by the reshuffling of ions in the intra- and extracellular fluids. This means that the nerve fibre is not a conductor of electrical current in the sense that a copper cable is, for the nerve fibre actually generates the current. The ionic exchange does not, however, occur to an equal extent all along the fibre, but only at specified intervals, and the sodium pump therefore only functions intermittently along the fibre, which explains the surprisingly small amount of energy required to work the pump when compared with the importance of the process of ionic exchange in nervous conduction.

In myelinated fibres, Erlanger & Gasser (1937) observed that conduction proceeded in a series of jumps, producing what is known as the saltatory wave. The internodal segments of the fibre (the sections between two nodes of Ranvier) seemed to be the units which regulated the speed of transmission. The nodes of Ranvier reacted to stimulation and to other factors in a different way from the internodal segments of the fibre. Tasaki (1948, 1952), when investigating a single nerve fibre with a microelectrode, found that a stimulus of threshold strength would excite the node but not the internodal segment, which showed that the node had the lowest threshold, and he suggested that conduction jumped from one node to the next and that the strength of the potential was maintained by reinforcement at each successive node. The threshold of a node is so low that a nervous impulse can bypass an anaesthetised node and excite the next (Tasaki & Takeuchi, 1941). Tasaki also observed that a dose of anaesthetic which affected the nodes and unmyelinated fibres alike did not depress conduction in internodal segments of the nerve. Changes of temperature affect the nodes very much more immediately and severely than the internodal segments; ultraviolet irradiation, when concentrated on the node, decreases its excitability, whereas the internodal segment is not affected, provided the myelin sheath is intact (Booth *et al.*, 1950).

The distance between the nodes of Ranvier can therefore be expected to have an important influence on the speed of conduction if the wave of excitation is propagated from one node to the next. The theory of saltatory conduction was discussed at length by Stämpfli (1954) who set out three points which had to be proved before the theory could be established. These were: (1) excitable structures (membranes) are confined to the nodes of Ranvier only; (2) internodes, insofar as conduction of the nervous impulse is concerned, are passive core conductors without any excitability; and (3) activity is transmitted from node to node through local circuits.

These three points, then, constitute the basis of saltatory conduction. It is now accepted that the action potential produced at a node initiates longitudinal electrotonic currents which, when they reach the next node, fire off new action potentials. The internodal segment temporarily affected has decreased resistance and is thus more permeable to sodium ions (this has been proved in the nerves of the frog by Tasaki & Freygang (1955), their evidence confirming earlier observations made by Hodgkin & Huxley (1945) on the squid giant axon). The zone of influx is called the 'sink' for the current flow. The neighbouring (inactive) parts of the membrane are the 'source' of the current flow. These electrotonic currents, or 'eddy currents', run along the internodal segments and, so to speak, set off the fuse in the next node, causing the depolarisation of the membrane which, in turn, initiates the same process at the following node. Since the longitudinal electrotonic current decreases in strength as its distance from the previous node increases, it might be thought that there would be a danger of its being too weak on arrival at the next node to excite it, and nervous conduction would therefore cease. According to Stämpfli, however, the strength of this action current is approximately five to seven times the stimulus threshold of the nodes, and he calls this the 'safety factor', for this means that the wave of excitation can, if necessary, skip over one or even two inexcitable nodes and still have suffi-

cient strength to continue the process of conduction.

It is due to the work of Hodgkin & Huxley, and Katz & Stämpfli, and to the studies of Grundfest, Shane & Freygang (1953), who found that a decreased concentration of sodium ions in the medium surrounding a nerve fibre depresses the action potential, that the ionic hypothesis of saltatory conduction has been fairly certainly established; the myelin around the nerve fibres appears to be a very efficient device which controls the inward and outward flow of sodium and potassium ions to the nodes.

Nerve impulses and brain waves

Having established the electrical nature of impulse transmission, the next problem to be solved is the code used by sense organs transmitting their messages to the centre. The experimental technique used is to listen into the active cable, tapping the conductors. This method was utilised predominantly by E. D. Adrian as early as 1928 and published in a classic and masterly monograph (Adrian, 1928). The sense organs distributed in the skin and in specialised positions in the head are constantly receiving outside stimuli and their transmitted series of nerve impulses were recorded electrically and acoustically. Impulses recorded from various sites – e.g. touch receptors, vision receptors – were propagated in a similar mode by action potentials or bursts of potentials, with any specific markings to identify their source. The sense organ discharges thus resulted in volleys of electric potentials and machine-gun like bursts were heard. In his monograph, *The basis of sensation*, Adrian compared the discharges (1) of the optic nerve after the eye was exposed to light and (2) of the sciatic nerve, produced by tension of a calf muscle. These records from very different sources look identical and do not betray their origins. The intensity of the stimulus was found to be expressed proportionately by the frequency of impulses.

Completely different electrical discharges can be recorded from the surface of the brain. These are wave-like oscillations and are not comparable to the spike discharges of active perpheral nerves. While the spike discharges can be compared to the electrical discharges of zig-zag flashes of lightning, the brain waves can be compared to flashes of diffused brightness seen in clouds in a hot summer night. These slow discharges were discovered by the German psychiatrist Berger (1929). To honour the discoverer, Adrian called the slow waves, of about 10 cycles/s, Berger rhythm (see Fig. 4.2).

Before the scientific significance of brain waves was well known, much clinical use was made of their recording. It was easy to record these electrical oscillations from electrodes attached to the skin of the scalp. This led to valuable *diagnostic findings* about brain maturation, neurological diseases, and various functional states such as awareness and sleep. Foremost early researchers were Kornmüller in Germany, Grey Walter (a pupil of E. D. Adrian) in Britain and Gastaut in France who recognised different wave patterns from different brain regions (Kornmüller, 1935; Walter, 1953) (Fig. 4.2). The occipital lobe of the human brain, for example, emits brain waves of 10 cycles/s, which are called α waves (Berger rhythm). The human frontal lobe, however, has a faster wave pattern of lower amplitude.

Maturation processes are also expressed in brain wave patterns and Man needs to reach the twelfth year of life before a uniform cortical wave pattern of electrical activity can be recorded (Fig. 4.3). In the first year of life the activity is seen as slow waves, about 3 cycles/s. The frequency increases up to 4–7 cycles/s after the fifth year. After puberty some brain regions can yield frequencies up to 32 cycles/s. The amplitude of all frequencies recorded from the scalp is very low (0.1–200 μV) and the scalp acts like a filter for the potentials from the cortex. Uniformity and amplitude of brain waves increase when the subject is resting and the eyes are closed (Fig. 15.7).

The electroencephalograph (EEG)
Neurophysiological basis

Creutzfeldt (1983) has devoted much of his research to exploring the clinical application of the EEG and has carried out fundamental experimental work to search for the electrical sources of the EEG. Creutzfeldt has shown that the cortical EEG (recorded directly from the surface of the cerebrum) and the discharge activity of neurons immediately beneath the EEG electrode can be very similar. This makes a causal relation most likely. A primary source for cortical potentials are the afferents from specific and non-specific thalamocortical connections, which in turn lead to post-synaptic depolarisation of neurons, mainly in layer IV of the cortex. In this context the rhythmic waves of the EEG are generated by thalamic projection nuclei. It appears now that the specific projection nuclei of the thalamus are more important for EEG maintenance than are the non-specific nuclei. These specific projection nuclei are activated by peripheral sensory stimuli but inhibited by ascending reticular activity from midbrain levels. These interplays of activity lead to either a synchronised or a desynchronised EEG. It seems certain that the activity of thalamo-cortical neurons determines the functional

Fig. 4.2. The main types of electrical recording of the brain's activity (EEG) in relation to age and degree of consciousness (from Bushe & Glees, 1968).

Definition	Wave pattern	Frequency (cycles/s)	Average amplitude (μV)	Physiological variation of potentials of:			
				EEG during wakefulness		sleep EEG	
				adult	child	adult	child
delta-waves	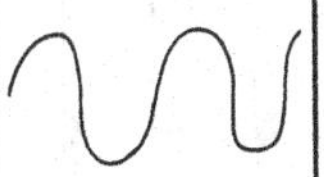	0.5–3	about 100 (5–250)	not present	dominating activity up to 18 months	can occur in all age groups	
theta-waves	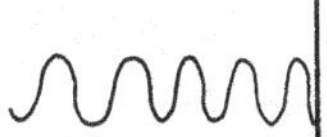	4–7	about 50 (20–100)	not always present	dominating 18 months to 5 years	normally present in all age groups	
alpha-waves	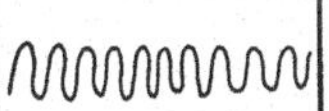	8–13	40–100 (20–120)	dominating activity	dominating from 5 years onwards	not typical for sleep	
beta-waves	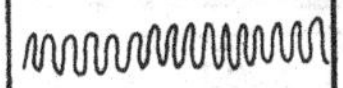	14–30	about 20 (5–20)	occurring in bursts frontally and pre-centrally	rarely occurring	β activity as 'spindles' in light sleep for all ages	

state of the cerebral cortex in conditions of alertness, its reduction and sleep. An EEG governed by α waves indicates relaxation. Disintegration of the rhythm and the appearance of slow waves means reduced attention and a state of consciousness lying between just being awake and falling asleep. Large slow waves of δ frequency indicate a state of unconsciousness, sleep or coma (Fig. 15.7). Depth of sleep is shown by an increase in very slow waves. A completely flat EEG indicates the cessation of thalamocortical activity.

Clinical significance

As is clear from the above, the EEG indicates the state of awareness, attention and sleep. This is the basis for its being an important diagnostic tool of the functional state of the cerebral cortex. Pathological states such as epilepsy and disturbances of cerebral regulation of activity can be easily recorded and allow the monitoring of drug application affecting the brain in the same way as the electrocardiogram allows the monitoring of heart treatment.

Sleep and its relation to the reticular function

Man spends about one third of his life sleeping. Generally speaking sleep is the arrest of specialised and orderly forebrain activity, while autonomic functions like respiration, circulation and digestion continue, though altered. From a general neurological point of view the state of consciousness varies in the

different degrees of sleep. We are all aware of the difficulty in waking someone from a very deep sleep and painful stimuli have to be strong causing a conscious reaction.

At first, brain researchers believed that sleep was caused by interrupting the afferent sensory flow, for this must be the conclusion watching a sleeper. His eyes are closed and he seems neither to hear or to feel. However this state is not due to an inhibition of sensory pathways. Sensory messages reach as usually their cortical destination, clearly to be seen as evoked potentials, but do not wake the sleeper. But some discrimination is left: a mother soundly asleep will wake up when her own child cries; a person deeply asleep will not respond to a series of names, but for his own. There is obviously a certain brain activity present and Berger (1929), the discoverer of the electric activity (EEG) of the brain, already showed characteristic slow potentials, so called spindle activity in different phases of sleeping. Illustrated in Fig. 4.4, four different stages of EEG activity can be discriminated:

I The first phase of going to sleep, lasting a few minutes, in which the sleeper is easily aroused show irregular electrical waves of low voltage

II The stage of spindle activity, showing marked discharges grouped together combined with slow eye movement

III The stage of slow waves of high voltage, almost 5× higher than when being awake, a slowing of pulse rate, blood pressure and temperature while the muscles show reduced tone

Fig. 4.3. Development of cortical activity and wave patterns (from Bushe & Glees, 1968).

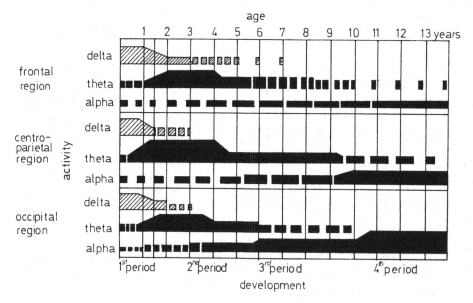

IV This is the phase of deep sleep, which can hardly be disturbed and usually predominant during the first half of the night.

After about 90 min of sleep special signs of sleep occur. The sleeper returns from stage IV to a phase characterised by very rapid eye movements (REM phase). In this phase marked dreaming occurs; depending on events during the day, dreams are of pleasant or menacing character. At the same time, respiration changes, body temperature increases, pulse rate and blood pressure elevate and the male will frequently show an erection combined with sexually explicit dreams. These REM episodes can appear several times at night or in early morning, when noises from beginning traffic 'creep into' dreams. It is not well known how far ageing changes this pattern and whether intense dreaming maintains or hinders a normal psychological life (Hess, 1964).

What is the essence of sleep? Instinctively, we reply that it is a necessary rest period for the brain exhausted by a day's activity. We all feel refreshed after a good night's sleep. However, the EEG recordings disprove the view that the brain 'sleeps' or is inactive, although the proportion of neurons awake is unknown. Hess in his experiments on the diencephalon (see above) assumed that mammals have a sleep centre and von Economo (1929) concluded from his neurological studies of encephalitis lethargica that Man has a centre for causing sleep in the periaqueductal grey matter of the midbrain. According to these views sleep is an active event, with its own rhythm, and is independent of day or night. Experiments on young volunteers housed in deep mines have shown that sleep and wakefulness are based on biological rhythms and not caused by outside events.

Another concept of sleep holds the opinion that the neurons need pauses to recharge their 'metabolic batteries' and that at the same time memory deposits take place while sleep prevents new recordings and provides the necessary periods of silence. If this were true the capacity for listening and recording of memories is limited, making teaching above a certain time limited an unwanted and unrewarding burden. The favourable fixation of memory in resting periods following learning seems to be proved by those pupils who claim a better retention of work before going to bed or early in the morning when the brain is said to be 'fresh'. Moruzzi, the Italian brain researcher, devoted much time to the study of sleep mechanisms and assumes that Pavlov's conclusions from his conditioning experiments concerning sleep were correct. Pavlov found that dogs fell deeply asleep when, in the course of an experiment, previously conditioned reflexes were evoked. Pavlov concluded that this led to a state of inhibition and spread over the whole cerebral cortex causing sleep. However, this cause of sleep only may be a special case for producing sleep.

The studies by Magoun (1958) and Moruzzi & Magoun (1949) of the reticular formation have given further support to the view that sleep and waking are regulated by the reticular formation of the brainstem, for this system regulates not only muscle tone but, with its ascending component, the state of consciousness, which in turn is integrated with the state of sleep (cf. Oswald, 1960, 1962). The significance of a switch on and off system already had been demonstrated by Bremer in his early EEG studies (1935) of the *encephale isolé* when his records showed alternating periods of wakefulness patterns and sleep patterns.

Fig. 4.4. Typical electroencephalographic records illustrating the states of wakefulness and sleep (after Jung, 1953). I: Frontal and occipital records show (*a*) alertness and (*b*) a drifting mental state. II–IV show stages of sleep: (*c, c*^{1}) spindles and frequent delta waves; (*d*) large delta waves (3 cycles per second); (*e*) large, very slow delta waves (0.6–1 c.p.s.). A, B: EEG records with very prominent alpha waves becoming more obvious in sleep.

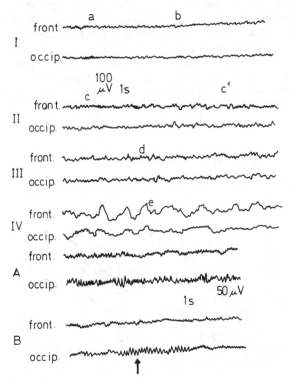

When Bremer (1954) eliminated parts of the activating reticular system the preparation showed all signs of sleep.

It would, however, be wrong to assume that sleep means a state of rest for the brain. Records from individual cortical cells show high activity while the overall oxygen consumption is high too. But individual brain regions when stimulated or executing commands (see p. 72) will show a much higher oxygen and glucose consumption. This clearly points out that the brain has *per se* a high metabolic maintenance metabolism. But the studies (in particular consult Jasper *et al.*, 1958) of the reticular formation apart from its influence on sleep, awakening and consciousness have been fruitful too in understanding drug action on the brain, e.g. the effects of anaesthetics, alerting drugs and tranquillisers (Silverstone & Turner, 1982). In summary we may conclude that Man needs 8 h of sleep, but the sleeping periods are independent of the rhythm of day and night, for polar expeditions report needing this amount of sleep whether working heavily or not. Sleep is an individual requirement and not a community activity. The human type of sleep is not necessarily the same as that seen in animals, where of course vast differences in mode of sleeping are present.

A baby may begin by sleeping almost continuously, deceiving the inexperienced mother about the future drain on her resources. In fact the baby has to be awoken to be fed. It is usually assumed that the baby is forced to blend into the day and night rhythm of its parents, but sleeping periods are independent of real time as outlined above. It seems that a short period of sleep in daytime – a nap – can restore fitness and it is important to give this to people, who are on a 24 h duty full of stress.

A brief word about snoring, which tells us of the presence of a sound sleeper, causing jealousy or anger in the still awake. It seems that snoring is an expression of an ageing reticular system or a reticular system lacking an adequate oxygen supply. Small sensory stimuli can restore the normal threshold without waking the sleeper. Snoring can only be afforded by people safe in their bed. Wild living animals have a lighter sleep and civilised human sleep is different from animal sleep, unless domesticated, for the animal can rest but not sleep deeply without being made a prey. For primitive type of living sleep means being defenceless and the sleeping animal has to hide, to survive. Animals sleeping in groups always have guards for protection, like soldiers sleeping in camps.

Finally, one brief comment on paradoxical sleep, a term introduced by Jouvet & Jouvet (1966) and referring to the observation, that after a period of orthodox sleep, characterised by slow EEG waves, periods of fast waves of low voltage occur. This is paradox sleep, active sleep or desynchronised sleep. R. Hess (1964) sees in these periods an attempt of the cerebral cortex to be prepared for the tasks of awakening, although the organism is on the whole in a state of sleep.

Synapses

This term defines the contact points between nerve cells, required to establish interconnection and sequences of communication. The term synapse was coined by Sir Charles Sherrington (1906), a physiologist, working first at Liverpool and later at Oxford, and includes not only the interconnection between each neuron but also between neurons and their 'servants' such as muscle cells and glandular cells. Considering a synapse from the constructional point of view it is best understood if we use as a model the neuromuscular junction, the motor endplate (Fig. 4.5). The synapse is large and shows its constructional details clearly. These consist of a neural portion, or pre-synaptic part, and a post-synaptic part, a specialised portion of the muscle membrane, the responding or the receptive part (Fig. 4.6). The latter sometimes forms a sub-synaptic web which is dark-stained under the electron microscope. Figure 4.5 illustrates the principal components of the endplate under very high power with the electron microscope. Two important components can be seen, namely the mitochondria (the energy producers) and the synaptic vesicles. These two are typical components and are always present in the peripheral synapses such as the motor endplate and in the synapses within the central nervous system.

Fig. 4.5. A motor endplate as seen with light microscopy and stained with silver (from Glees, 1971). n.m. = nuclei of striated muscle; n.m.e.pl. = nuclei of the motor endplate.

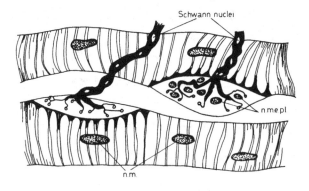

It was originally thought that the electrical impulses, when reaching the nerve fibre ends, were sufficient to cause depolarisation and muscle contraction. We now know that an electrochemical process operates in order to effect the contraction by making the post-synaptic membrane permeable. The chemical component in the case of cross-striated or voluntary muscle is acetylcholine, while the synapses of the post-ganglionic sympathetic nerve fibres utilise adrenaline or noradrenaline. The liberation of acetylcholine by the motor endplate appears to be regulated by impulse duration. The vesicles are filled with the neurotransmitter substance and allow for the liberation of small quantities (this also occurs, on a much smaller scale, during the resting state of the muscle). Studies on the neuromuscular junction are the most successfully performed on the electric fish, *Torpedo* (Fig. 4.7(*a*),(*b*)). Recently, the fine molecular details

Fig. 4.6. Diagrammatic representation of a motor endplate as viewed with an electron microscope. Note that the endplate has all the characteristic elements of synapses in the CNS. b.m. = basal membrane; m = mitochondria; m.f. = muscle fibres; pos.m. = post-synaptic membrane; prs.m. = pre-synaptic membrane; s.v. = synaptic vesicles.

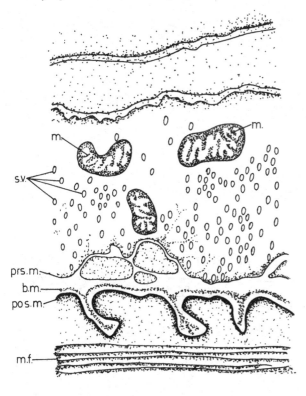

of the receptive substance, the acetylcholine receptor, have been worked out (Brisson & Unwin, 1985).

The motor endplates can be classified as cholinergic synapses and can be made visible with silver stains and with a specific cholinesterase-staining technique. Histochemical reactions can also be applied to reveal sympathetic or adrenergic nerve fibres and their endings after fixation in formalin and then using fluorescence microscopy. The intense fluorescence of adrenergic amines can readily be used for their detection and location.

While neurotransmitter substances in the peripheral nervous system – acetylcholine and noradrenaline – were discovered early, starting with Otto Loewi's work on the heart, where he found that vagal stimulation liberated acetylcholine (Loewi, 1921), chemical transmission in the CNS was recognised later. This is partly due to the fact that the synapses in the CNS are minute, requiring the resolution power of the electron microscope before they could be fully understood. It became apparent that the central synapses contained vesicles, suggesting the presence of a transmitter substance. The main types of central synaptic connections are illustrated in Figs 4.8–4.10. A detailed discussion of synaptic morphology can be found in Jones (1975) and Uchizono (1975).

Synapses in the CNS are of two types: excitatory and inhibitory. The neuromuscular junction is a typical excitatory synapse, while inhibitory synapses sometimes contain GABA as the neurotransmitter substance (Fig. 4.11). In excitatory synapses, the neurotransmitter causes an increase in sodium and potassium ion permeability. The membrane potential increases to about 0 mV, and this increase is spread electronically to trigger the propagation of an action potential in the axon hillock of the post-synaptic neuron (see Aidley, 1978). In inhibitory synapses, the neurotransmitter causes an increase in chloride ion (and in many cases potassium ion as well) permeability. The membrane potential is 'clamped down' to the chloride ion reversal potential, about −80 mV, preventing any voltage changes that would lead to the propagation of an action potential.

A neuron receives about 10^4 neuronal inputs on its surface (see Carpenter, 1984). The state of a particular neuron depends on the combined effects of excitation and inhibition at any time. The excitation effects are summed temporally and spatially. Spatial summation is arithmetic when the excited patches of membrane are far apart, but when they are near, the summation is less than expected: this is occlusion.

Excitatory and inhibitory effects cancel each other out. When they occur near each other, current

Fig. 4.7. (*a*) *Torpedo marmorata*, an elasmobranch fish, opened to show electric organ (after Dowdall, 1981). e.l. = electric lobe with emerging nerves entering the organ on one side and containing the motor cells (see (*b*)); o.l. = electric organ.
(*b*) Specialised motor endplates innervate the *T.*

marmorata electromotor system. The electrocytes of this electric fish are derived from myoblasts. The synapses are anologous to those in the skeletal muscle of vertebrates and are also cholinergic. Their pre-synaptic terminations were called terminal sacs by Dowdall (1981).

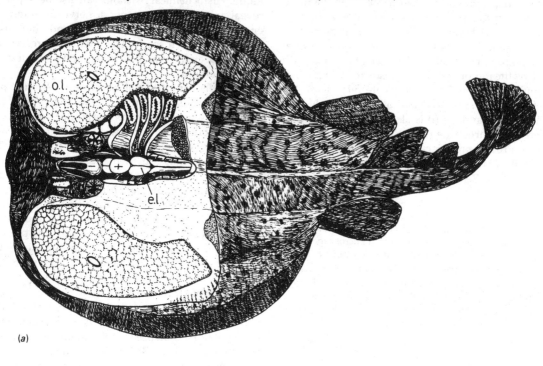

(*a*)

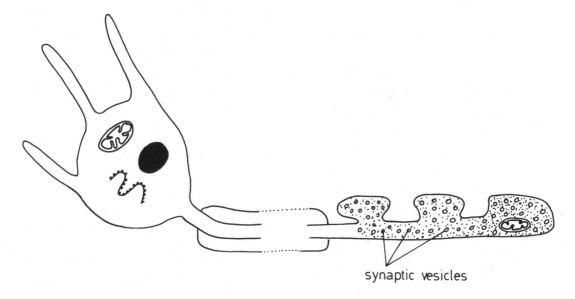

synaptic vesicles

(*b*)

inhibition occurs: the opposing currents cancel each other out. When they occur far from each other, there is voltage inhibition: the membrane potential is clamped at $-80\,$mV and the excitatory currents are 'drained' away.

The advantages of chemical synapses over electrical synapses are obvious. Electrical synapses only allow for the passage of one type of electric current, but the chemical synapses allow for a large variety of chemicals to influence the post-synaptic neuron to different degrees. There are two broad categories of neurotransmitters: the peptide neurotransmitters and the simple-molecule neurotransmitters. The peptide neurotransmitters include the opioid peptides, substance P, cholecystokinin, etc. It takes a lot of time and energy for the body to produce these substances, and these metabolically 'expensive' compounds are used to modulate long-term physiological effects. On the other hand, simple-molecule neurotransmitters such as monoamines and acetylcholine are used to modulate short-term physiological effects, e.g. fight,

fright and flight response. They are metabolically less 'expensive', and can be broken down easily.

Synpatic transmission allows for the integration of information. Each neuron receives input from many other neurons, and weighs all the excitatory and inhibitory input from the cells to determine its own activity: to fire or not to fire. This is the basis of the integrative action of the nervous system.

Selective excitatory and inhibitory action is important in the coordination of motor activity, e.g. in the withdrawal of the limb, the agonist muscles have to be excited to contract while the antagonist muscles must be inhibited. This is also essential in enhancing contrast of sensory input, e.g. lateral inhibition. These pathways exist for visual, touch and pressure inputs.

Lastly, the inhibitory output prevents the set-up of 'reverberating circuits' in the brain. Its great importance can be demonstrated in convulsions when the inhibitory output is deficient.

Fig. 4.8. (*a*) Neurons and their main types of synaptic connections (from Glees, 1971). a. = axon with one terminal making direct contact with the dendritic shaft; a.d. = axo-dendritic synapse in contact with a 'spine', a specialised post-synaptic formation; a.s. = axo-somatic synapse; d. = dendrites.

(*b*) In the olivary pre-tectal nucleus, the dendritic appendage of the retinal afferent enters the glomerular neuropile and synapses with the post-synaptic neuron (R to P). The post-synaptic neuron then synapses on to a 'conventional' dendrite (P to D) (after Campbell & Liebermann, 1979).

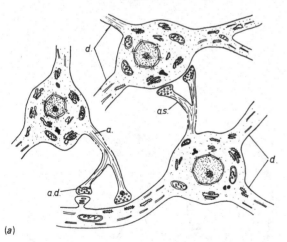

(*a*)

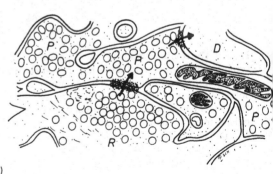

(*b*)

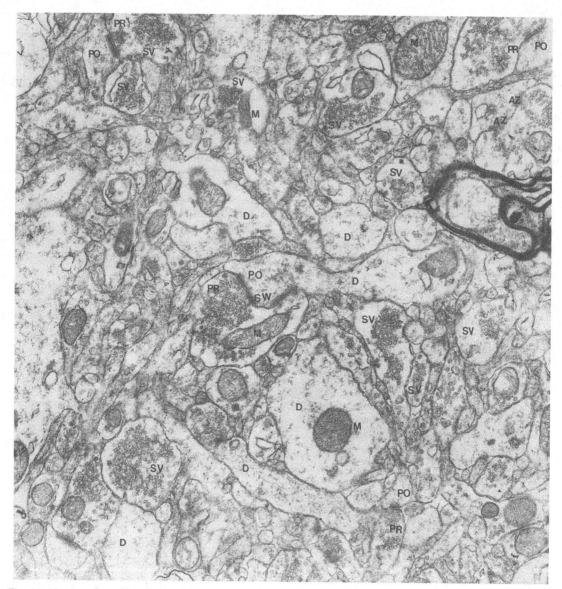

Fig. 4.9. The complex arrangement of synapses in the cerebral cortex is apparent in this high power electron micrograph. Synaptic vesicles of the agranular spherical type are abundant (SV) measuring 40–50 nm in diameter. AZ = active zone or vesicle release area; D = dentritic profiles; M = mitochondrium; PO = postsynaptic part; PR = presynaptic part; SW = synaptic web or postsynaptic thickening.

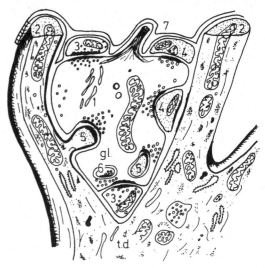

Fig. 4.10. Accumulations of various types of synapse are referred to as glomeruli and are numerous in the lateral geniculate body. gl. = glomerulus; t.d. = theca dendrite; 1 = main axon; 2 = main dendrites; 3 = secondary axon terminal; 4 = smaller dendrites; 5 = dendritic spine; 6 = axonal spine; 7 = part of the glial sheath of the glomerulus.

Fig. 4.11. Electron micrograph of GAD-positive (dark) terminals (axo-somatic synapses on pyramidal tract neurons). GAD is a neurohistochemical stain for GABAergic synapses, revealing the presence of inhibitory amino acids. Photograph kindly supplied by Dr Kiichiro Saito, University of Tsukuba, Japan.

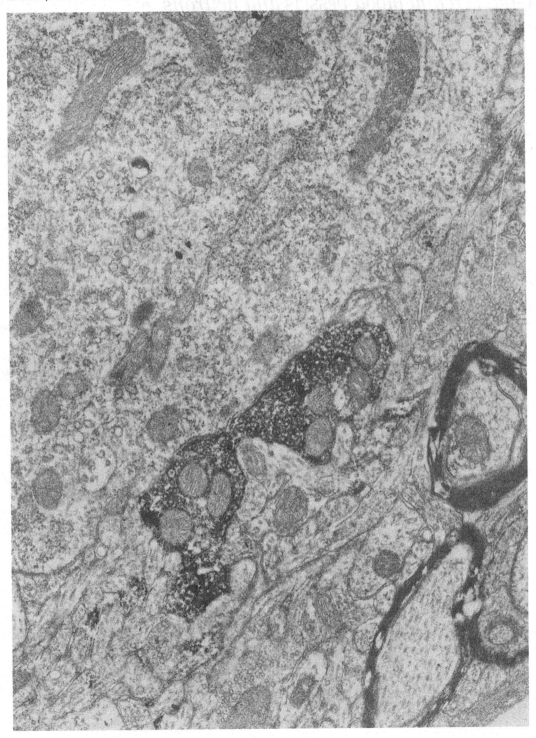

5
Glia, cerebral blood vessels and neurons

Both neurons and macroglia develop from the matrix of the ventricular zone of the neuroectoderm (see Fig. 2.22). Due to its origin from neuroectoderm the macroglia, consisting of astrocytes and oligodendrocytes, is referred to as ectodermal glia (Figs 5.1 and 5.2) in contrast to the microglia (mesoglia) which migrates from the mesodermal bone marrow via the blood vessels to the brain (Fig. 5.3).

In view of the density of the glia around the vascular tree and the number of glial processes attached to the vessel wall early in development, the connection between glia and the cerebral vessels must be regarded as very close and presumably of great functional significance. Although all forms of macroglia and microglia are found near the cerebral blood vessels, the connection between the astrocytes and

Fig. 5.1. Non-specific stains for neuroglia show only the nuclei. (A) Astrocytic nuclei (*a*) in the white matter and oligodendroglia nuclei (*b*). (B) The same kinds of nuclei in the neighbourhood of a pyramidal cell of the grey matter. c = transitional type of nucleus. (after Glees, 1955).

Fig. 5.2. Diagrammatic cross-section of the developing neural tube. The neuroectodermal cells give rise to ependymoblasts which either differentiate into astrocytes, with their vascular endfeet, or from glial membranes on the external side of the neural tube (after Kershman, 1938). a.b. = astroblast; a.s. = apolar astroblast; astro = astrocyte; e = ependymal cells; e.b. = ependymoblast; n.e. = neuroectoderm; o.b. = oligodendroblast; oligo = oligodendrocyte; p.s. = primitive spongioblast; s. = spongioblast; s.p. = protecting spongioblast.

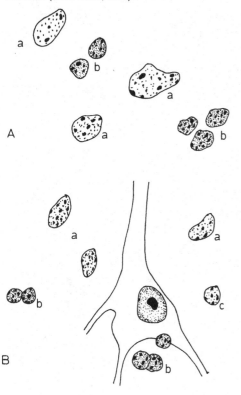

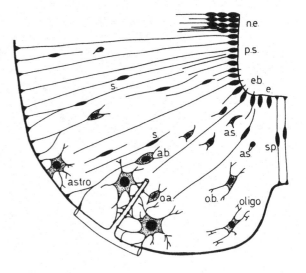

Fig. 5.3. Development of microglia from cells of the capillary wall (redrawn from Kershman, 1939). *A*, *B*–pericapillary amoeboid cells. *C*–microglia cells in mitotic division. *cap.* = capillary. *D*, *E*–more mature forms of *C*. Section from diencephalon of 8 week human embryo.

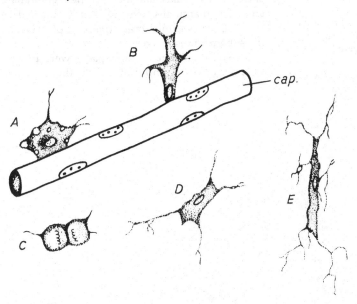

Fig. 5.4. Drawing of glial end feet attached to a cerebral vessel in the grey matter of area 9 of the frontal lobe of a monkey.

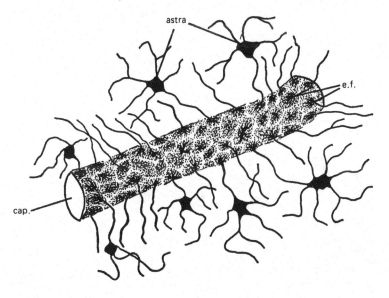

vessels is particularly close. Each astrocyte sends a process, terminating in a little endplate, to the vascular wall, and one or more astrocytic processes encircle the vessels for a considerable distance (Fig. 5.4). The envelopment of the vascular wall by astrocyte pro-

cesses and vascular endfeet is referred to as a glial barrier; the multitude of endplates is known as the membrana limitans gliae perivascularis. The glia cells also form a border against the surface of the brain (the marginal glia of Held) and with their processes and terminal enlargements form the membrana limitans gliae marginalis, which is firmly attached to the connective tissue membrane (limitans piae) bordering the subarachnoidal space.

These subarachnoidal spaces were previously supposed to communicate with the perivascular

Fig. 5.5. Electron micrograph of a longitudinal section through a capillary. Numerous astrocytic glial endfeet (A) are attached to the multi-layered basement membrane (B) by fusion (F).
E = endothelium; J = tight junction of two endothelial cells; m = mitochondria; P = peri-capillary microglia cell; RB = red blood cell: S = P. synapse.

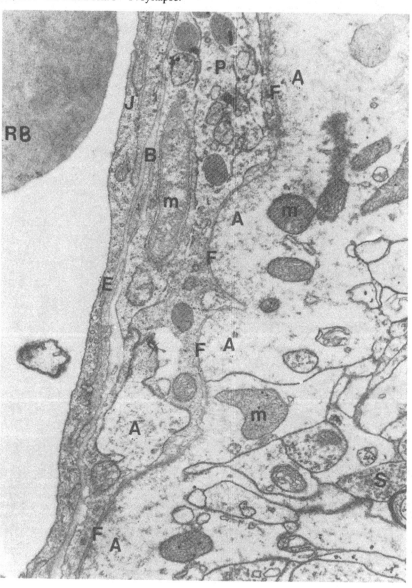

spaces (Virchow–Robin spaces) between the adventitia and the membrana limitans gliae perivascularis, but these are most likely artefacts caused by fixation. All cerebral blood vessels lie within the cerebrospinal fluid (CSF) spaces of the pia-arachnoidal tissue before they enter the brain. This tissue, which covers the surface of the brain, also accompanies the vessels for a short distance into the substance of the brain, where it fuses with the perivascular adventitia. Thus fusion leads to the formation of pial funnels and produces a pial ring of connective tissue which narrows considerably and separates the subarachnoidal spaces from the perivascular spaces.

The ensheathing of capillaries by glial endfeet (Fig. 5.5) prevents the direct contact of neurons with the vascular system. Furthermore, light microscopy shows that glial processes appear to seal off not only the internal mesenchymal areas of the blood vessels, but also the external surfaces of the brain from the pia-arachnoid (Fig. 5.6). In this way, the neurons and their processes are suspended within an enormous sponge of neuroglia. In this sponge, the major pillars are the blood vessels, while the neuroglia, in particular the astrocytes, interconnect the vascular tree by means of processes. This arrangement suggests a supporting function of glia and, on account of glial envelopment of capillaries, a metabolic transport function. These two functions appear especially important in the Müller cells in the retina, a modified neuroglial cell (Fig. 5.7).

Physiological significance of the blood–brain barrier

Because glucose (Fig. 5.8) is an important metabolite of the brain, the maintenance of a constant glucose concentration in the extracellular fluid of the brain is essential. This concentration is maintained by an active transport system effecting homeostasis of the brain glucose level at a concentration some 35% below the plasma level. Davson (1967) points out that this is achieved by a carrier-mediated system which becomes saturated at above-average plasma levels, so that in severe hyperglycaemia transport is reduced and in hypoglycaemia it is favoured. This regulating system must be located at the blood–brain barrier – in the cerebral capillaries. These capillaries have one special morphological feature: they are enveloped by

Fig. 5.7. The retina contains a special type of neuroectodermal glia cell called the Müller cell after its discoverer. Müller cells extend the whole width of the retina, bordering the vitreous body on one side and the pigment cells on the other (see Fig. 13.8). A = matrix; B = germinal cell; C = retinal receptor; D = Müller cell; E,G = developing neurons. The neuron F has contact with the capillary K via cell J. The cell H provides the glial sheath for the axon of neuron F. The functions of cells J and H can be transferred to G by the Müller cell (from Glees & Meller, 1968).

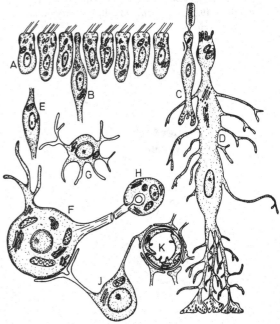

Fig. 5.6. The ectodermal neural frame is separated from the mesodermal frame of the pia-arachnoid (p.a.) by a limiting glial membrane of astrocytes in a manner similar to that of the glial endfeet attached to vessels (see Fig. 5.7) (from Glees, 1955).

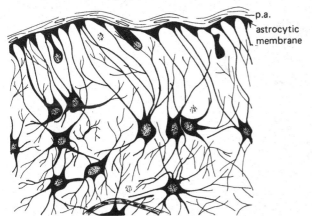

Fig. 5.8. Diagram of a cerebral capillary illustrating the glucose transfer route. Arrows indicate possible transfer routes or storage in endfeet (from Glees, 1985). b.m. = basement membrane; e.f. = glial endfoot; endoth. = endothelial lining; g = gap in membrane; M = mitochondria.

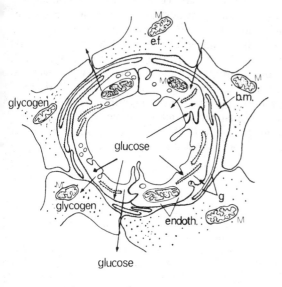

terminal expansions of the astrocytic processes. This glial envelope might account for the low degree of permeability of cerebral capillaries. However, Brightmann (1965a,b) pointed out that large molecules such as ferritin, which are used as tracers in electron microscope studies, pass between the gaps of these glial processes. This shifts the capacity for a selective permeability onto the endothelial cells of the cerebral capillaries, provided they possess special features discussed below.

The origin and distribution of microglia

The history of microglia cells has been reviewed by Glees (1955) and, more recently, by Cammermeyer (1970), who stressed the comparative aspect, and by Peters *et al.* (1970) in electron microscope studies. There is general agreement among neurohistologists that normal microglia cells, when stained by Hortega's silver carbonate method, have very distinct characteristics, for example a polar branching of tortuous processes, scanty cytoplasm and an elongated, deeply staining nucleus. They occur in the brain when vascularisation begins and their most widely accepted origin is considered to be the bone marrow. Their precursors, white blood cells (the monocytic cells of Roessmann & Friede (1968)), migrate through the vessel walls (Fig. 5.3) into the brain. These cells are called by Cammermeyer (1970) extravascular or juxtavascular mitotic cells, and they give rise to the microglia cells proper. Fleischhauer (1960a,b) has demonstrated, throughout the brain and pia-arachnoid, perivascular cells containing fluorescent material and appearing to be microglia differing in no way

Fig. 5.9. Mature microglia cells changing into compound fat granule cells after injury (redrawn after Penfield, 1928). *a* = unaltered cell; *d* = compound granular cell.

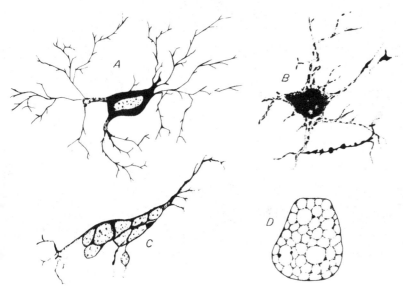

from pericytes and macrophages. The final appearance of resting microglia is determined by the shape of clefts of the extracellular space. Resting microglia cells are still capable of dividing, as has been shown convincingly by Kreutzberg (1966) (Fig. 5.9). Microglia cells may either migrate to the vessels or settle down to their usual arrangement after neuronal 'disturbance' (for example cutting the axon) has subsided.

Microglial proliferation leads to a detachment of pre-synaptic terminals from the cell body of facial neurons (Blinzinger & Kreutzberg, 1968), an important neurobiological finding confirmed in the hypoglossal neurons of the rabbit by Hamberger *et al.* (1971). Zimmermann *et al.* (1972), reviewing the relevant literature, described the sequence of neuronal reaction to axonal amputation, and the subsequent perineuronal glial behaviour, as an interrelation of neuronal stress and glial response. However, these authors were unable to cause a perineuronal glial re-

sponse by metabolic neuronal stress of spinal ganglia caused by colchicine injection, and concluded that perineuronal proliferation represents a response to an increase of the neuronal volume rather than a reaction to an increase of neuronal metabolism. Furthermore, Kreutzberg & Barron (1978) could show that perineuronal microglia cells show a high enzymatic activity (5-nucleotidase) when reacting to chromatolytic events occurring in facial nerve neurons after axotomy. Some authors stress the migratory activity as disclosed by autoradiographic means and consider that microglia cells are only temporary limited guests in brain tissue (Cammermeyer, 1970). However, in normal and pathological studies of the CNS it seems advantageous to take their presence for granted and to keep the term microglia cell rather than replace it by the term macrophage or histiocyte. In particular, Cammermeyer has shown the presence of microglia in germ-free rats, and has pointed out that their existence in the brain is not caused or activated by immunological processes. In the electron microscope studies, accompanied by excellent photomicrographs, of Vaughn *et al.* (1970) and Vaughn & Pease (1970), these authors prefer the name 'multipotential glia cell'

Fig. 5.10. Electron micrograph of a microglia cell (M) in fusion with a neuron. (N) Note that the cell borders of the neuron are fused and allow the passage of lipids from the neuron into the microglia cell. G = Golgi tubes; L = lipid (from Glees, 1985).

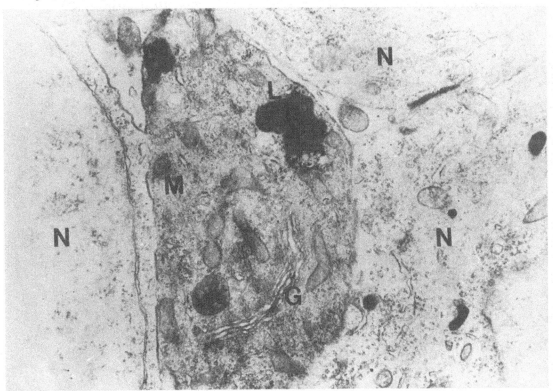

to characterise the phagocytic cells removing débris in the degenerating optic nerve following retinal destruction. The faculties of these cells are identical to those of microglia. These cells arise either from local stock or originate from numerous sources as discussed by Cammermeyer (see above). Cammermeyer (1970), reviewing the literature and adding extensive material of his own, stresses not only the ubiquitous distribution but also shape differences in various locations. Generally, microglia cells are found in the grey matter among perineuronal satellites, close to neurons and blood vessels, and in the white matter following the course of myelinated fibres. They account for about 10% of neuroglia cells. Microglia cells can be located close to the ventricular wall where their processes radiate underneath the ependyma. Altman (1969a,b) and Altmann & Das (1964, 1965) conclude from their autoradiographic studies in rats (newborn to adult) that cell production of neuroglia and of microneurones

continues throughout life. The removal of horseradish peroxidase by microglia and the importance of the perivascular route taken by these cells has been described by Wagner *et al.* (1974).

Function of microglia in the normal brain

Having studied microglial reactions and behaviour in experimental and normal brain material over a period of some years with both light and electron microscopy, I have found microglia cells in extremely close apposition to neurons (Fig. 5.10). Both cells have large communicating gaps in their respective cell walls and osmiophilic material appears to have been ferried from the neuron to the interior of the microglia cell. Microglia cells filled with osmiophilic granules make their way to the blood vessels (Fig. 5.11). The mode of ingestion and route of transportation is illustrated in Fig. 5.11. The uptake of interneuronal débris by microglia would assign a definite function for micro-

Fig. 5.11. Composite diagram to illustrate transport and uptake of lipids by microglia (M₁, M₂) (from Voth & Glees, 1985). (A) Immature nerve cell. (B) Mature and ageing neuron in fusion with microglia cell. (C) Astrocyte. (D) Capillary. Ax = axon; adS = axo-dendritic synapse; asS = axo-somatic synapse;

B = basement membrane; D = dendrites; e = endothelium; EF = endfoot; ER = ergastoplasm; FL + MT = filaments and microtubules; G = Golgi apparatus; L = lumen of capillary; Li = lipid; LiM = lipid in mitochondrion; M = mitochondrion; N = nucleus; Nt = neurotubules.

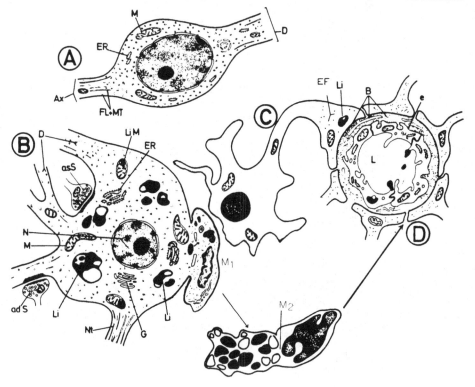

glia in the normal brain, a function which seems not to be limited to the removal of dying nerve cells and their processes. With this concept in mind, the migration of microglia through normal neural tissue, studied by Cammermeyer, would illustrate the real significance of the great number of microglia cells present in normal brain tissue. These cells would not have to wait for the occurrence of infections or traumatic injuries to the nervous tissue but would already carry out the removal of waste material, which the specialised neuron is not capable of doing.

Innervation of cerebral vessels and blood flow

Although the astrocytes provide an additional coat to the cerebral vessels it is unlikely that they have any direct influence on the regulation of blood flow unless this were possible at capillary level (see below). A monograph by Purves (1972) on cerebral circulation points out that Willis (1664) was one of the first to refer to nerve fibres accompanying cerebral vessels. For historical interest it should be mentioned that the German anatomist Stöhr began his histological career by giving a very clear description of the innervation of larger cerebral vessels (Stöhr, 1928a,b), but denying the innervation of intraparenchymal vasculature. With this statement a great controversy was started; this controversy still exists in the sense that it is debated whether vascular spasm causing a migraine attack or malfunction of the brain is confined to those large cerebral arteries obviously supplied by autonomic fibres and whether the small and terminal vessels of the microcirculation are capable of autoregulation. This poses the question as to whether contractility of cerebral capillaries is feasible; actin and myosin are located in endothelial cells and supporting electron microscope studies show a capillary adrenergic innervation (Rennels & Nelson, 1975).

Ultrastructure of neuroglia

The great advances in ultrastructural analysis of glial cells are clearly apparent when studying major reviews like those of Mugnaini & Walberg (1964) and the ultrastructural atlas of Peters *et al.* (1970). By 1964, electron microscopy of nervous tissue had improved technically sufficiently to be related to the results of light microscopy, a necessary step stressed by Glees (1958a) at a conference on the biology of neuroglia at the National Institutes of Health in Bethesda. The admirable work of Mugnaini & Walberg (1964) on newborn, young and adult rats and cats established the criteria for differentiating fibrous and protoplasmic astrocytes from oligodendrocytes and microglia. Their studies enabled histologists to compare the cell types

seen in electron microscopy with the classical pictures of silver impregnation. A useful table prepared by Mugnaini & Walberg summarises the differences between the major types of glial cells and stresses the distinct differences between astrocytes and oligodendrocytes (Fig. 5.12). The latter have both a dense cytoplasm and nucleus and an abundance of granular endoplasmic reticulum (ergastoplasm), while the fibrous astrocytes possess a relatively clear filamentous cytoplasm with little endoplasmic reticulum. When attempting to prepare (on the basis of richness in ultrastructural organelles) a graded scale of metabolically active neuroglia, using the criteria of Mugnaini & Walberg, of Peters *et al.* (1970) and of Glees & Meller (1968), one is led to conclude that the most metabolically active neuroglia cell is the perineuronal oligodendrocyte. Then follows the protoplasmic astrocyte, the fibrous astrocyte and, last, the microglia cell. Taking into account the ultrastructural appearance of astrocytes, their ability to produce a wealth of intracellular filaments in pathological conditions and their early embryological association with blood vessels, a supporting function seems likely. In addition, their framing of capillaries points to some metabolic function. Early in their development, the oligodendrocytes are closely associated with neurons. Glioblasts can be discriminated eventually from neuroblasts since they turn into oligodendrocytes (Fig. 5.12), which have a very electron-dense nucleus and fewer ribosomes and ergastoplasm.

Quantitative data

The morphological complexity of the nervous system and its dense packing of neurons, glia and vessels can best be seen from the electron micrograph in Fig. 5.12, where one capillary seems to serve seven cell bodies and a wealth of non-myelinated fibres. Recent reviews concerning the relationship of neurons and neuroglia by Blinkov & Glezer (1968) and by Wolff (1965), are based on electron microscope studies of the occipital cortex and cerebellum in the rat. The use of electron microscope techniques has the advantage that neuronal and glia tissues are equally well stained in the same picture (Fig. 5.12), whereas the selective stains for nervous tissue used in light microscopy show either neurons and their processes or only neuroglia. Electron microscope studies, however, have little chance of a major sampling of neurons and glia, and the inherent difficulty of differentiating the very fine glial processes from those of the dendritic profiles not entering a synaptic relationship is apparent in sections treated with the available techniques. Wolff (1970) has carried out a very detailed electron microscope study of the structure and shape of astrocytes in relation to capillaries and to neurons, and to their distribution in the neuropile, a plexus of very fine nervous fibres. Wolff discriminates two types of astrocytic processes: long ones, detectable in light microscopy, and very short ones, referred to as lamellae, seen only in electron micrographs after good fixation and with high resolution. Wolff estimates the percentage volume of astrocytes in the neuropile of the rat to be between 22 and 27% and quotes an estimate of astrocytes in Man to be between 15 and 30 cells/0.1 mm³. Friede (1954) assumes that 50% of the vertebrate CNS tissue volume is made up of neuroglia. Furthermore, Wolff assumes that 60–80% of the astrocytic surface area is due to laminated expansions

(10–40 cm²/mm³ of neuropile). Thus Wolff believes that the astrocytes control the tortuous intercellular spaces by lining 45–50% of it. The best way to assess the relationship between neuroglia and neurons is the use of one of the customary Nissl stains, which reveal neurons clearly and stain neuroglia nuclei distinctly. Counting is most easily achieved by interposing a suitably divided grid between the lenses of the eyepiece. To express the data in volume percentage, the methods of Haug and Heider are recommended. Heider has investigated the quantitative increase of neuroglia in the human pyramidal layer after birth. Between birth and the second month of life the number of glial cells per unit volume decreases by 25%, a further reduction of 24% occurring by the age of 12 years. This seems to indicate that for the final number of pyramidal axons already present at birth, a proportionate amount of glia is already allocated. For it is only after birth that myelinisation of the axons occurs. Their final size and degree of myelinisation reach adult conditions during childhood when the distribution of

Fig. 5.12. Electron micrograph of an oligodendrocyte. Note the large, round nucleus full of chromophilic substance, surrounded by richly organised cytoplasm, containing ribosomes, endoplasmic reticulum, Golgi apparatus and lipid inclusions.

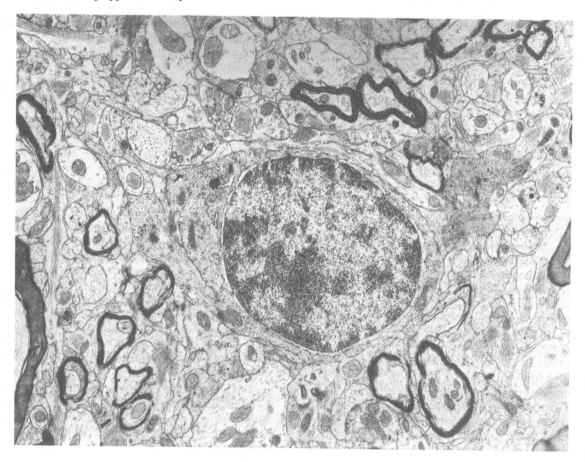

glia achieves its final state. Brizzee & Jacobs (1959) examined the glia index (number of glia cells divided by the number of neurons) in the motor cortex of maturing cats. The glia index increased rapidly from a value of 0.83 in the youngest animals, to 1.00 in animals of 1 kg body weight, to 1.4 in the 2 kg group. The authors concluded that the glia index is determined by the functional complexity of the cortex as well as by brain weight. A developmental study on similar lines was made by Hillebrand (1966), who investigated the postnatal changes of glia in the corpus callosum of cats aged 2 days to 11 years. Soon after birth the number of glial nuclei increased rapidly to four times the number at birth. This process was concluded at the end of the first month and was then followed by a decrease in cell number. This decrease in cell number was accompanied by an increase in volume due to myelinisation of callosal fibres. Myelin formation in the corpus callosum of the cat starts at the end of the first month. Joseph (1954) investigated the changes in the glial population in the degenerating posterior columns of the spinal cord of the rabbit, allowing for degeneration times of 10, 20, 50 and 100 days. The glial population increased about threefold after 20 days, reaching a level of 4.5-fold after 100 days. Joseph discriminated between large pale and small dark nuclei without specifying the type of glia, but it is obvious from his pictures that the large nuclei were those of astrocytes and the smaller nuclei were probably those of microglia. The reaction to fibre degeneration appears to involve both types of cell. Diamond *et al.* (1966) examined the interesting problem of whether the cortical cell population differs in rats living in enriched (stimulated) and impoverished (isolated) surroundings. The authors reported a 14% increase in neuroglia in the rats in an enriched environment. The visual cortex of these animals extended 6.4% more in depth compared with those of isolated rats. The increase in neuroglia was absolute and not relative to the increase in neurons. Diamond *et al.* confirmed the glial increase following behavioural manipulation seen by Altman & Das (1965) using autoradiography to quantify cell proliferation. Diamond *et al.* (1966) believe that the increase in glia must be due to increased functional requirements in rats living in an enriched environment, using more extensive synaptic connections and having a higher cerebral metabolism. They find that the normal ratio of neurons to glia in the visual cortex is 1:2.6, having previously reported a ratio of 1:1, like Brizzee *et al.* (1964), in contrast to Hydén (1960) who found a 1:10 ratio.

Brownson (1960) made a careful study of the glia–neuron relationship for the guinea-pig at various ages from 1 to 62 months. The purpose of this study was to assess whether X-irradiation would alter the number or type of perineuronal satellites in the course of ageing. Brownson found a significant increase with increasing age in the percentage of neurons with satellites. As a percentage of perineuronal glia cells he found 62.8% oligodendroglia, 26.5% astroglia, and 10.8% microglia. The average number of glia cells per neuron was 0.88 at 1 month and 1.24 at 62 months.

Functional considerations in relation to morphology

The presence of glycogen granules in astrocytes, in particular in their vascular processes, suggests their participation in carbohydrate metabolism. This view is supported by radiation studies reviewed by Haymaker (1969): a dose-dependent increase in glycogen content was established and an accumulation of glycogen in cortical astroglia seen within a few hours after radiation. On exposure to large doses, excess glycogen can be found in the astrocytes and oligodendroglia cells of the white matter. In addition to glycogen increase, Maxwell & Kruger (1965) reported a great increase in the number of mitochondria, an increase in the extent of the Golgi apparatus and nuclear changes. These authors believe that the radiation effect acts on the metabolically active ultrastructure. According to Haymaker (1969), oligodendrocytes have various reactions to radiation: the cortical oligodendrocytes can be made necrotic, while on the whole this cell type responds less severely in the white matter. However, survival time and changes in dose can alter the picture drastically and there can be striking differences between species. Haymaker draws attention to vigorous mitotic division of neuroglia in the rat's cerebral cortex within a day or two after high-dose exposure. The metabolic consequences related to dose and survival time are of a complex nature due to the various tissue components of the CNS involved, and the authoritative review of Haymaker should be consulted. It is of interest to refer here again to Brownson (1960) who found no significant alterations in the normal appearance of the neuron–neuroglia relationship in the guinea-pig cerebral cortex following units of 1600 r of X-irradiation in any of the following age groups: 1 month, 6 months, 15 months, 38 months and 62 months.

To study the ultrastructure–function relationship of the various types of glia, Wendell-Smith *et al.* (1965) have chosen an interesting strategic point of attack, the exit of the optic nerve in the cat. In the cat, as in Man, the optic nerve appears to acquire a myelin sheath after its exit from the eye, behind the lamina cribrosa. The post-laminar part contains both astrocytes and oligodendrocytes. Only the latter contain a conspicuous number of ribosomes and orientated endoplasmic reticulum. The authors compare the structural differentiation of the oligodendrocyte with the Schwann cell of peripheral nerves and believe the oligodendrocyte to be the metabolically more active cell. But neither astrocytes nor oligodendrocytes participate in the removal of degenerating optic nerve fibres. This activity is carried out by microglia or multipotential glia, a term used by Vaughn *et al.* (1970) in a comprehensive study of degenerating rat optic nerves. A metabolic interaction of glia and neurons has been reported by Hansson & Norström (1971) in studies of colchicine interference with the axoplasmic transport mechanism of neurosecretory neurons of the rat hypothalamus. After a few days the astrocytes show a marked increase of glial filaments and of perinuclear organelles. Oligodendrocytes situated between colchicine-affected neurons show extensive folding of the nuclear membrane, an increase of polyribosomes and other organelles and the appearance of parallel membranes resembling myeloid bodies. The authors interpret these changes to mean an increase in glial metabolic activity, similar to that in supraoptic neurons. Cytochemical localisation of 5-nucleotidase in glial cell membranes by Kreutzberg *et al.* (1978) was taken by them to suggest that glia cells contribute to neuronal metabolism by being involved in adenosine production affecting calcium ion fluxes. Much thought has lately been given to the vasodilatory action of calcium; further confirmation of this view could support a more active role for neuroglia in the regulation of microcirculation.

Chemical composition of the brain

About 80% of the brain tissue consists of water; 40–75% of the dry weight consists of lipids of which 41% are cholesterol, 16% glycolipids, 14% ethanolamine phospholipids and 5–6% sphingomyelin. The remainder of the dry weight is made up of proteins, mainly contained in neurons, their processes and neuroglia cells. Myelin, the ensheathing coat of long axons, is made up of 21% protein (proteolipids, basic myelin protein) and 79% lipids. Some of the proteins of the neurons are in association with lipids and compose the many membranous structures of the brain cells. While for short-term neurophysiological considerations the nerve cells appear to be simple bags filled with salt solutions, metabolic, clinical neurological and neuropathological studies have to pay full attention to the membranous neuronal structures so clearly seen with the electron microscope. With high-power resolution, the complex membranous organelles of the neuron are revealed. The nerve cell contains a wealth of mitochondria, indicating the high metabolic demands on the cells.

Brain metabolism

The significance of glucose for the brain is dramatically apparent: lowering the level of blood sugar leads to unconsciousness and consciousness can be restored quickly by giving glucose intravenously. This is used clinically in the treatment of schizophrenia by insulin injection, a metabolic shock therapy which lowers the glucose levels suddenly. The brain utilises 5 mg glucose per 100 g brain weight in 1 min. Storage of glucose or glycogen is negligible and other sources of energy are hardly utilised; this makes the brain completely dependent on a secure and continuous supply of glucose. The passage of metabolic products through the blood–brain barrier is described on p. 59. Oxidation of glucose is thus the primary source of energy.

The amino acids glutamate and aspartate are present in the brain in high concentrations and have an excitatory influence on neuronal activity. Glutamate is involved in intermediary metabolism but does not seem to be involved directly in the production of neurotransmitters (Cooper *et al.*, 1978). The protein metabolism of the neuron is directed towards the production of neurotransmitters. This is very obvious in the case of neurosecretion by hypothalamic neurons. Labelling these cells with radioactive amino acids shows very clearly that the nucleus and the Nissl substance are concerned with neurotransmitter biosynthesis.

6
Cerebral blood and cerebrospinal fluid systems

Fig. 6.1. Arterial blood supply to the head and brain, lateral view. The aortic arch (a.a.) is the main feeder, The two main vessels emerge on the left side: the left subclavian artery (l.s.a.) and the common carotid (c.c.a.). The vertebral artery (v.a.) emerges from the l.s.a. and enters the transverse vertebral foramen, between vertebrae IV and VII, and usually at vertebra VI. The v.a. enters the skull through the foramen magnum and supplies the brain (see Fig. 6.3) The c.c.a. divides at the level of the hyoid (hy.b.) into the external (e.c.a.) and internal (i.c.a.) carotid arteries. The i.c.a. is exclusively for taking blood to the brain. At the level of the base of the brain, the i.c.a. and the vertebral circulation join at the circle of Willis (c.a.W.) (from Glees, 1971). b.a. = basal artery; c.c. = cricoid cartilage; clav. = dorsal nasal artery; e.a. = ethmoid artery; f.a. = facial artery; m.a. = maxillary artery; o.a. = ophthalmic artery; S.s = Sylvian sulcus; th.c = thyroid cartilage; t.g. = thyroid gland; tr. = trachea; I^{rst} c. = first rib.

The blood supply to the brain
Introduction
As already emphasised in the section on brain metabolism, the supply of nourishment originating in the liver reaches the brain via the vascular system. It is carried by four large arteries, two internal carotid and two vertebral arteries (Figs 6.1 and 6.2). The inter-

Fig. 6.2. The base of the skull, illustrating the main entrance openings for arterial vessels and exits for venous return and cranial nerves (from Glees, 1971). 1 = frontal sinus; 2 = foramen caecum; 3,4 = cribriform plate and openings for olfactory nerve bundles; 5 = optic canal; 6 = superior orbital fissure; 7 = foramen rotundum; 8 = foramen lacerum; 9 = foramen ovale; 10 = foramen spinosum; 11 = internal auditory meatus; 12 = jugular foramen; 13 = anterior condyle foramen; 14 = hypoglossal foramen; 15 = emissary vein; 16 = foramen magnum.

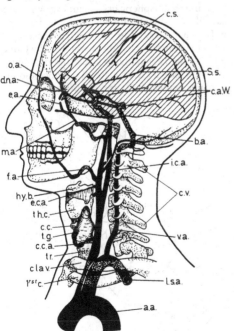

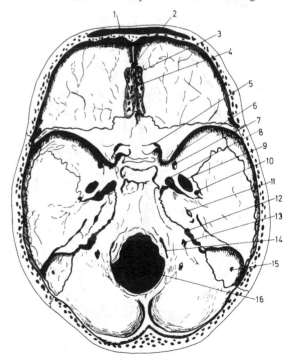

nal carotid arteries supply essentially the forebrain, while the midbrain and hindbrain are fed by the vertebral arteries. This arrangement is found in Man and other primates but varies considerably in other mammals. In primates the common carotid divides into two large vessels, one supplying the face and the other directed solely towards the brain. The internal carotid, however, is in some animals (e.g. the dog) a much smaller branch of the common carotid or a branch of the internal maxillary artery (e.g. the cat). In Man this vessel branches from the external carotid but does not supply the brain; instead it gives off branches to cranial nerves. For developmental reasons the internal carotid reaches the base of the brain by a complicated

route, entering the skull through the external carotid foramen and passing into a bony canal about 1.5 cm long; when leaving and piercing the dura the artery enters a venous sinus (the cavernous sinus). Inside, the vessel usually runs at right angles running forward along the body of the sphenoid bone, bending sharply again and running upwards, leaving the cavernous sinus behind the emergence of the optic nerve. The artery surrounded by the internal carotid sympathetic plexus bends backwards again, and divides into the anterior and middle cerebral arteries. The S-shaped bends of the artery are referred to as the carotid siphon. It has been suggested that the siphon has a damping effect on systolic blood pressure which can remain relatively normal for long periods in hypertensive states. As Platzer (1956a,b) pointed out, the degree of the U- or S-shaped bend of the carotid varies a great deal; it may not be present at all and seems not to be important. The positioning of a strongly pulsating artery inside a venous cavity might produce

Fig. 6.3. The base of the brain. The large brain arteries approach the areas they supply from the ventral surface of the brain, joining as arterial ring vessels. In the diagram, the tip of the temporal lobe has been removed on the left side to show the course of the middle cerebral artery. The left cerebellar hemisphere is not shown to allow the posterior cerebral artery to be illustrated (from Glees, 1971). f.p. = frontal pole; o.b. = olfactory bulb; o.p. = occipital pole. 1 = anterior cerebral artery; 2 = ant. communicating a.; 3 = internal carotid a.; 4 = post. communicating a.; 5 = post. cerebral a.; 6 = superior cerebellar a.; 7 = basilary a.; 8 = left vertebral a.; 9 = ant. inf. cerebellar a.; 10 = post. inf. cerebellar a.; 11 = ant. spinal a.

Fig. 6.4. The blood supply of the basal ganglia and thalamus seen in a frontal plane (from Glees, 1971). The shaded areas show the territories of the anterior (ter.ant.ce.a.) and posterior (ter.post.ce.a.) cerebral arteries; the area in white is the territory of the middle cerebral artery. cl. = claustrum; c.n. = caudate nucleus; corp.cal. = corpus callosum; corp.forn. = fornix; gl.pal = globus pallidus; i.f. = interhemispheric fissure; int.cap. = internal capsule; l.n. = lentiform nucleus (putamen); m.b. = mamillary body; S.f. = Sylvian fissure; th. = thalamus. 1 = middle cerebral a.; 2 = branch of mid. cerebral a. supplying insula and putamen; 3 = lenticulo-striate branches; 4 = lenticulo-optic or thalamic branches; 5 = ant. cerebral a.

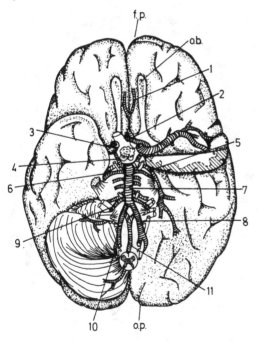

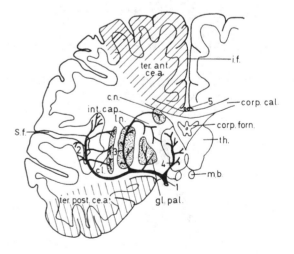

a pumping action on the venous return or may allow heat exchange between arterial and venous flow.

The topographical position of the artery inside the cavernous sinus is important because of its topographical relation to the cranial nerves, e.g. ophthalmic, oculomotor, abducens and trochlear. The close packing of arterial, venous and nervous structures explains a number of disease processes, such as those caused by pressure on these nerves by the dilatation of the carotid walls (aneurysm), or the rupture of the vessel causing pulsating arterial blood to enter the tributaries of the cavernous sinus, thus causing exophthalmic pulsations. The vertebral arteries branch off the subclavian and ascend in the transverse foramina of the cervical vertebrae, entering the brain cavity through the foramen magnum. After fusing into one large basiliary vessel, this vertebral circulation forms, through communicating channels with the carotid arteries, an arterial shunt, the arterial Circle of Willis (Figs 6.3–6.7).

Evolutionary aspects of the cerebral arteries

In 'lower' animals (see pp. 11–12) the brain is a somewhat refined cranial portion of the spinal cord, supplied by spinal or vertebral arteries. In mammals, whose forebrain is considerably enlarged, additional vessels contribute to the cerebral circulation, stemming from the common carotid; an example is the dog where the small internal carotid, the ascending pharyngeal and an anastomising branch from the middle meningeal (Steven, 1981) all contribute. The dog has communications between meningeal and cerebral vessels which do not normally occur in primates, which favour a separate brain circulation and possess large internal carotids. Comparatively speaking, the vertebral circulation in Man supplies the evolutionarily older brain, the brainstem, while the carotids supply the newer brain, the cerebral hemispheres.

Each carotid artery transports 600 ml of oxygenated blood to the brain per minute; each vertebral artery transports 200 ml of blood per minute. This difference shows either the greater demand for oxygen of the cerebral hemispheres in contrast to the brainstem, or the existence of a larger capillary net in the hemispheres. There are marked differences in regional blood flow. The total blood flow through the carotid artery and its return through the jugular vein takes 7 s, while the blood of the vertebral artery needs 9 s to return (Toole & Patel, 1967). Arterial filling and venous return can be studied in radiographs after

Fig. 6.5. Arterial supply of the medial aspect of the left cerebral hemisphere (from Glees, 1971).

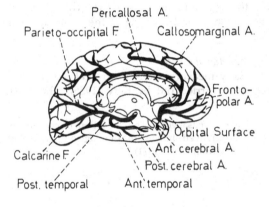

Fig. 6.6. Arterial supply of the lateral aspect of the left cerebral hemisphere (from Glees, 1971).

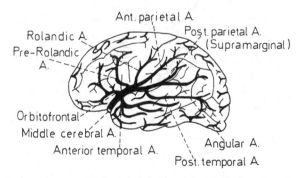

Fig. 6.7. Vascular territories of the cerebral arteries, lateral view (from Glees, 1971).

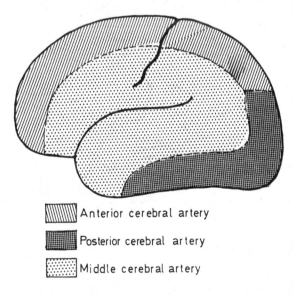

Fig. 6.8. A clinically orientated diagram of the main functional brain areas are their supply by the middle cerebral artery (m.c.a.) of the dominant left hemisphere, with special reference to sensory-motor areas (from Glees, 1971). a.a. = angular artery; a.c. = auditory cortex; a.p.a. = ant. parietal a.; a.t.a. = ant. temporal a.; B.c. = Broca motor centre of speech; i.m.c.a. = inferior part of the m.c.a.; l.g.b. = lateral geniculate body; l.o.f.a. = lat. orbito-frontal a.; o.r. = optic radiation; p.p.a. = post. parietal a.; pr.R.a. = pre-Rolandic a.; p.t.a. = post. temporal a.; R.a = Rolandic a.; s.m.c.a. = superior part of the m.c.a.; t.p.a. = temporpolaris a.; v.c. = visual cortex; W.c. = Wernicke sensory centre of speech.

intra-arterial injection of radiocontrast medium through the carotid or vertebral artery (angiography).

Excessive head movements such as may occur in disco dancing can occlude the blood flow through the vertebral arteries causing permanent damage to brain-stem structures (pp. 125–8). Although the arterial Circle of Willis appears to compensate for a sudden occlusion of one or more main arteries, this is not so in practice. The communicating arteries are normally of unequal diameter, and are sometimes missing altogether. The time factor allowing for a gradual dilatation of these ring vessels is of course a very important consideration. If the compensatory action of the anterior communicating artery is insufficient or absent, a compression of the carotid feeding the dominant hemisphere causes a very impressive failure of sensory–motor power in the leading arm and/or impairment of speech (Fig. 6.8).

Venous drainage

The outflow of cerebral blood occurs via superficial and deep cerebral veins, all of which enter specially constructed non-collapsible intradural veins, called sinuses (Figs 6.9 and 6.10). The venous blood is collected by two internal jugular veins emerging from the sigmoid sinus (Fig. 6.11), which is usually larger on the side belonging to the dominant hemisphere.

Functional aspects

Early measurements of cerebral blood flow in Man were carried out by Kety (1955). The subject

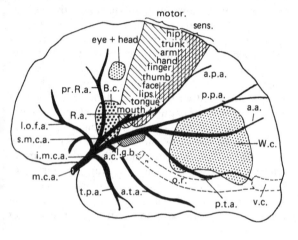

Fig. 6.9. Superficial cortical veins entering superior sagittal sinus (from Glees, 1971).

Fig. 6.10. Basal veins. The cerebellum on the left has been removed showing the drainage into the vein of Galen (from Glees, 1971).

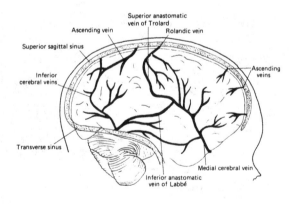

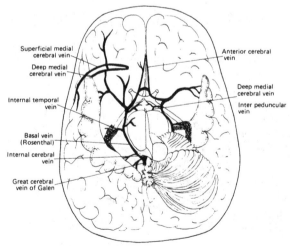

Fig. 6.11. The veinous cerebral blood returns via large sinuses built into the dura preventing their collapse. Superficial cerebral veins enter the sagittal sinus, the basal cerebral veins into the superior petrosal sinus and the ophthalmic vein into the cavernous sinus. Most cranial nerves, the internal carotis and the optic nerves are also shown (from Oertel & Glees, 1949). 1 = superior sagittal sinus; 2 = superior cerebral veins; 3 = falx cerebri; 4 = middle meningeal vessels; 5 = inferior sagittal sinus; 6 = cavernous sinus; 7 = internal carotid artery; 8 = optic nerve; 9 = pituitary stalk; 10 = inferior petrosal sinus; 11 = spheno-parietal sinus; 12 = cavernous sinus; 13 = superior petrosal sinus; 14 = inferior cerebral vein; 15 = abducens nerve; 16 = hypoglossal nerve; 17 = foramen magnum; 18 = falx cerebelli; 19 = tentorium cerebelli; 20 = occipital sinus; 21 = trigeminal nerve; 22 = 9, 10, 11 nerves; 23 = sinus rectus; 24 = trochlear nerve; 25 = 7.8 nerves; 26 = tentorium cerebelli; 27 = transverse sinus.

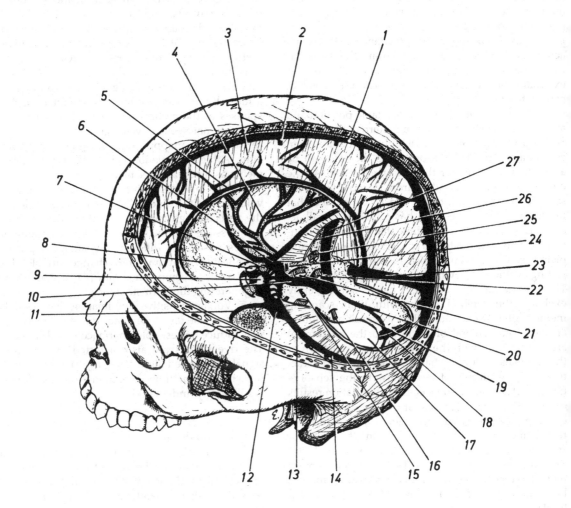

inhaled 15% nitrous oxide for 10 min. Arterial and venous saturation measurements allowed determination of average blood flow, about 50 ml of blood per 100 g brain tissue per minute, while average oxygen consumption was found to be 3.5 ml per 100 g cerebral tissue per minute.

In 1961 a Danish group of research workers (Lassen *et al.*, 1978), using radioactive isotopes, were able to measure the blood flow in circumscribed regions of the human brain and applied this method (radioactive xenon-133) to clinical diagnostic problems. The inert gas xenon dissolved in sterile saline is either injected into a large artery feeding the brain, or is inhaled by the patient. The appearance of the radioactive substance at, and removal from, the brain surface is recorded by a gamma-ray camera fed by 254 externally placed detectors, each scanning 1 cm^2 of cortical tissue.

A normal subject in a comfortable position and at rest does not show a uniform pattern of blood flow, for the frontal cortex receives a higher blood flow than central and occipital portions. This increase can be as much as 30% higher than the mean flow. As the density of capillaries and neurons is most likely the same in the whole cortex, it can be concluded that the frontal part of the brain has a higher overall activity. Lassen *et al.* (1978) assume that this higher frontal lobe activity is related to conscious awareness and planning of behaviour which is going on also in a resting position, reviewing constantly past and future. The Scandinavian authors have subsequently explored the cerebral cortex with their scanning method after visual and auditory stimuli and found an increased cerebral blood flow to the anatomical areas concerned with the reception or elaboration of these signals. Voluntary hand movements are characterised by an increased blood flow to the sensory–motor cortex, confirming electrical stimulation results (p. 94). Similarly, injections of a radioactive isotope of oxygen while hand movements are performed, reveal increased oxygen uptake in the relevant somato-sensory and motor areas (Raischle *et al.*, 1976). The increased blood supply to the supplementary motor area when voluntary movements are performed has been explained by Lassen *et al.* (1978) as an aid to planning motor performance or, to express this in computer language, as a programmer for movements. Their findings for the non-dominant hemisphere are discussed on p. 102. Although we assumed above that the mean blood supply of the cortex was the same everywhere, it is however important to realise that the rate of blood flow and capillary density are different, not only in the grey and white matter but also in individual layers of a particular cerebral area. The density of the blood supply as far as microcirculation is concerned depends on the wealth of synaptic contacts and on the metabolic requirement of neuronal cell bodies, which is governed by the activity required. Metabolic activity can be assessed in electron micrographs by counting the relative density of mitochondria in the neurons; this density varies considerably.

Metabolic activity of the brain can also be assessed by imaging with voltage-sensitive dyes in the intact brain. The changes in membrane potential of CNS neurons, and hence their activity, can then be followed in an anaesthetised animal preparation (Orbach *et al.*, 1985). Recently, an even less invasive method has been developed (Grinvald *et al.*, 1986). This involves measuring the reflected light from the intact brain (the 'intrinsic signal') using photodetector arrays. By appropriate sensory stimulation, the responses of the cortical neurons are measured using conventional electrophysiological recordings, voltage-sensitive dye mapping and imaging with reflected light. A high correlation is found between measurements using these three methods.

The time resolution of optical mapping using voltage-sensitive dyes is less than 1 ms, while that of the reflected light signals is in the order of seconds. It is possible that the bases for the two imaging techniques arise from different physiological processes: in reflected light imaging, changes in blood flow and/or blood composition may play a significant role in generating the intrinsic signals.

Voltage-sensitive dye imaging has the advantage of a fast response time, but it is invasive and may induce undesirable pharmacological side-effects. The dye signals are also distorted by the intrinsic signals. Reflected light imaging, however, is non-invasive but the time resolution is low, and its basis is still poorly understood.

Comparative organ data

In one minute, the brain receives 750 ml of blood and claims 14% of the heart's output (the liver receives 28% and the kidneys 23%). The brain's consumption is used mainly for maintenance of function, while the liver uses the blood flow for laying down storage material such as glycogen and the kidneys spend most of their energy on excretion and reabsorption.

Blocking the blood supply to the brain for more than 15–20 s at normal body temperature will lead to permanent neuronal damage; hypothermia may delay this effect.

The energy demand of the brain is essentially

supplied by glucose made available by the liver from stored glycogen. This explains the great vulnerability of the brain to disturbance of carbohydrate metabolism due to failure of liver function or if a sudden and marked increase in insulin occurs, causing a steep fall in blood sugar which in turn impairs brain metabolism. Prolonged or massive doses of insulin will cause permanent damage to neurons relying on a continuous and constant supply of glucose.

The distribution of energy supplies and the uptake of metabolites to and from the brain by the brain capillaries deserves special attention, as the brain capillaries are specially structured and layered. The basement membrane of capillaries is sizeable and multilayered and lined by the glial endfeet of the astrocytes, which provide an additional cellular sheath. This special blood–brain barrier is discussed and pictured on pp. 57, 58, 79.

The cerebral stroke

Having discussed fully the blood supply of the brain, some mention of circulatory disturbances and failures is appropriate. Old age is often brought to

Fig. 6.12. Evolution and development of cerebral ventricles. Cerebral ventricles are an inherent part of the neural tube. At the cranial end of the tube the lumen enlarges allowing for folding of the cerebral mantle in particular at the level of the hemispheres and act as bio-mechanical watercushion for growth processes (from Glees, 1971). LV = left hemispheric ventricle; RV = right hemispheric ventricle; III = interthalamic ventricle; IV = rhombencephalic ventricle.

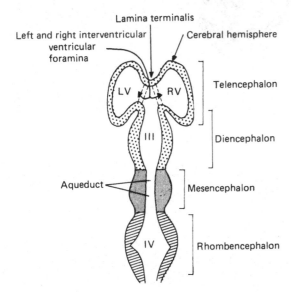

a sudden end by a vascular catastrophe, when the hardened, fragile brain vessels rupture and cause infarction (loss of blood to a given vascular bed). Depending on the area of disturbed supply, sudden cessation of a particular function, such as loss of motor power and / or loss of speech, may result (Fig. 6.8). This dramatic event will demand special care of the patient and a well-planned approach to rehabilitation by considering the age of the patient, whether the dominant hemisphere has been 'hit', and the degree of motivation for recovery.

As the larger brain arteries are situated in the cerebrospinal fluid (CSF)-filled spaces of the pia-arachnoid (Fig. 7.4), the rupture of the diseased vessel bleeds into the subarachnoidal spaces, contaminating the CSF with blood, spreading over wide areas. The disintegrating blood corpuscles liberate substances which in turn cause vascular spasm and worsen the clinical neurological picture. A reduction of vascular spasm is a primary aim in treating a cerebral haemorrhage, but it must be kept in mind that the neurosurgical repair of the bleeding vessel has to be carried out as soon as possible (Voth & Glees, 1985). In the event of a subarachnoidal haemorrhage, a lumbar puncture (Fig. 8.1) will yield blood-stained CSF because of the communication between the subarachnoidal spaces of the brain and the spinal cord.

Ventricular cavities and cerebrospinal fluid

The origin of the nervous system from the neural tube shows an inherent relation to a fluid-filled inner space. Inside the cranial cavity, surrounding the head process of the neural tube, the fluid space enlarges into larger ventricular cavities (Fig. 6.12) of which the cavities of the rapidly developing cerebral vesicles are the most impressive.

Sources of the CSF

The fluid in these cavities is largely produced by the vascular tufts of the choroid plexus which invaginate the cerebral cavities at certain strategic places. In view of their similarities with chorionic villi of the placenta, these tufts are called choroid plexuses.

The plexus consists of rich vascular loops which are covered by ependymal epithelium derived from the cells of the primitive neural wall (Fig. 6.13(a),(b)). In the foetus the choroid plexuses are especially large in order to fill the rapidly expanding cerebral hemispheres with fluid (Fig. 6.14). The site for invagination by the externally situated capillaries into the lateral ventricles is a specialised portion of ependymal epithelium in the medial wall of the cerebral vesicles (Fig. 6.14) and was termed the area choroidea by His, the

Fig. 6.13. (*a*) Low power histology of choroid plexus.
Cubical cell line free surfaces (Ep.) str. = stroma;
b.v. = blood vessels.
(*b*) E.M. view of the epithelium shown in (*a*) and
Fig. 6.14(15). Note the high microvilli seen in electron
microscopy.

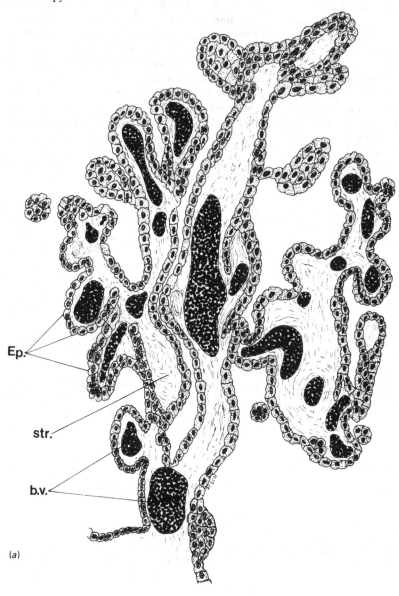

Ep.

str.

b.v.

(*a*)

Fig. 6.13(*b*) contd.

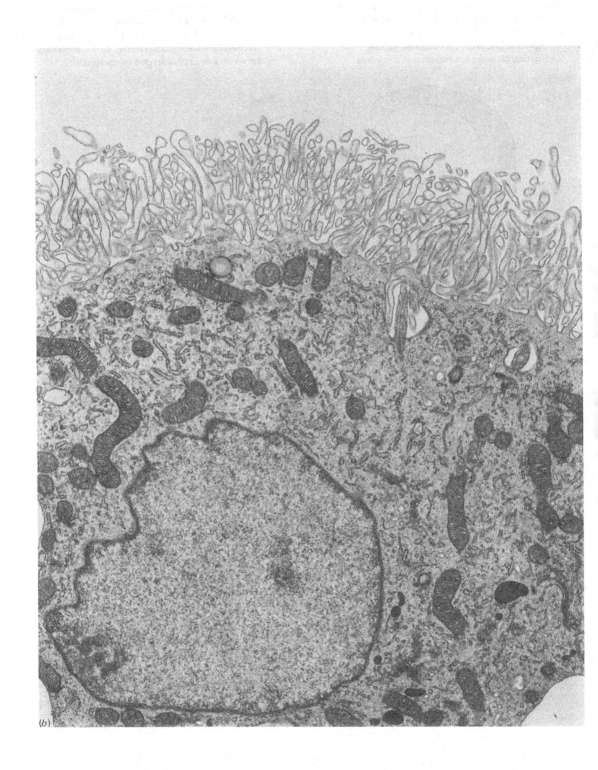

Fig. 6.14. In development the ventricular cavities harbour large choriod plexuses secreting sufficient fluid to keep the expanding cerebral mantle under tension (from Glees, 1971). 1a = cerebral mantle; 1b = future cerebral cortex; 2 = corpus callosum; 3 = hippocampal area; 4 = caudate nucleus; 5 = internal capsule; 6 = putamen; 7 = globus pallidus; 8 = temporal lobe and amygdaloid complex; 9 = thalamic nuclei; 10 = hypothalamic nuclei; 11 = 7; 12 = interventricular foramen; 13 = ependymal choroid stalk; 14 = hippocampus; 15 = choroid plexus; 16 = choroid vessels; 17 = origin of pyramidal tract and its descending course; 18 = adhesion between diencephalon and telencephalon.

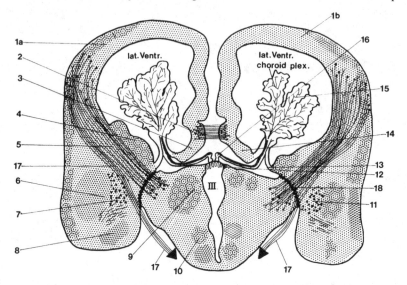

Fig. 6.15. Medial aspect of the ventricular system (from Oertel & Glees, 1949).

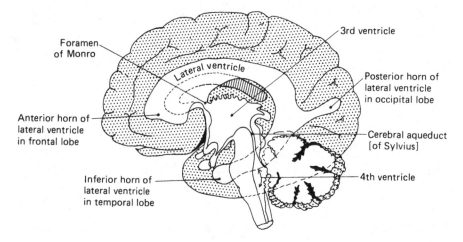

eminent embryologist of the late nineteenth century. The choroid plexus of the third and fourth ventricle derives from vascular invagination of the embryonic ependymal roof plate. At the end of the second month of human foetal development, the choroid epithelium changes into a single layer of cuboidal cells rich in glycogen and similar to developing astrocytes.

Beneath the epithelial lining a rich capillary plexus develops, surrounded by connective tissue fibres (Fig. 6.13(*a*)). When viewed with the electron microscope (Fig. 6.13(*b*)) the epithelial cells can be seen to possess microvilli and cilia towards the lumen, while the cellular border towards the capillary wall exhibits a row of complicated folds. The similarity of the electron microscope picture of the choroid plexus with that of the proximal tubules of the kidney suggests a major role in water transport, but the tubular kidney cells are engaged in water reabsorption while the choroid cells are assumed to secrete a watery fluid. A logical conclusion solely from the electron micrograph appearance of the choroid plexus would favour the absorption of CSF, but this would contradict the present prevailing view of a secretory role.

A possible further source for fluid collection in the ventricular cavities could be seepage from the brain tissue via the ependymal ventricular lining. This fluid would have the function of lymph, for the brain has no separate lymphatic channels. Extra-choroidal formation of CSF has been discussed extensively by Milhorat (1972), who has produced convincing evidence that extrachoroidal sites may be equally important for CSF production.

CSF composition

The CSF consists of 99% water; when compared to blood plasma, it contains a higher percentage of sodium, a minimal amount of protein, and two-thirds the amount of glucose (Davson, 1967). The CSF may thus represent the extracellular fluid of the brain.

CSF pressure

When examined for clinical diagnosis, the CSF is usually tapped at lumbar level (Fig. 8.1) and its pressure is found to compare to a column of saline of 150 mm, when the patient is in a lateral lying-down position. The CSF pressure is somewhat higher than

Fig. 6.16. Escape and drainage routes of cerebrospinal fluid (from Oertel & Glees, 1949).

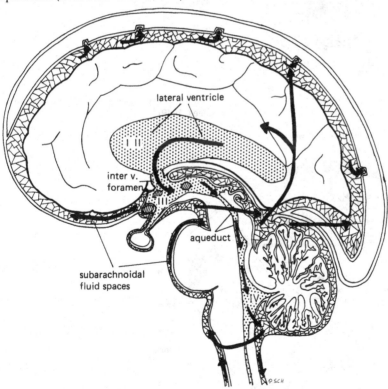

Fig. 6.17. At the level of the IV ventricle. The CSF can escape through lateral foraminae of Luschka, marked by arrow (from Oertel & Glees, 1949). v.a. = vertebral artery.

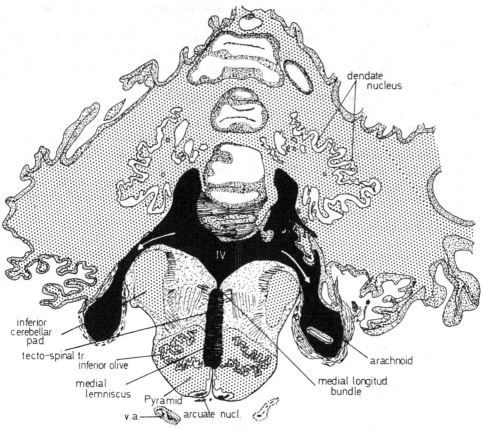

Fig. 6.18. Diagram of the arachnoid granulations (AG) assumed to filter CSF into the venous circulation of the superior sagittal sinus (from Oertel & Glees, 1949).

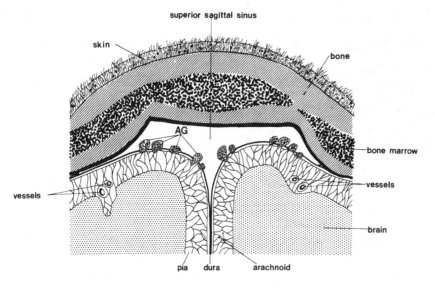

the venous pressure in the dural sinuses, thus facilitating drainage and absorption.

CSF flow direction

The CSF flows from the large internal cavities of the brain (the lateral ventricles) through the interventricular foramen of Monro into the third ventricle and through the Sylvian aqueduct into the fourth ventricle (Fig. 6.15). From the fourth ventricle, the CSF can escape through the lateral foramina of Luschka and through the median foramen of Magendie (Fig. 6.16 and 6.17). From these openings the CSF enters the subarachnoidal basal spaces around the brainstem, which are called cerebello-pontine and pre-pontine cisterns. These spaces communicate caudally with all subarachnoidal spaces of the spinal cord. Cranially the fluid enters the subarachnoidal spaces laterally and frontally to the hemispheres and medially through the cysterna ambiens and the surrounding spaces of the great cerebral vein of Galen, to ascend medially and posteriorly to the cerebral hemispheres. Most likely a considerable amount of fluid is absorbed by vessels in the arachnoid spaces while the rest enters the arachnoid granulations in the superior longitudinal venous sinus in order to be taken up by the bloodstream (Fig. 6.18). This generally accepted view of directional CSF flow is supported by ultrastructural experimental evidence (Fig. 6.19). Obstruction of the

Fig. 6.19. Schema of blood, brain, and cerebrospinal fluid relationships in the mouse (redrawn from Brightmann & Reese, 1969). A, astrocytic process. C, choroid plexus epithelium. Cs, choroid plexus stroma. E, endothelium of parenchymal vessel. EC, endothelium of choroid plexus vessel. Ep, ependyma. GJ, jap junction. N, neuron. P, pia. S.CSF., cerebrospinal fluid of subarachnoid space. TJ, tight junction. V.CSF., cerebrospinal fluid of ventricles. The dashed line follows two typical open pathways connecting ventricular cerebrospinal fluid with the basement membrane of parenchymal blood vessels and with the basement membrane of the surface of the brain. Peroxidase is seen within these pathways. Where peroxidase cannot cross cellular layers such as the parenchymal vascular endothelium (E) and the epithelium of the choroid plexus (C), the component cells are joined by tight junctions. The thick arrow (top) indicates a 'functional leak' whereby substances crossing the fenestrated endothelium of the choroid plexus can pass along the choroidal stroma to enter the parenchyma of the brain at the root of the choroid plexus. A 'leak' in the opposite direction could also occur, as indicated by the arrow point.

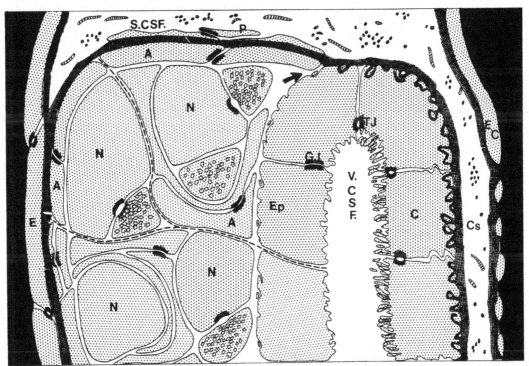

cerebral aqueduct, the connection between the third and fourth ventricles, causes dilatation of the lateral ventricles and results in internal progressive hydrocephalus. Similarly, failure of absorption can cause an external hydrocephalus.

The rate of CSF formation in man is estimated to be about 500 ml/day, while the available volume is about 140 ml, making a renewal of the fluid every 4–5 h probable. The fluid pressure varies between 150 and 180 mm saline, depending on posture and the level of the neuraxis at which the pressure is measured. Furthermore, the fact that the closed system of CSF circulation is independent of atmospheric pressure allows venous volume and pressure to influence the overall pressure of the fluid. The biochemical and microscopical analysis of the fluid is of crucial clinical importance, and a number of neurological diseases can thus be diagnosed. Brain haemorrhages spill over into the CSF and the number and types of blood cells signal the severity of brain vascular injury or infection. Metastatic brain tumours spread their malignant cells into the fluid and can be identified; pathogenic organisms (viral, bacterial and others) can be cultured and the therapeutic approach specifically directed.

For the regulation of acid–base balance of CSF see Kazemi & Johnson (1986).

7

The cerebral hemispheres

Following the evolutionary and developmental lines taken in previous chapters, a division of the adult brain into medulla, pons and cerebellum, midbrain and diencephalon (composed of thalamus and hypothalamus) will be adhered to (Fig. 7.1). However, a description of the hemispheres is given first as they have overgrown the earlier developed and older portions in primates, particularly in Man.

These hemispheres are often assumed to be the whole brain due to their enormous size, covering diencephalon, midbrain and to some extent the cerebellum as well. The left and right cerebral hemispheres are divided by a deep, longitudinal cerebral fissure. If we enter this fissure and push the hemisphere laterally we see that the bottom of the fissure is formed by a thick plate of white fibres interconnecting the two halves of the forebrain and serving the exchange of information between the hemispheres (Figs 7.1 and 7.2).

Fig. 7.1. The divisions of the brain shown diagrammatically and from a medial aspect. The cerebral cortex (in white) shows the most important sulci and fissures (from Glees, 1971). c. = cerebellum; c.c. = corpus callosum; c.h. = cerebral hemisphere; f. = frontal pole; hyp. = hypophysis of pituitary; o. = occipital pole; o.c. = optic chiasma; th. + hypoth. = thalamus plus hypothalamus, together called diencephalon.

Fig. 7.2. Horizontal section through the brain, with emphasis on the position of pathways in the internal capsule. Arrows indicate the locations of the fronto-thalamic and thalamo-frontal pathways. In the genu of the internal capsule, the cortico-bulbar and cortico-spinal fibres are followed by the thalamo-cortical connections (from Glees, 1971). a.c.v. = anterior cerebral vessel; ac.r. = acoustic radiation; c.c. = corpus callosum genu; cl. = claustrum; c.n. = caudate nucleus; c.s.p. = cavum septi pellucidi; e.c. = external capsule; f = fornix; fr. = frontal pole; g.p. = globus pallidus; i.c. = internal capsule; i.c.c. = intercollicular commissure; ins. = insular cortex; l.g.b. = lateral geniculate body; l.v. = lateral ventricle; m.g.b. = medial geniculate body; m.c. = branches of the middle cerebral artery; m-t.t. = mamillo-thalamic tract; o = occipital pole; p.b. = pineal body; pu. = putamen; s.c. = superior colliculus; o.r. = optic radiation; IIIv. = third ventricle; t = thalamus.

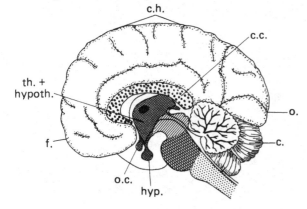

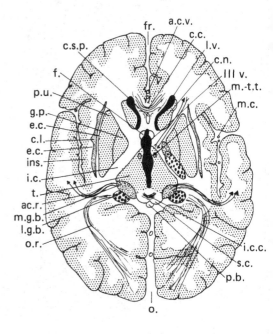

Fig. 7.3. The position of the brain inside the skull
(from Oertel & Glees, 1949). Note the relatively
posterior location of the sensory-motor cortex
indicated by the central sulcus (c.s.). c. = cerebellum;

c.sut. = cranial suture; ext.m. = external meatus;
f.p. = frontal pole; m.f. = mental foramen;
o.p. = occipital pole; o.-p.sut. = occipito-parietal
suture; S.f. = Sylvian fissure; sp.c. = spinal cord.

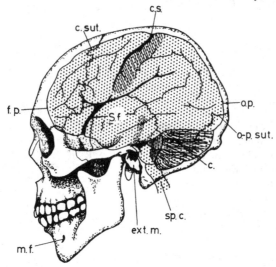

Fig. 7.4. A nuclear magnetic resonance image of the
living brain. Such investigations provide important
information on disease processes. The brain divisions

are clearly outlined. (Photograph kindly supplied by
Dr F. Koschorek, University of Kiel, Federal Republic
of Germany.)

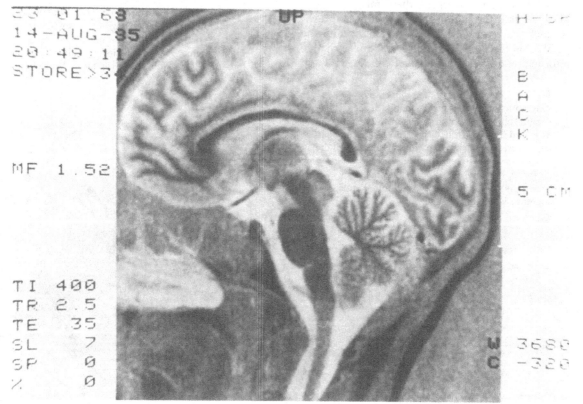

Each hemisphere has an upper (dorsal), a lateral, a medial and a basal surface. In contrast to submammalians, mammals – in particular higher primates and Man – have a highly developed and complicated pattern of foldings which are the expression of an enormous increase in cortical surface intimately related to an extensive and orderly blood supply.

The development of the cerebral cortex is thus closely linked with a highly efficient blood supply and is different in arrangement from the supply to subcortical centres. The raised cortical folds are called gyri and the separating narrow grooves called fissures and sulci (Figs 7.3 and 7.4).

Usually the name fissure is reserved for the large dividing grooves of which the lateral cerebral fissure is the most impressive, dividing the frontal and parietal lobes from the temporal lobe. This deep fissure starts at the basal surface and can be followed laterally and posteriorly into the parietal area (Fig. 7.5). A further obvious groove is the central sulcus or fissure, situated dorsally in the middle of each hemisphere (Fig. 7.5). This runs obliquely from the medial aspect of the hemisphere and transversely towards the lateral fissure but not joining it. The parieto-occipital sulcus can only be seen clearly on the medial aspect of the hemisphere (Fig. 7.6) and separates the parietal from the occipital lobe. This sulcus connects with the calcarine sulcus, which separates the upper and lower lips of the primary visual cortex. The sulcus cinguli terminates close to their meeting point, running parallel with the corpus callosum and bordering between them the gyrus cinguli, which is the cortical portion of the limbic system (p. 98), a central regulating system for the autonomic nervous system (Fig. 7.6).

Essential divisions of the hemispheres

The fissures and sulci allow a delineation of cerebral lobes, e.g. frontal, parietal, occipital and temporal lobes (Fig. 7.6). In the depth of the lateral cerebral fissure lies a fairly extensive convolution of cerebral cortex, the insula. This cortical area is hidden by overcrossing portions of the frontal, parietal and temporal cortex, a process normally concluded towards the end of pregnancy (Fig. 7.7). The evolutionarily oldest portion of the forebrain serving mainly olfaction is greatly

Fig. 7.5. Brain regions (from Glees, 1971). c.s. = central sulcus; S.f. = Sylvian fissure. The frontal lobe (f.l.) shows the inferior (i.f.g.), middle (m.f.g.), and superior (s.f.g.) frontal gyri and the precentral gyrus (pr.g.). The parietal lobe (p.l.) shows the angular (a.g.), post-central (po.g.) and supramarginal (s.g.) gyri. The occipital lobe (o.l.) is separated on its medial aspect by the parieto-occipital sulcus (p.-o.s.). The temporal lobe (t.l.) shows the inferior (i.t.g.), middle (m.t.g.) and superior (s.t.g.) temporal gyri.

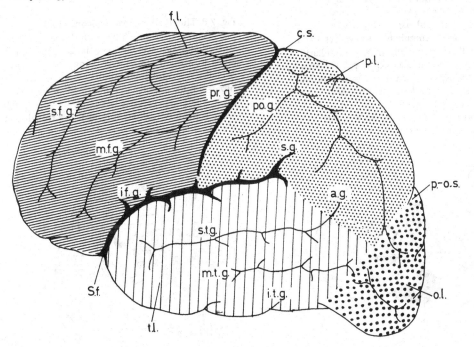

reduced in primates and is separated from the neo-cortical convolutions by the rhinal fissure (Fig. 7.8). However, mammals possessing an acute, highly developed sense of smell still have a fairly large olfactory cortical portion, referred to as the pyriform lobe (Fig. 7.8).

The frontal lobe stretches forward from the central sulcus to the frontal pole and laterally to the Sylvian or lateral cerebral fissure. The dorsal and lateral surface is formed by three parallel gyri running in a sagittal direction (Fig. 7.5) – the superior, middle and inferior frontal gyri. The inferior gyrus can be divided into an opercular, a triangular and an orbital portion. The basal part of the frontal lobe is formed by several convolutions collectively called orbital gyri.

The pattern of the temporal lobe is characterised by the parallel running gyri, the superior, medial and inferior temporal gyri. On the basal surface the fusiform gyrus and the hippocampal gyrus are prominent features in addition to a hooklike convolution, the uncus. The most important convolutions of the parietal lobe are the post-central gyrus, the supramarginal gyrus and the angular gyrus, while the most important region of the occipital lobe, the visual area, is located in the lingual gyrus around the calcarine fissure on the medial side of each hemisphere.

Fig. 7.6. Sagittal section through the left hemisphere, medial aspect (from Glees, 1971). a.c. = anterior commissure; c. = cerebellum; c.a. = cerebral aqueduct; cal.s. = calcerine sulcus; c.c. = corpus callosum; c.s. = central sulcus; e. = epiphysis; f. = fornix; g.c. = gyrus cinguli; h. = hypophysis and infundibular stalk; m. = medulla; m.i. = massa intermedia; m.b. = mamillary body; m.i. = massa intermedia; o.c. = optic chiasma; o.g. = orbital gyrus (gyrus rectus); o.n. = oculomotor nerve; p = pons; p.c. = posterior commissure; p.o.s. = parieto-occipital sulcus; quad.pl. = quadrigeminal plate; s.cin. = sulcus cionguli; IV.v. = fourth ventricle.

Fig. 7.7. Frontal brain section. This low-plane section of a medial aspect shows how many divisions of the brain can be combined in one section. The arrows indicate callosal connections (from Glees, 1971). c.c. = corpus callosum; c.ex. = capsula extrema; cl. = claustrum; c.m.n. = centre median nucleus; c.n. = caudate nucleus; d.-l.n. = dorso-lateral nucleus; d.-m.n. = dorsomedial nucleus; e.c. = external capsule; f = fornix; g.h. = gyrus hippocampi; hip. = hippocampus; i.c. = internal capsule; ins. = insular cortex; l.n. = lentiform nucleus; l.g.b. = lateral geniculate body; p. = pons; p.-l.n. = postero-lateral nucleus; p.-v.l.n. = postero-ventral lateral nucleus; p.-v.m.n. = postero-ventral medial nucleus; r.n. = red nucleus; s.n. = substantia nigra; III v. = third ventricle.

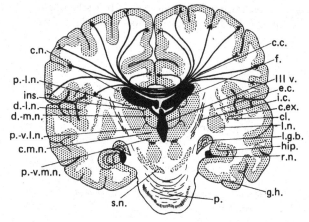

Fig. 7.8. The relation of the neocortex to the palaeocortex (pyriform lobe) in the hedgehog (Insectivora: Erinaceidae). The thalamic projection areas are seen in a transverse plane (after Diamond & Hall, 1969). aud.c. = auditory cortex; hip. = hippocampus; i.c. = intermediate cortex; l.g.b. = lateral geniculate body; p.l. = pyriform lobe; p.l.n. = posterior lateral nucleus R.f. = rhinal fissure; v.c. = visual cortex.

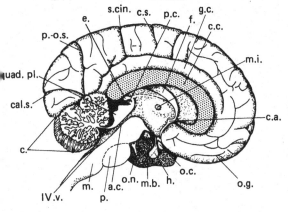

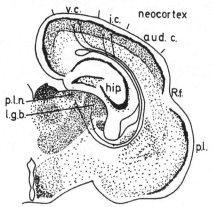

Evolutionary and developmental aspects of cerebral organisation

The organisation of the forebrain leading to the elaboration of a layered cortex must be studied in relation to the sensory channels terminating in the forebrain. The primary and oldest sensory channel of the forebrain is the olfactory sense. This sense, relayed in the olfactory bulb, conveys chemical clues about the environment to the primitive vertebrate brain. Although the sensory cells are highly sensitive receptors, their information content about the direction of food or danger is very limited. The intensity of the sense of smell, like the sense of taste, is very dependent on the varying directional forces of its solvent, water or air. This makes precise location of the source impossible, although it raises the level of alertness in the animal.

Vision, however, using the straight propagation of light, can provide topographical data about the outside world for precision localisation. We must therefore assume that sense organs can be divided into two main classes: those serving mainly to increase attention to the outside world and alertness; and those providing reliable data for the position of the individual in space. It is the latter information which reaches the cerebral cortex for classification, associational content and memory deposition. To compute these data, the cerebral cortex, with its highly organised structure and enormous number of synaptic contacts, seems highly suitable for this task.

Cortical evolution

The neocortex appeared in vertebrate evolution with the 'arrival' of primitive mammals, although recent reptiles have signs of a neuronal organisation within the forebrain which could be considered a forerunner of the mammalian cortex.

The reduction of the olfactory brain and an elaboration of neocortical organisation, including a reconstruction of the diencephalon, started effectively with the evolution of mammals.

We will follow now the concepts of cortical evolution laid down by Edinger (1904), Ariens-Kappers (1920), Elliot-Smith (1919) and in particular Diamond & Hall (1969). Diamond & Hall used the brain of the hedgehog as a model for illustrating the early evolutionary development favouring the neocortex in relation to the (evolutionarily) older cortex of the pyriform lobe (Fig. 7.8). The dorsal part of the diencephalon developed simultaneously, dividing into separate neuronal groupings called collectively the thalamus. These thalamic nuclei send axonal processes called cortical afferents (Fig. 12.5) to circumscribed cortical areas (Figs 7.9–7.10). There is a very close interdependence of the thalamus and the cortex, especially in Man (Fig. 9.25), and a further advance in cerebral evolution from a smooth non-convoluted brain to a

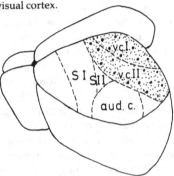

Fig. 7.9. Thalamic projection areas in the hedgehog (from Diamond & Hall, 1969). aud.c. = auditory cortex; S I = primary somato-sensory cortex, S II = secondary somato-sensory cortex; v.c.I. = primary visual cortex; v.c.II. = secondary visual cortex.

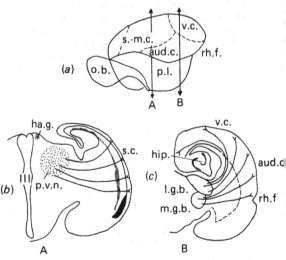

Fig. 7.10. (*a*) In a lateral view of the brain of a primitive mammal the neocortex lies above the palaeocortex (p.l., pyriform lobe). The two cortices are divided by the rhinal fissure (rh.f.). (*b*) Cortical projection areas in the platypus. The numerous sensory inputs from the bill are received by the large thalamic relay nucleus (p.v.n., posterior ventral nucleus). (*c*) Cortical projection areas in the opossum. (From Diamond & Hall, 1969) aud.c. = auditory cortex; ha.g. = habenular ganglion; hip. = hippocampus; l.g.b. = lateral geniculate body; m.g.b. = medial geniculate body; o.b. = olfactory bulb; s.c. = sensory cortex; s.-m.c. = sensory-motor cortex; v.c. = visual cortex; III = ventricle.

convoluted one is illustrated in Figs 7.11 and 7.12, showing a comparison between the smooth-surfaced brains of *Tupaia* and the squirrel monkey with the highly advanced brain of the cat, which has a gyrated convoluted neocortex.

The main advance in cerebral development must therefore be seen in the elaboration of the neocortex, receiving projections of sensory channels via the thalamus, the projection areas of the cortex and their connections with adjacent cortices, the association areas, allowing the collection of experiences and learning, leading to an 'intelligent' use of these experiences. In those animals largely depending on the senses of smell and taste, food and danger signals can be noted but not located exactly. The information quality lacks a direction parameter, forcing the organism to verify the source of the signals by coming into close contact with the source and thus neglecting the inherent danger of a close contact.

Quite different however is the information content of the visual receptor. The visual signals radiate for a considerable distance in straight directions and the object can thus be analysed from a safe distance: identification can be coupled with spatial parameters. The vastly superior visual sense, when finally ascending in evolution to forebrain levels, together with cortical projections of skin and joint receptors, led to a reconstruction of the forebrain, whose loosely arranged cortical cells changed to a multilayered structure functionally arranged in vertical columns, allowing for a very precise and orderly wiring-up process. Thus the neocortex of the forebrain not only has rows of horizontally arranged cells, of the same morpho-

logical type, but these cells also have a definite polar arrangement by having dendrites reaching into layers above and basal dendrites extending horizontally and contacting lower layers. Parallel to these evolutionary changes in the forebrain, a new relay and mixing station was constructed at diencephalic level, the thalamus. The thalamus appears to have taken over some forebrain functions, such as converging of impulses and feedback circuits, allowing the cortex to allocate more neurons for precision recordings of external signals and memory deposition.

Histological structure of the cerebral cortex and functional aspects

The cellular arrangement and the course of the afferent and efferent fibre systems exhibit a high

Fig. 7.12. The projection areas of the thalamic nuclei on to the neocortex in the cat. Note the large auditory connection. l.g.b. = lateral geniculate body; m.g.b. = medial geniculate body; p.l.n. = posterior lateral nucleus; p.v.n. = posterior ventral nucleus; v.l.n. = ventral lateral nucleus; v.m.n. = ventral medial nucleus.

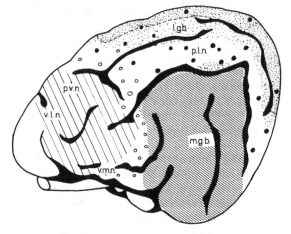

Fig. 7.11. Comparative lateral views of the brains of (left) an insectivore (Soricidae) and (right) a rodent (Sciuridae), illustrating the similarities in thalamo-cortical projections (from Diamond & Hall, 1969). aco.c. = acoustic cortex; a.t. = area temporalis; v.I = primary visual cortex; v.II = secondary visual cortex.

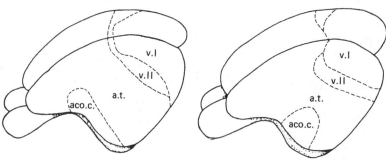

degree of orderliness, not seen below cortical level, where neurons are lumped together in scattered groups referred to as nuclei. This arrangement is clearly visible in a diagrammatic representation illustrated in Fig. 7.13 in reference to the classical stains in neurohistology.

The similarity of the cortex to a microcomputer circuit is very obvious and based on the principle of microunits of transistors and printed circuits. Although the latest 'edition' – the neocortex – uses a six-layered cortex (Fig. 7.14), there is an earlier stage in development, seen in the hippocampal structure, a three-layered organisation. These three basic layers consist of a polymorphic, a pyramidal and a molecular layer, of which the pyramidal layer is the most obvious. In order to explain the cellular arrangement and their synaptic connections, I use the excellent studies of the late anatomist Hamlyn (1962) and refer to Figs 7.15–7.19. We can learn from this pattern that a vertical or polar configuration in particular when

Fig. 7.13. Appearance with light microscopy of the cerebral neocortex treated with the classic stains. The Weigert stain reveals the criss-cross pattern of vertical and hoirizontal myelinated nerve fibres. The Golgi method brings out the cellular pattern of large and small branching neurons. The Nissl stain shows up the general cell pattern and has been used for classification of the human cerebral cortex by Brodmann (1909) and von Economo (1929).

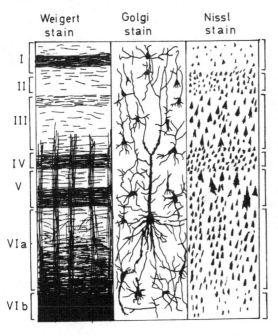

seen three-dimensionally, provides the best possible way of wiring up complex circuits. The hippocampal cortical organisation, in contrast to the 'modern' six-layered cerebral cortex, has a further primitive feature: the main outgoing system of myelinated axons is collected superficially close to the ventricle and referred to as the alveus, and bundled together in its further archlike course as a fornix to reach the hypothalamus. The neocortex, evolutionarily speaking, utilises mainly smaller pyramidal cells and extensive branching of both dendrites and axons. This arragement is most suitable for extensive convergence, mutual excitation or inhibition of arriving impulses. All neurons are arranged uppermost to the outgoing and incoming fibres to form the grey matter, while the underlying fibres are called white matter on account of the white appearance of the myelinated ensheathing. It must be emphasised again that this arrangement suits the vascular supply coming from the pia-arachnoid admirably well, as the grey matter, in contrast to the white matter, is the main oxygen consumer. The extensive dendrite arborisation of the cortical neurons account for about 30% of the grey matter and for 90% of the neuronal surface. This fact is not immediately apparent when we stain cortical brain sections for cell bodies with the Nissl stain (Fig. 7.13). The branching is best revealed by a Golgi stain or by intracellular injection with a dye spreading through the whole neuron such as Procion Yellow or by injecting the enzyme horseradish peroxidase (HRP) which can 'fill' the whole neuron.

The vertical anatomical arrangement of neuronal organisation is also expressed functionally, namely in the physiological distribution of incoming stimuli, in a vertical pattern of synaptic activity, as one might expect from the anatomical branching (see Fig. 7.20) of afferent fibres. I refer here to the early findings of Mountcastle (1967) in the sensory cortex and of Hubel & Wiesel (1977) in the visual cortex (see Fig. 13.13). This vertical cellular arrangement appears to be most suitable for the perception of movement and direction in the visual space.

While morphology can describe the cortex only according to cell types and layers and study the synaptic pattern, physiology has made considerable advances in understanding some aspects of cortical function by analysing the surface electrical potentials, such as the EEG slow waves (see Figs 4.2 and 4.3) or the arriving waves of impulses coming from subcortical levels (Fig. 7.20). Additional advances were made with microelectrodes (extra- and intracellular), which can be located in a given cell layer by micromanipulators.

Microelectrode recording and injections of HRP, both anterogradely and retrogradely, have greatly increased our knowledge of neuron interconnectivity in the last years. The new techniques of labelling with HRP or radioactive amino acids have increased the amount of detailed information on neuronal location and connectivity. This recently acquired information, particularly regarding the concept of cortical organisation, will be incorporated in the following account.

The primary sensory cortex

The territory of this receiving cortex in primates consists of the post-central gyrus, posterior to the central sulcus behind the motor cortex. A separation in a motor or pre-central area and a somato-sensory cortex are present in higher primates; the central sulcus

Fig. 7.14. Based on the Nissl technique (see Fig. 7.13). Brodmann separated the human brain into a number of different areas. This classification is still in use in neurological science: (*a*) lateral view; (*b*) medial aspect. (From Brodmann, 1909.)

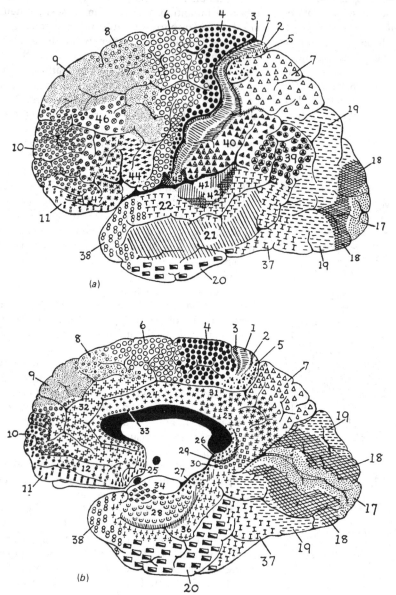

Fig. 7.15. Diagrammatic representation of the hippocampus (cornu ammonis). The large pyramidal cells have a distinct polar arrangement and can be divided into segments (C.A.1, C.A.2, C.A.3, C.A.4). These segments are selectively involved in disease processes of the brain such as epilepsy or susceptibility to neurotoxins. The cells of the dendate gyrus (d.g.) envelop the hippocampal segment C.A.4. The alveus is formed by the myelinated fibres from the hippocampus which, in turn, form the fornix. (From Glees, 1971.) f. = fimbria hippocampi (the beginning of the fornix); h.s. = hippocampal sulcus; s. = subiculum; t.d.a. = tractus dendato-ammonis.

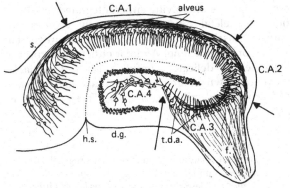

can be called a limiting sulcus between sensory and motor areas in Old World simians but not in small New World simians, according to Carlton & Welt (1980). The post-central gyrus – the primary sensory cortex – receives as a main input posterior column nuclei of Goll and Burdach and the posterior ventral nuclei of the thalamus.

The density of sensory innervation must be seen in relation to the animal's way of life in a particular environment. Mammals such as Man, using their fore-limbs for exploring their environment, have a specially large receiving area for the hand, in particular for the thumb and index finger and especially the finger pads. Adrian, in his comparative classical papers, made us aware that the boar using the snout for searching receives its sensory information at cortical level mainly from this peripheral region (Figs 7.21 and 7.22). Similarly, horses and cows have cortical representation mainly from the snout and nasal area and the peripheral forelimb area. From the results of comparative neurology it is obvious that the cerebral cortex is 'engaged' in discriminatory activity, while reflex actions of these peripheral areas are dealt with at subcortical levels.

Fig. 7.16. The general patterns of neurons and some of the fibre connections of the hippocampus seen in Golgi preparations (after Cajal, 1928). Arrows indicate direction of conduction. Only a few of the neurons are shown to allow a clearer overall picture. (See Figs 7.17 and 7.18 for synaptic organization.) a. = alveus; B = fibres entering tangential layer; d.g. = dendate gyrus (fascia dendata); f. = fimbria;

hip. = hippocampus; l.v. = lateral ventricle; s. = subiculum; s.g. = stratum granulosum; s.h. = sulcus hippocampi; s.lac. = stratum lacunore; s.m. = stratum moleculare; s.luc. = stratum lucidum (stratum pyramidale); s.oriens = stratum oriens; s.p. = stratum polymorphum; s.r. = stratum radiale; t.f.s.m. = tangential fibres embedded in stratum moleculare.

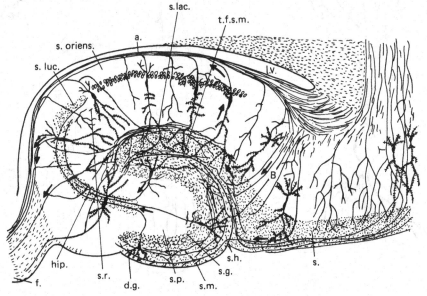

With this general conclusion in mind we further can assume that one of the tasks of the cerebral cortex is the storage of information in order to compare acute sensory signals with those of the past. Subcortical centres will store stereotypic instinctive behaviours, while the cortex acquires new sensory information, comparing this with stored 'material' to achieve an adapted behavioural response.

The post-central gyrus is usually referred to as a primary somato-sensory region, receiving mainly crossed sensory body projections, according to clinical and experimental evidence. However, in the last 20 years neurophysiological experiments showed additional areas receiving peripheral sensory signals besides the post-central gyrus (Fig. 7.23). These cortical areas receive crossed and uncrossed connections.

The input to the secondary sensory cortex (Sm II) comes, like the one to Sm I, from the ventral posterior nucleus of the thalamus and not, as was originally suspected, from the primary sensory cortex or from callosal fibres. The primary sensory cortex is not only larger but functionally divided in relation to the anatomical subdivision in Areas 3, 1 and 2. These subdivisions are related to different receptors of the body, e.g. in the case of joint receptors which are directed exclusively to Area 2.

The neocortical motor system

At each level of the neural axis, motor responses are encountered involving either integrated reflex action of skeletal muscles or aimfully coordinated smooth muscle action in the sphere of the urogenital system or the intestine. A motor outlet at neocortical level serves delicate, aimful, precise, modifiable movements which are often the summation of years of learning and critical correction. These conditions

Fig. 7.17. Individual cells of the hippocampus (Golgi impregnation). Different parts of the cells occupy various hippocampul layers modulated by different synaptic inputs. The axons of these large pyramidal cells emerge as thin processes entering the alveus. The axons also give off collateral fibres to the upper layers (after Hamlyn, 1963). a. = alveus; c.f. = collateral fibre; s.lac. = stratum lacunare; s.m. = stratum moleculare; s.o. = stratum oriens; s.pyr. = stratum pyramidale; s.r. = stratum radiale.

Fig. 7.18. Diagrams from electron micrographs of large pyramidal cells (see Fig. 7.17), showing the different types of synapse in various layers (after Hamlyn, 1963). A – G. pre. = pre-synaptic; post. = post-synaptic. Layers as in Fig. 7.17. n. = nucleus.

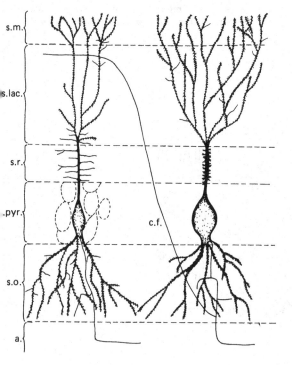

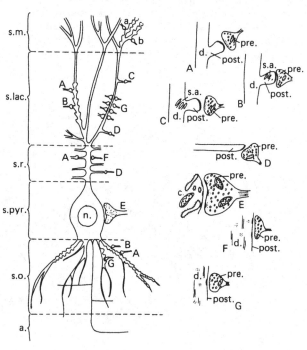

Fig. 7.19. Synaptic organisation of a mossy fibre termination in the hippocampus. Many active points are present and the spine contains the so-called spine apparatus of flat vesicles (from Hamlyn, 1963).
a.s.v. = accumulation of synaptic vesicles;
d. = dendrite; i.s. = intersynaptic space;
m. = mitochondrion; mt. = microtubules;
n. = neurofilaments; n.m.a. = non-myelinated axon portion; pre. = synaptic area; s.a. = spine apparatus;
sp. = spine; s.v. = synaptic vesicle;
s.w.(a) = subsynaptic web in active point;
s.w.(d) = subsynaptic web in denorite.

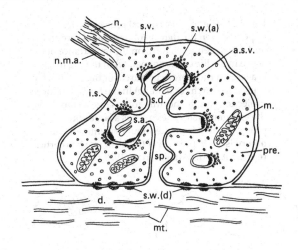

Fig. 7.20. Evoked potential methods for tracing interconnections have conformed the connections found anatomically. These electrophysiological methods are still in use in clinical neurology and can provide fast information on intact and non-functional pathways in patients. 1. Tracing ascending connections by stimulation of sensory nerves or the posterior spinal column. The surface potential recording is shown in 1a. 2. Antidromic stimulation of the pyramidal tract in the spinal cord or at higher levels will result in potential 2b. 3. The callosal potential (3c) is recorded by stimulating one hemisphere and recording from the other. 4. Stimulation of the ascending reticular system results in a change in the EEG (4d). AVN = anterior ventral nucleus; CMN = centre median nucleus; CN = caudate nucleus; DLN = dorso-lateral nucleus; DMN = doso-medial nucleus; i = indifferent electrode; PVN = posterior ventral nucleus. (From Glees, 1961a.)

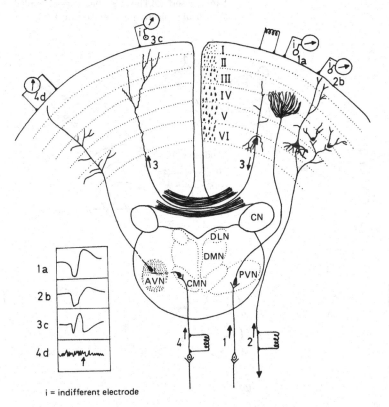

i = indifferent electrode

Fig. 7.21. The size of a cortical projection area depends upon the density of peripheral receptors and this depends, in turn, on the importance of the sense in the life of the animal. (*a*) In the pig there is a large cortical projection area for the snout which is used to search for food. (*b*) In the horse the cortical projections for the nostrils are as large as those for the extremities. (*c*) The cow has a large cortical projection area from the snout (trigeminal) but otherwise only the skin of the front feet has cortical representation. (After Adrian, 1928.)

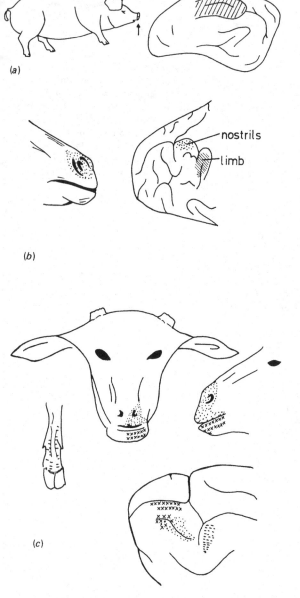

are fulfilled at the cortical level in Man by the pre-central gyrus (Fig. 7.24). Histologically the pre-central gyrus shows a special arrangement of neurons (Figs 7.13 and 7.20) in layer V, the large or giant cells of Betz, named after the nineteenth-century anatomist who described them for the first time (Betz, 1874, 1881). The Betz cells occur in clusters and serve as a sample of very large pyramidal cells (see Fig. 3.3). The large and long descending axons form parts of the descending cortical pathway, called the pyramidal tract from its appearance in cross-section at the medullary level. Neuroanatomical studies, neuro-physiological experiments and clinical observations all confirm that this large and conspicuous fibre tract, emerging mainly from the pre-central gyrus or area 4, is responsible for the execution of willed, aimful delicate movements (Fig. 7.25). The early concept that this fibre tract represented the axons of Betz cells was disproved by Lassek (1940, 1941a,b; 1942a,b; 1943), who counted the total number of these large pyramidal cells in one hemisphere and found not more than 34 000 cells, whereas the number of fibres in this human pyramidal tract was about 1 million at the

Fig. 7.22. (*a*) The sensory cortical projections in the cat are crossed. (*b*) The dog's head has a detailed and rich cortical projection. (After Adrian, 1928.)

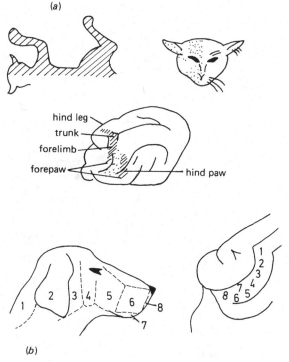

Fig. 7.23. Somato-sensory regions in the squirrel monkey (Cebidae) (from Blomquist & Lorenzini, 1965). Cortical evoked potentials were recorded after stimulation of the peripheral nerves or nerve trunks.

Four different somato-sensory regions were detected: Ms I, Ms II, Sm I, Sm II. A = arm; F = face; L = leg; T = trunk; * = Penfield's supplementary sensory area.

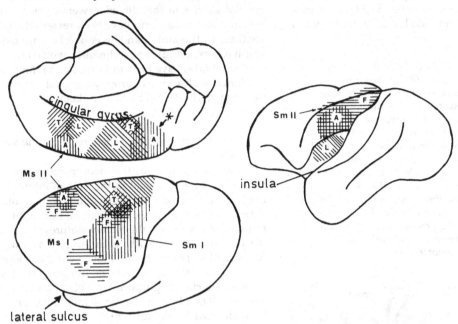

Fig. 7.24. Diagrammatic lateral view of the human brain illustrating the main sulci and gyri, and the isolation of the frontal lobe, anterior to the lateral ventricle, by classic bilateral leucotomy – a technique of psychosurgery. The primary motor cortex is stippled.

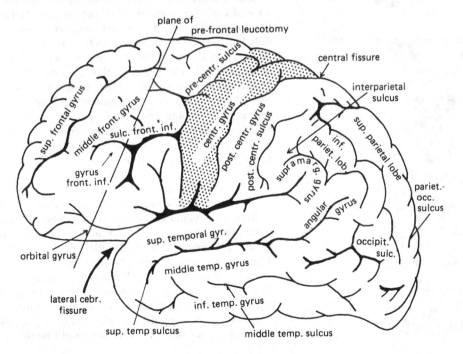

medullary level. It is improbable that the 34 000 axons branched in their descending course to reach this large number of fibres. It is more likely that smaller neurons of the pre-central gyrus contribute substantially to the cortico-spinal population of fibres. The cortico-spinal tract is present in all mammals but is especially prominent in primates.

Fig. 7.25. Diagram of the pyramidal tract (cortico-spinal, cortico-medullary fibres) illustrating the proportional innervation of the body. The most important areas, such as the face and hand motor neurons, have very large innervation areas, as shown in Man by Penfield & Boldrey (1937) and Penfield & Rasmussen (1950). A. Cortical level. a1, a2, a3, a4, a5 cortical motor fibres for areas as illustrated. c.c. = corpus callosum. B. Position of motor fibres in internal capsule. g.p. = globus pallidus; p = putamen. C. Position of motor fibres in cerebral peduncle. III = oculomotor nerve. D. Pontine level. Vm = motor root of trigeminal nerve. E. Medullary level. X = vagus nerve; XII = hypoglossal nerve. F. Level of decussation for 90% of fibres.

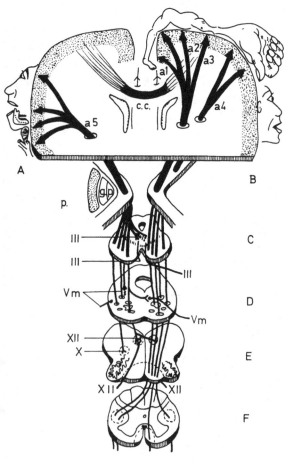

Functional significance

The number of cortico-spinal fibres in different mammals appears to be related to the range of movements in particular to those of the human hand. Experimental studies in this direction were carried out in primates and in cats and have been reviewed including those by this author and his co-workers in a monograph (Glees, 1961a). The techniques evolved by Cole & Glees (1961a) have been improved and refined and combined with direct neurophysiological recordings by Kuypers (1981) and by Lemon (Lemon *et al.*, 1983; Lemon & Muir, 1983).

The development of the voluntary, purposeful motor system

The maturation of this neocortical system can be studied in great detail in the human infant, both in normal development and in pathological conditions when the cerebral cortex has been injured at birth or by infection. Normally the system matures slowly and the baby moves aimlessly with all the limbs in the first months. These chaotic movements, accelerated by emotional states, distress or hunger, are slowly gaining directional purpose; an object lowered into the cot will first be aimed at by all four limbs, grasped by both arms by a young baby and by one arm by an older baby. The all-purpose limb movements become arm movements exclusively and progress towards a controlled one-hand pattern, the first sign of lateralisation and cerebral dominance. This guidance of voluntary movement usually occurs after the first year of life. The neocortical guidance system not only has to learn to use messages from the peripheral sensors but also to dominate the older motor system at subcortical levels. The cortical over-ruling is flexible and dynamic if the cortical system is damaged experimentally by tumours or by injuries in clinical cases, the older, involuntary motor pattern reappears. Highly skilled hand movements are normally best performed when sitting down to prevent overloading of the cortical guidance system.

Number and fibre size

The pyramidal system certainly has the number of fibres one would expect for the range and delicacy of movement required. Man has about 1 million fibres in each pyramidal tract and the fibre size ranges from 1 μm to 11–22 μm. About 90% of all fibres are around 1–4 μm in diameter. These different diameters indicate that the system sends its impulses with varying speed to the various levels of motor execution. The big fibres might serve to prepare for the arrival of impulses mediated by smaller fibres or they might be directed to strategically important neuron pools of muscle groups, used for rapid eye movements or hand and finger movements. The late myelinisation of the cortico-spinal system, one year after birth, confirms the view taken by Flechsig (see p. 1) that evolutionarily recent neuronal systems acquire their myelin sheath after birth, while old established pathways mature *in utero*. After myelinisation the pyramidal tract area doubles its size.

The area of origin for cortico-spinal and cortico-bulbar fibres is not limited to Area 4 of the pre-central gyrus. Area 6, in front of Area 4, and the post-central and parietal areas also contribute to the fibre population, but the numbers of these fibres vary according to the species. In Man, Areas 4 and 6 contribute about 80% of the pyramidal tract fibres (Glees, 1961a; Kuypers, 1981; Dawnay & Glees, 1986).

Neurophysiological observations in relation to voluntary movements

Disturbances in motor performance are normally the first signs of a disease process in the afferent vessels of the sensory–motor cortex or of a tumour developing in this region. Such disturbances are very marked in encephalitis lethargica and Parkinson's disease, characterised by rigidity and tremor. Treatment with Levodopa will relieve symptoms but reveals in post-encephalitis patients archetypal movements of subcortical mechanisms; these were demonstrated by Sacks (1982) who also made other interesting observations on motor assistance by sensory stimuli in this pathological condition.

Electrophysiological recordings show that about a second before voluntary movements start, the cortical DC potential undergoes a negative shift. This potential shift is referred to as the preparatory potential for the following muscle action. A positive surface potential appears, 30–90 ms after this, caused by the ascending discharges from the thalamus and resulting from the firing of muscle and joint receptors. In view of the surface position of the cortico-spinal tract at medullary and spinal cord levels it has been possible to apply electric shocks to the tract and to record from the neurons of the motor cortex antidrocmically conducted discharges from cells of cortico-spinal tract origin. In this way resting potentials and modes of discharge of these cells have been studied in detail (Phillips, 1955). These pyramidal tract neurons (PTN) served as a useful model for analysing the effects of converging impulses from different sensory sources (hearing, vision, touch and deep sensations). The behaviour of PTN is different from that of neurons in the sensory cortex, as PTN respond mainly to certain peripheral receptors. The PTN of a monkey previously trained to a particular pattern of movement after visual awareness of a light signal show a discharge 70 ms later. Within this 70 ms, the pattern of electrical registration from the motor cortex indicates that a voluntary decision is in preparation to execute the learned and purposeful movement.

Independent skilled finger movements as developed to the high degree seen in musicians, are an expression of cortical motor control. This control is brought about by *direct* excitatory influence on motor neuron pools of intrinsic hand muscles (Muir & Lemon, 1983a,b) and not indirectly. Surveying all the experimental data from work on motor performance over the last 100 years one is tempted to say that this direct stimulation was to be expected. But the road to this insight was a tortuous one as most experiments were on subprimates, where the pyramidal system is less well developed and 'works' more in dependence on other spinal systems. Upright gait, greater visual precision and the need for greater precision of quick hand movement enabled the cortico-spinal projection to over-rule spinal and bulbar reflex mechanisms. Further details of connections at the spinal level will be discussed in Chapter 8.

The frontal lobes

The frontal lobes include all the brain tissue in front of the central sulcus and include the motor region of the pre-central gyrus. Using Brodmann's terminology, the frontal lobes include granular (small cells) Areas 9, 10, 11, 12, 13, 45 and 46, but exclude Area 4, the primary somato-motor area, while Areas 6 and 8 are referred to as granular cortical and extra-pyramidal areas, although they also contribute to cortico-spinal fibres. The marked development of a granular frontal lobe is most apparent in primates and particularly in Man. While in such mammals as dogs and cats the motor regions occupy the most frontal regions of the brain, in primates a considerable portion of the neocortex lies in front of the primary motor cortex (Fig. 7.24). In Man about one-third of the cortical surface belongs to frontal lobe tissue.

Clinical observations on frontal lobe functions

About 50 years ago the prevalent view was that the pre-motor areas of the frontal lobe were silent areas and associative in character, without a clear circumscribed function. A further interesting point emerged, which is still valid today: diseases of the frontal lobes, especially if unilateral, are without any distinct signs in children, as I observed recently (Fig.

7.26). A large tumour located in the right frontal lobe was present in a girl of 14 years without causing physiological or intellectual deficits. This case supports the view that frontal lobe function is not lateralised. Careful clinical observations of mature people suffering from bilateral trauma or from tumours involving both sides of the frontal lobes show personality changes, such as lack of inhibition, failure of moral judgement or carelessness; these changes are only clearly revealed when both sides are diseased.

Frontal leucotomy

Essential knowledge of frontal lobe function has been gained from certain neurosurgical interventions which gained wide public interest some 40 years ago. Two types of surgery were used: (1) classical leucotomy, the severence of frontal lobe fibre connections (white matter); and (2) the selective removal, by suction or undercutting, of frontal dorsal or orbital gyri. The operation of leucotomy was carried out for the first time by Moniz & Lima (1936) in Portugal with a view to altering social and moral behaviour by psychosurgical intervention in areas of the frontal lobe. Psychosurgical operations have been attempted not only in the frontal lobe but also in man in the hypothalamus to alter sexual drives (Orthner, 1957)

Fig. 7.26. Right frontal (F) tumour (GT) in a girl of 14, without clinical signs. The butterfly figure is that of the anterior horns of lateral ventricles and part of the left lateral ventricle. Computer-tomographic picture.

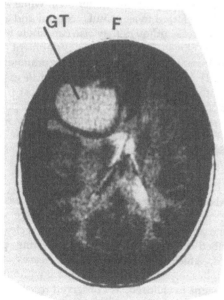

and in the connections of the basal ganglia with the thalamus, with a view to alleviating motor disturbance in Parkinson's disease (p. 108). Due to progress in treatment with psychotropic drugs, however, brain surgery of this kind has been superseded; drug treatment offers in these cases a more controllable condition than after an irreparable surgical intervention.

The early observations by Fulton & Jakobsen (1935) in higher primates inspired much of the human research and enriched considerably our insight into cortical function. The neurophysiologist Fulton, himself a trained neurosurgeon, and the psychologist Jakobsen found that chimpanzees subjected to difficult test situations displayed conflict behaviour when they received no reward after the tests. If a chimpanzee was unable to solve any problems in a series of tests, it would withdraw into a corner of its cage and refuse to take food. Its behaviour would become neurotic and further test runs would be impossible. As such animals could not be used for further experiments, Fulton removed the frontal lobes for final neuroanatomical experiments and found, to his great surprise, that the chimpanzees had lost their anxious and neurotic behaviour and submitted fully to renewed test trials. These experimental results were communicated by Fulton and Jakobsen in 1935 at an international congress attended by Moniz and Lima. After returning home, Moniz and Lima leucotomised withdrawn schizophrenics, hoping that their contact with the outside could be re-established. Not being trained in neurosurgery, they were afraid to remove the frontal lobes but assumed that severance of the connections should give the same effect. These incoming and outgoing frontal connections were located in the white matter and a special instrument, the leucotome was constructed; in this way the psychosurgical operation of leucotomy was born (Fig. 7.24). Leucotomy was aimed at two mental diseases – obsessional neuroses and schizophrenia; but patients with anorexia nervosa, a juvenile condition resulting in the refusal of food and leading to extreme cachexia, have also been leucotomised. Ploog *et al.* (1981) have recently discussed the neurobiology of this disease in relation to the limbic system (p. 98). The obsessional neurotic patient suffers from compulsive ideas, such as a continuous need for washing and cleaning, or a fear of infections, being in a big crowd or walking across large empty spaces, while the schizophrenic has personality changes, characterised by disturbances of mentation, faulty sensations and emotional withdrawal. Leucotomy causes a previously introverted patient to become more open to the outside world. In the same way a young female suffering from anorexia nervosa will start to eat and to respond to contacts. However, all patients show diminished self-criticism and reduced perseverance and concentration. A particular disadvantage of leucotomy is the loss of social responsibility, especially noticeable in a mental institution, where discipline in behaviour is essential. These behavioural changes are even more noticeable when the patient returns home, when he neglects his social duties and offends family members by tactless and frivolous remarks. This disinhibition is especially obvious in obsessional neurotics, who had been pedantic and very conscientious in their behaviour before the operation. The impression is gained that frontal lobe-damaged patients (accidental or leucotomised) show no interest in their past or in their future and live in a continuous aim-free present. Psychological tests are performed quickly but superficially; at first impression one could believe that an increase in intelligence has taken place after operation, but in fact the quick action is based on diminished criticism. In conclusion, leucotomy and frontal lobe injury indicate that the normal function of the frontal lobe is the control of emotional life, starting in childhood with control of emotionally motivated motor responses. From an evolutionary point of view, the frontal lobe seems to be a superimposed inhibitory centre for motor cortex activity, starting with restraining the spontaneous motor activity of the infant and gradually controlling drive-motivated behaviour. Frontal lobe function is aimed at making primates submit themselves to living together in an ordered social group. This process starts in early childhood, reaches a plateau after puberty and decreases towards old age, when the loss of the frontal lobe's critical overall control is the most obvious sign among the features of diminished cortical function caused by general neuronal atrophy.

Neuroanatomical connections of the frontal lobes, both granular and agranular, were revealed in human post-mortem studies of leucotomies and in animal experiments. The most important two-way pathway is the connection with the dorsomedial nucleus of the thalamus (Fig. 9.25). This neothalamic nucleus, connecting with the hypothalamus and with the cortex, has a direct link with the limbic system. Other pre-frontal (granular cortices) areas connect with the basal ganglia, tegmentum, midbrain and pons.

The temporal lobes

The temporal lobes of Man and other primates are clearly separated from the frontal lobes and the parietal lobes by the lateral cerebral fissure, the Sylvian fissure. Three different areas can be defined: (1) true neocortex, phylogenetically of recent development; (2) the olfactory or rhinencephalic portion; and (3) the hippocampus. Histologically these three portions are very different: the neocortical areas are six- to seven-layered cortex; the basally situated rhinencephalon (or paleocortex) is composed of irregular groups of neurons; while the hippocampus consists of three layers of cells and is referred to as the archicortex. The temporal lobe gains an early clinical significance when in childhood a middle-ear infection extends into the temporal area above and causes a brain abscess, an event much feared before the advent of antibiotics.

Connections of the temporal lobe

The neocortical Areas 22, 21 and 20 correspond to the superior, middle and inferior temporal gyri (Fig. 7.24). Although temporo-pontine connections do exist, their exact origins and terminations are not yet defined. The best-known ascending pathway originates from the medial geniculate body and carries auditory signals to a small part of the superior temporal gyrus (Area 22), the area supratemporalis granulosa (Areas 41 and 42) of Brodmann (see Fig. 7.14). This auditory projection area, the primary auditory cortex, is somewhat hidden away as it branches off the superior temporal gyrus into the depth of the insula and is also referred to as the transverse gyrus of Heschl. The inferior temporal gyrus (Area 21) has visual function, while the temporal pole (Area 38) receives mainly association fibres from the frontal lobe and temporal areas but no fibres from the thalamus. Due to the paucity of thalamic connections, the whole temporal lobe, as far as the neocortex is concerned, is referred to as an association cortex in contrast to a projection cortex, receiving its main input from thalamic nuclei (see Fig. 9.25). This associational character is brought out by the recent demonstrations of widely distributed efferent and afferent connections of the infero-temporal cortex with the frontal cortex (Kuypers *et al.*, 1965). While the functions of Areas 41 and 42 are obviously those of a sensory projection area, one wonders what is the functional significance of the other large temporal regions. Clinically, unilateral lesions can be silent unless secondary signs of epilepsy and distinct abnormalities in the electro-encephalogram are present. These temporal lobe epilepsies result in complicated psychological abnormalities and disturbed motor behaviour and vary in relation to the involvement of deeper structures such as the amygdaloid nuclei and hippocampus. Penfield & Rasmussen (1950) startled the neurologists by publishing his observations on electrical stimulation of the temporal lobe in epileptic patients. These patients, stimulated under local anaesthesia, reported chains of memory recall, suggesting that the temporal lobe is a store for past events (Mahl *et al.*, 1964). It must be emphasised, however, that stimulation of a normal temporal lobe does not produce these recall phenomena. On the other hand one might argue that the epilepsy can cause a sensitisation to make neuronal circuitry respond more easily when stimulated electrically.

The phylogenetically older portions of the temporal lobe

It has been noted above that the temporal lobe includes phylogenetically older portions of the forebrain which derive from the olfactory brain, so much reduced in primates. These portions stem from the non-layered palaeocortex, showing no cortical plate in the embryological stages (Fig. 2.32). As well as the

palaeocortex, the archicortex, referred to as the hippocampus, is included (Figs 7.15 and 7.11). Comparative neurological work, starting with that of Papez (1937, 1958), attempted to delineate a functionally interdependent system which gives the hippocampal and amygdaloid parts of the temporal lobe a prominent significance, the *limbic system* (Fig. 7.27). The palaeocortex, archicortex and some portions of the temporal neocortex, together with the gyrus cinguli, amygdaloid nuclei, septal area and area entorhinalis, are major portions of this system. Their relative contributions and size vary considerably among mammals. In Man the limbic system is best visualised by dissection from the medial surface of the brain. The hippocampus is laid free by opening the temporal horn of the lateral brain ventricle; from it emerges a large fibre tract, the fornix, so called because it arches over the diencephalon, descends to the hypothalamus and loops posteriorly to terminate in the lateral nucleus of the mamillary body. The medial nucleus of the mamillary body has a very conspicuous myelinated fibre connection with the anterior nucleus of the thalamus, the mamillo-thalamic tract or bundle of Vicq d'Azyr. From the anterior thalamus nucleus fibres can be traced to the cingular gyrus. Many of these fibre tracts are two-way connections or feedback circuits. The amygdaloid nuclei lie in the temporal pole in front of the hippocampus and are divided into lateral, central and medial parts. To some extent the amygdaloid nuclei

Fig. 7.27. The right cerebral hemisphere, medial aspect, illustrating the limbic system and its components (dotted). The hippocampus is covered by the hippocampal gyrus and the amygdaloid nucleus or complex lies deep in the anterior part of the temporal lobe, frontally to the descending horn of the lateral ventricle (from Glees, 1971);
forn.a = ascending pillar of fornix;
forn.d = descending pillar of fornix, terminating in the mamillary body (m.b.).

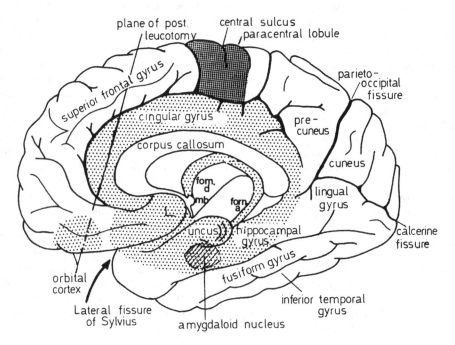

can be compared with thalamic nuclei and their relation to the cerebral cortex. The amygdaloid complex projects to the orbito-frontal cortex, receives fibres from the olfactory cortex and sends fibres to hypothalamic nuclei. Clinical signs observed in temporal lobe epilepsy such as smacking the lips or olfactory hallucinations are most likely not due to discharge of the neotemporal cortex but to involvement of the amygdaloid complex and/or orbito-frontal–temporal–basal involvements. The Klüver–Bucy syndrome, which includes extreme tameness and lack of aggression and is seen after bilateral removal of the temporal lobe, is most likely to be due to destruction of the amygdaloid area. This syndrome includes psychic blindness, an inability to recognise objects visually or by touch and to fall back on the early infant's oral reconnaissance system, the lips and tongue. This finding illustrates that the temporal lobe cortex supports the visual cortex in identification problems and also in remembering things, as we (Glees & Griffiths, 1952) observed in a patient suffering from bilateral destruction of the hippocampus and the fornix system. We see from these reports evidence for wide connections between the amygdaloid system, hippocampus, hypothalamus and reticular formation of the midbrain, interconnected by the medial forebrain bundle, stretching from the olfactory regions, amygdaloid area, mamillary body and central grey matter of the midbrain in a sagittal plane.

The hippocampus. On account of its special three-layered structure, the archicortex or allocortex has attracted the attention of many neurobiologists and clinicians. The fields covered range over electrophysiology, pharmacology, histochemistry and electron microscopy. Jung (1949) and a number of co-workers pointed out that electrical stimulation of the hippocampus leads to very marked epileptic discharges in the hippocampus, explained by the lack of inhibitory circuitry in a more primitive three-layered cortex. This concept furthered the research into inhibition and gave some evolutionary reason for the development of a six-layered cortex. However, localised hippocampal discharges did not change the behaviour of an awake non-restrained animal with implanted electrodes.

Ultrastructurally, the hippocampus was analysed by Hamlyn (1962) who revealed complex synaptic relations (Figs 7.17–7.19). These investigations showed how many afferents converge on the large pyramidal cells but on different portions of the neuron. The row of hippocampal cells can be divided into segments (Fig. 7.15) which behave differently

under stress. We found that the cellular segment CA4 (Fig. 7.21) ages much more rapidly, indicated by its increased lipofuscin content, than the other segments (Continillo & Glees, 1985).

Akert (1963) was able to show that a cat continued lapping up milk while being stimulated in the hippocampal area. However, the spread of epileptic discharges, particularly after discharges in the reticular formation and cortical association cortex, led to confusional states, resembling psychomotor attacks in epileptic patients, who may act in a completely irrational manner in this state. Feldberg & Sherwood (1954) and Fleischhauer (1963) attempted to study hippocampal activity by neuropharmacological means. Due to the anatomical position of the hippocampus, in the ventricular cavity of the inferior horn, injection of active pharmacological substances into the cerebrospinal fluid can be made close to the free surface of the hippocampus. Neurophysiological examinations of human post-mortem material has increased our knowledge of hippocampal function (Grünthal, 1948; Glees *et al.*, 1950; Ule, 1950; Glees & Griffiths, 1952; Conrad & Ule, 1951). These papers implicate hippocampal function in the process of memory deposition or fixation. In cases of hippocampal destruction, diminished emotional reactions and dementia are apparent, including 'oral behaviour' seen also in schizophrenics. This oral behaviour is also a part of the Klüver–Bucy syndrome described above.

Akert (1963) and his co-workers saw a similar syndrome in male cats, which exhibited an abnormal sexual behaviour after lesions in the amygdaloid complex. The limbic system was also implicated in self-stimulating experiments carried out in rats by Olds & Molner (1954), who reported that implanted electrodes within the limbic system's septal nuclei caused the animals to give themselves electric shocks regardless of pain or being offered food. It appeared that the region stimulated initiated an obsessional urge for repeating the stimulus, even if it meant starving or dying of thirst. This behaviour resembles the urge of a drug addict to achieve drug satisfaction at all costs (see Chapter 15).

Figure 7.27 shows the inclusion of the gyrus cinguli in the limbic system although it is a neocortical element composed of six-layered cortex. To eliminate a portion of the limbic system in certain mental illnesses, some neurosurgeons followed the concepts laid down by leucotomy research and removed anterior portions of the cingular gyrus. However, the surgical approach to this gyrus is difficult. The cortical veins entering the superior sagittal sinus have to be cauterised in order to retract the medial aspect for surgical approach (Fig. 6.11). The gyrus is surrounded by branches of the anterior cerebral artery which may be injured by sucking out the cerebral tissue. These concomitant injuries make it difficult to obtain selective results, although the aim of surgery was to achieve reduction of the cortical control of the limbic system in order to alter pathological behaviour. Electrical stimulation of the cingular gyrus in the conscious patient due to be cingulo-ectomised revealed no behavioural responses or disturbances in hand movements or of awareness, as had been claimed by some authors, and the assumption that the cingular gyrus was in control of the limbic autonomic system could not be verified. Clinical results following the removal of the cingular gyrus on both sides resembled those of a mild frontal injury. Post-mortem neurohistological examination showed that the connections to the anterior nucleus of the thalamus were interrupted, confirming for Man an observation made in primates (cf. Glees *et al.*, 1950).

The parietal cortex

The parietal lobe lies between the primary visual cortex and the motor cortex and is well separated in primates by two deep fissures, the lunate sulcus posteriorly and the central fissure anteriorly. Due to the close functional relation of the anterior portion of the parietal lobe (the post-central gyrus) with the motor cortex, this somato-sensory part has been discussed on pp. 92–4. It should be mentioned here that clinical neurophysiology has benefited greatly from experimental findings that peripheral nerve or skin stimulation produces evoked potentials in the somatosensory cortex. These evoked potentials are important tools for the clinician to look for and aid him to localise neurological deficits (Desmedt, 1971).

The posterior parts (see Fig. 7.14), Brodmann's Areas 5, 7, 39 and 40, achieve their greatest extension in Man, particularly Areas 39 and 40 which are concerned with human verbal ability. Areas 5 and 7 were assumed to be associative in character and their connections were thought to be mainly transcortical, but recent techniques using labels such as horseradish peroxidase (HRP) show thalamic afferents from the lateral posterior nucleus to Area 5 and from the pulvinar thalamic to Area 7. Intralaminar thalamic nuclei, paracentral and lateral central nuclei seem to project as well to the parietal cortex. The pulvinar has no direct sensory input from the periphery but receives incoming stimuli from the anterior colliculi of the midbrain, the pretectal region and from the visual cortex, in the same way as the posterior thalamic nucleus which receives impulses from the spino-thalamic fibres. Areas 5 and 7 furthermore receive intracortical association fibres from the posterior central gyrus and from the non-striated visual cortex, respectively. Efferent fibres from Areas 5 and 7 terminate in the pontine nuclei and the reticular nucleus of the pons. These connections have been established by recent tracer methods and have revealed that the parietal lobe occupies an important role in skilled and complex movements needing sequences of planned and thoughtfully aimed movements. These findings have been further extended by evoked-potential recordings after stimulations of the auditory, visual and somatosensory systems. To exclude the effects of anaesthetics, behavioural experiments were carried out, combined with single-neuron recordings from the parietal lobe (from implanted electrodes). It was found that the neurons of Area 5 were fired from somatosensory neurons, while neurons of Area 7 (Fig. 7.14) could be excited by visual or somato-sensory stimuli. Two-thirds of Area 5 neurons were stimulated contralaterally by joint receptors and about 10% of the neurons by cutaneous stimuli from large receptive fields (see Creutzfeldt, 1983 for further details). Creutzfeldt draws attention to the fact that neurons of Areas 5 and 7 fire more strongly or exclusively when the experimental animal executes goal-motivated aimful hand movements.

This confirms some early observations by Glees & Cole (1954) presented to the International Neurological Congress in Lisbon in 1953. Glees & Cole compared the effects of anterior (Areas 3, 1 and 2) and posterior (Areas 5 and 7) in well-trained *Macaca nemestrina* monkeys. The results can be summarised as follows.

Motor power. None of the monkeys with lesions in Areas 5 and 7 showed any impairment of motor power in either the contra- or the ipsilateral hand, whereas the loss of motor power was considerable after lesions had been made in the sensory cortex.

Dexterity. We were particularly interested to see the effects of parietal lobe lesions on dexterity, as the test we used required some oculomotor coordination. We found that after bilateral lesions in Areas 5 and 7 the time taken to pick up six baits in our dexterity test increased by about 0.5. This defect, which was recorded for a month, may well be attributed to impairment of oculomotor coordination rather than to loss of simple motor ability.

Tactile and visual discrimination

Blum, Chow & Pribram (1950) reported that their tests had revealed no loss of ability to make tactile or visual discriminations in the one monkey of their series with bilateral lesions confined to the parietal lobes. The results of our own tests confirm this. In the two monkeys trained to discriminate between a cone and a pyramid hidden in a bag by touch only, no loss of this skill was recorded, although they both had difficulty in finding the opening of the bag in the early post-operative period. They also tended to feel in only half the bag and to ignore the other half, a habit we had not noticed before operation. Two monkeys were tested after operation for the retention of colour and form discriminations learnt when intact. They also showed no defects. However, in one of these two animals and in one other monkey we did find some indication of post-operative impairment in the learning of visual colour and form discriminations, an observation which confirms the work of Harlow *et al.* (1952) on monkeys with lesions involving not only bilateral destruction of the parietal and temporal lobes but also unilateral destruction of the frontal and occipital areas.

Visual appreciation of spatial structure

By far the greatest effects of lesions in the parietal lobe were seen in our test using the transparent glass or the non-transparent zinc tube. After operation on the non-dominant hemisphere, the monkey tended to reach the bait through the opening of the tube which he had not used before. For instance, if he had used only the opening on his right when intact, after operation he changed to the frequent use of the opening on his left. This change, however, was only temporary and in most cases a gradual return to the pre-operative behaviour occurred within a week.

In two of the monkeys we later made second and similar lesions in the dominant hemisphere with the result that the change of approach to the bait reappeared, but this time, instead of gradually disappearing within a week, it became more firmly established, for at least a month. What occurs in the later survival period we are not in a position to say, because the monkeys had to be killed fairly soon after operation so that the histological studies could be made.

Our observations on monkeys bear some resemblance to the clinical reports of parietal lobe lesions given by McFie, Piercy & Zangwill (1950), Gilliatt & Pratt (1952) and Goody & Reinhold (1952, 1953). The right–left confusion and the neglect of one half of space reported by these authors are similar to the uncertainty and variability of the monkey's approach

to the bait in the tube, his difficulty in finding the opening of the bag, and his tendency to feel in only one half of it. Further evidence of defective oculomotor control was seen in the results of our tube test: in the early post-operative period some monkeys had difficulty in finding the opening of the tube and often reached out beyond or above it or even tried to reach the bait through the glass. This is perhaps comparable with the disturbances in the perception of spacial relationships and in the execution of constructional tasks under visual control, which McFie, Piercy & Zangwill (1950) recorded in their patients.

We also noticed that when the glass tube was replaced by the metal one, so that the bait was not visible, the operated monkey sometimes used one opening to obtain the bait, and sometimes the other. This behaviour bears a striking resemblance to that of Gilliatt & Pratt's case (1952), whose neglect of the left half of space was noticed only when the eyes were open. This might mean that our lesions in the parietal lobe also disrupted the organisation of visual stimuli after they had reached cortical level. Another observation which supports this view is that one monkey, very skilful in catching pieces of apple thrown into his cage, showed a marked defect in this ability for a few days after operation.

Neuroanatomical findings

Histological studies of monkey brains with lesions in the sensory cortex were made with the Marchi technique. These showed a close connection between Areas 3, 1 and 2 and Area 4, i.e. between the pre- and post-central gyri; few fibres could be traced into the more posterior Area 5 and the fact that no fibres were traced into Area 7 is remarkable as the connection with this area is generally assumed to be much stronger. Subcortical fibres from the post-central gyrus were distributed to the thalamus and to the spinal cord by joining the pyramidal tract. The histological investigation of brains with lesions in Areas 5 and 7 showed a strong fibre connection with Areas 3, 1 and 2 and with Areas 4 and 6. We also found that the occipital lobe projects into Areas 5 and 7. These histological findings, particularly the small number of fibres connecting the post-central gyrus with the posterior parietal lobe, and our observations on trained monkeys, indicate that the posterior parietal lobe is not concerned only with the organisation of tactile impulses but also appears to be a link between visual stimuli and the activity of the sensory-motor cortex, while the anterior parietal lobe is chiefly linked with the motor cortex (Area 4).

In Man, operative or traumatic lesions in the parietal lobe show a slowing down of contralateral head and body movements concerned with turning and a diminished ability for purposeful movements (parietal lobe ataxia, cf. Creutzfeldt, 1983). Creutzfeldt also discusses the clinical literature and special terms coined by the neurologists, such as constructive apraxia, when the patient is unable to solve a puzzle, and idiomotor apraxia, when tools are not used purposefully. Furthermore, large lesions on one side can produce a 'neglect' of objects in the contralateral visual space leading to spacial disorientation. In all clinical cases of parietal injury, attention must be paid to whether the lesion involves the dominant hemisphere or not (p. 107), as the dominant hemisphere also carries the ability for language and small lesions in the posterior parieto-temporal area can cause distinct deficiencies in the use of the native or primary language or in a secondary language acquired at a later stage (Glees, 1961a,b,c). The whole complex integration of various cerebral functions in receiving signals from sensory channels and assembling these in co-ordinated motor actions, especially in language formation, is well illustrated in considering parietal lobe functional aspects. For further reference on human parietal function consult Critchley (1953).

Hemispherectomy – anatomical and physiological aspects

The removal of one half of the forebrain is a radical brain operation; it can be carried out for the removal of a diffusely growing tumour or to alleviate an epileptic state, and poses several fundamental neurobiological questions. The first question is: Why is the brain a bilateral symmetrical structure? The obvious answer will be that most body organs are organised bilaterally, e.g. two kidneys, two lungs, but we see also a tendency for fusion, e.g. the heart or a fused or horseshoe-type kidney, even the absence of one kidney is seen. Similarly, considerable brain function can be exercised by one half of the brain due to partial crossing over of pathways. One wonders whether the bilateral representation of both body halves in each hemisphere can be considered to be an evolutionary attempt at simplifying the forebrain by aiming to give control to only one large hemisphere and not two. On the other hand, two separate hemispheres allow for a safety factor, the deficits occurring from injuries to one hemisphere could be compensated for by the other if still intact. If this were the aim of evolution, crossed and bilateral connections to the halves of the forebrain would be the basis for recovery of function after a unilateral trauma. Glees

(1967) has followed up some human cases who had undergone the removal of a hemisphere and has also surveyed the literature. Glees & White (1958) have studied such cases while back at their work. It was astonishing to see how well integration into the work process of assembling simple accessories, such as rear lamps for motor cars, could be achieved. In spite of the removal of the diseased hemisphere made unusable by severe epilepsy and the ensuing spasticity of one side, the remaining hemisphere could be trained to exercise some control of the side deprived of its motor centre, such as the voluntary adduction of the thumb. From the study of these cases it emerged that in Man, other body areas besides the head region are represented bilaterally in each hemisphere. The ipsilateral sensory information appears to have larger peripheral fields and is less precise in localisation, but additional post-operative training can improve the situation.

In childhood, as soon as language and a centre for a dominant hand in one hemisphere (usually the left) have been established, this particular hemisphere becomes the leading or dominant hemisphere. This means that a removal of the non-dominant hemisphere does not cause such severe functional losses in Man as does removal of the dominant one. The dominance of one hemisphere is normally established around the tenth year of life. Between the two hemispheres is a very large commissure referred to as the corpus callosum.

Brain weight and intelligence

Brain weight in the human foetus, very low in the first month of gestation, reaches about 4 g in the third month and about 100 g in the seventh; at birth the human brain weighs around 280–300 g (Fig. 7.28). Neurological, neurophysiological and biochemical maturation has been reviewed by Joppich & Schulte (1968), while valuable data on foetal brain growth, including myelination, can be found in Gilles *et al.* (1983). During the first 9 months the infant doubles its brain weight; by 3 years the brain weighs about 900 g; by the fifth year of life the final brain weight of 1300–1400 g may have already been attained. In childhood, brain weight is relatively high compared to body weight.

The question arises as to whether there is a minimum adult brain weight necessary for average human intelligence. Here, I can quote from Feremutsch (1955), who studied a patient in a mental institution over a considerable period and then at post-mortem, when he discovered a microcephalic brain of about 395 g in weight (Fig. 7.29). The brain was structurally normal but much too small and had not matured beyond the stage of a 3 year old. I had the opportunity to examine this patient when I visited the institution and could only admire his enormous dexterity and skill in moving and climbing, and his pleasant, friendly behaviour. From this case I should like to speculate that a brain weight of 800–900 g, in the absence of disease and abnormalities and reduced only in size, is the lowest limit for human intelligence.

It is wrong to assume, however, that a high brain weight automatically ensures a high degree of intelligence. At birth, the cerebral cortex can be likened to a blank tape or an unprogrammed computer. In contrast to the brainstem, which is genetically fully programmed and ready to function at birth, the telencephalic brain requires early social, cultural and educational training in order to develop its full capacity.

The absolute brain weight of Man is exceeded by those of whales and elephants, both mammals of high intelligence; we might ask why these animals have been unable to match the development of Man.

Although life in water has led to limb reduction and a fish-like form of propulsion, whales are mammals with highly developed social systems, living in family or larger groups, tending their offspring, and communicating by high-frequency sound. Elephants also show a social order within their groups and show great care for their young (and those of other females within the group). They help each other in emergencies, communicate by sound, and are capable of orderly cooperative work, for example in teak forests.

The brain weight of a very large whale can be almost 10 kg. A blue whale with a body weight of 100 tonnes has a brain of 5.5 kg (Fig. 7.30). In Man, brain weight is about 2% of body weight, whereas in the blue whale this relation is 0.007% (see Table 7.1). However, the main part of the whale's body weight is blubber, fatty insulation from the cold sea water, and this makes the usual brain:body weight comparison meaningless. It would be better to relate brain weight to the proportion of the skin area having a distinct sensory function (see p. 92). Similarly, one

Fig. 7.28. Infant development and increase in brain weight.

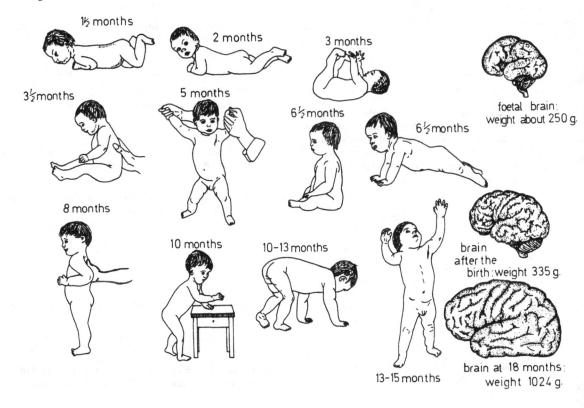

should relate muscle weight to spinal cord and not to the brain itself.

Portmann (1965) defined three steps in mammalian encephalisation; the 'highest' group includes toothed whales (e.g. dolphin), elephants and Man, while the 'lowest' group includes insectivores, bats and rodents. The decisive factor for intelligence is the size of the telencephalon. Man chooses animals from his 'group' to help him in a number of complicated tasks. For example, trained dolphins can be used to dive for and recover underwater objects and elephants are trained to help in forestry, felling trees and moving logs.

Anatomically a high brain weight implies a high density of neurons. The telencephalon is the part of the brain which gives Man his dominant position in the animal kingdom. The telencephalon is responsible for cultural and social behaviour. If we refer again to Figs 2.32 and 2.33, we see that the telencephalon is largely identical with the cerebral cortex. The brain-stem, responsible for autonomic functions, is the housing for the inherent 'primitive' brain; the telencephalon, tightly folded to increase its surface area, is the individual part of the brain, ready to be 'programmed' by sensory input. The human learning process is discussed on pp. 106–7; further comparative data on learning in fish, amphibians, birds and mammals can be found in Macphail (1982).

Table 7.1

Class and family	Species	Body weight (kg)	Brain weight (g)
Primates	*Homo sapiens*		
Hominidal	Negro (USA)	73	1365
	Caucasian (USA)	67.78	1319
Pongidae	*Pan troglodytes*	52.16	440
Cerco-pithecidae	*Macaca mulatta*	3.292	91.7
	Papio cyno-cephalus	19.51	175
Cebidae	*Cebus capucinus*	3.101	72.18
Lorisidae (Lori)	*Galago senegalensis*	0.2	5
Lemuridae	*Lemur catta*	1.725	21.8
Artiodactyla			
Bovidae	*Bos taurus*		
	Guernsey	472	425
	Holstein	916	458
Giraffidae	*Giraffa camelopardalis*	1220	700
Cervidae	*Odocoileus virginiamus*	65.22	210
Hippo-potamide	*Hippopotamus amphibius*	1351	723
Perissodactylae			
Equidae	*Equus caballus*	485.31	706.7
Proboscidae			
Elephantidae	*Loxodonta africana*	6554	5712
Carnivores			
Felidae	*Felis capensis*	9.555	66.74
Canidae	*Canis familiaris*	24.49	105.9
Cetacea			
Balaeno-pteridae	*Balaenoptera musculus*	58.059	6800
	Megaptera nodosa	39.311	6439
Mono-dontidae	*Delphinapterus leucas*	447.03	2349
Insectivores			
Talpidae	*Scalopus aquaticus*	0.0396	1.16
Soricidae	*Blarina brevicauda*	0.0188	0.352

After Altman, L. & Dittmer, D. S. (1962). *Growth*. Biological Handbooks. Fed. Amer. Soc. Exp. Biol. Washington.

Fig. 7.29. The brain of a true microcephalic (case of Feremutsch, 1955). Note that the insular cortex is still open to the outside and that the brain hemispheres do not overlap the cerebellum. A further sign of retarded development is the failure of the temporal lobe to rotate fully (see Fig. 7.5).

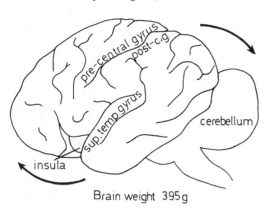

Brain weight 395 g

Fig. 7.30. The common dolphin (*Delphinus delphis*) and its brain. The brain is large with a well-developed cerebral cortex and large areas associated with hearing and vision, while the sense of smell is rudimentary. (Photo and drawing courtesy of D. McBrearty.)

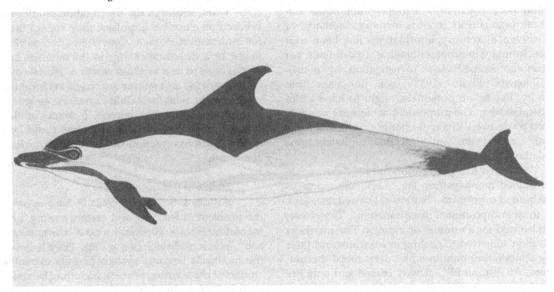

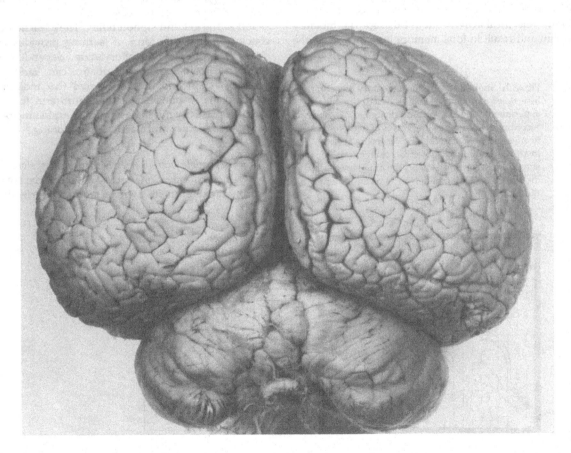

Learning and memory

Learning is an event which takes place after sensory messages have reached cortical centres, with or without motor reactions. The preservation of the sensory message and its recall is memory. Memory, or the storage of sensory information, has been examined in many neuropsychological experiments but has so far escaped close investigation by neurophysiologists. Eccles (1953) took the view that memory, like action potentials, ought to have a bioelectrical basis and he proposed that memory was preserved by neuronal chain discharge and had its functional expression in electroencephalographic oscillations.

We tested this proposition during experiments with trained monkeys (see Fig. 7.31). The monkeys were trained to perform a battery of learned tests (colour, form and positional discrimination). These tests were learned for a number of months. The monkeys were then subjected to cooling in ice water and their body temperature monitored by deep rectal thermometers. At 19 °C all EEG activity ceased and only the heart ECG was recordable. According to the theory of electrical memory maintenance, cessation of the brain's electrical activity should disrupt the memory circuit and result in total memory loss. However, the monkeys in our series showed no such loss, being able to perform tasks learned both before and after body cooling.

Thus, although the propagation of information is based on electrical impulses, they are not the basis for information storage. One alternative mechanism might be a structural change in the neurons but this would need to be a very fast reaction. Models of information storage and release are found in chromosomal nucleic acids, with their ability to release genetic information on the morphogenesis. It seems unlikely at present, however, that such a model could be used for the quick information service needed for learning and recall.

Molecular biology of learning

Kandel & Schwartz (1982a,b) have approached the problem of learning and memory using a fundamental molecular biological model, the marine mollusc *Aplysia californica* (see p. 20). They believe that the mollusc's nervous system permits experimental studies of the learning process, including behavioural, morphological, biochemical and neurophysiological aspects. Their work has focused on short-term sensitisation of the gill and siphon reflex. They reached the conclusion that this form of learning provides evidence that protein phosphorylation, dependent on cyclic adenosine monophosphate, can modulate synaptic action and they suggested that molecular mechanisms responsible of this short-term form of synaptic plasticity might be helpful in explaining both long-term memory and classical conditioning.

The possible location of the human memory store

One basic question is posed immediately: is each neuron capable on its own of storing information?

Fig. 7.31. Short- and long-term memory preservation in a cooled monkey (see text for description of experiment). The EEG records change from a normal recording (1), through slow waves of high voltage, to an isoelectric recording (4). Recording 5 shows heart beat and muscle potentials from bursts of shivering. Recording 6 shows the time-base: each division is 1s. A = amplifier; r.t. = rectal thermometer.

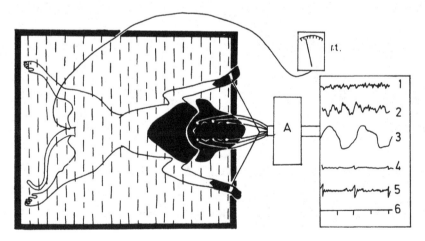

From a morphological point of view, the answer is 'yes', provided that a particular neuron is part of a sensory receptive system. Exceptions are the spinal and cranial nerve ganglia; they are designed solely for receiving and conducting information and their cell bodies are used only for maintaining structural integrity. A further cell type excluded from information storage would be the motor neuron, which is designed to execute commands but cannot modify its performance, which is governed only by synaptic interplay. These considerations appear to me to preclude that a study of reflex pathways can advance our understanding of memory phenomena; sensitisation in a reflex pathway is synaptic–ionic in nature and, though it may play a role in learning and memory, it is unlikely to be the essence of memory.

Clinical observations clearly point to the cerebral cortex as the seat of learning and memory, and one might wonder whether the cortex contains special memory cells and memory circuits. To some extent the corpus callosum system is certainly involved as far as information exchange is concerned, but it is not a memory system *per se*.

The acquisition of memory is based on learning. A human infant recognises first its mother's face and then begins to remember the faces of other members of the family. To remember seems to be a satisfying act, for a baby smiles happily when recognising a person. Memory has a built-in reward system as it confirms the identity and continuity of an individual. Personality is built up of individual experiences and life without memory has probably lost much of its value to the individual.

Memory loss covering a short period may occur with head injuries and is called retrograde amnesia. Memory loss in these circumstances may not throw light on memory function as such, however, since the memory loss may not be due to a direct impact on memory cells or circuits but may be the expression of simultaneous cerebrovascular spasm (see Voth & Glees, 1985) and the ensuing general metabolic interference. Such a loss may, however, indicate that acute or recent phases of memory storage processes are in a 'fluid' condition before becoming more firmly 'engraved' or deposited. Clinical evidence indicates that early and acute preservation seems to occur, or to be facilitated, in the hippocampus (Glees & Griffiths, 1952).

Integrated memory, originating from various sensory inputs, is certainly a general function of the cerebral cortex and is most likely carried out by the circuitry of the upper two or three layers. The storage and retrieval of sensory information are the real neuro-science problems of the future. The extension of our knowledge of connections, made possible by the refinement of modern techniques, will not advance our understanding of the fundamental problem of how we remember and 'replay' past events. Without memory and learning, enabling the comparison of present and past events, the nervous system would be only a reflex machine – intelligence, planning and foresight would be impossible.

The corpus callosum

This large intercerebral neocortical commissure reaches its highest development in primates, especially in Man. The interconnecting fibres grow out late in ontogenetic development at a time when both hemispheres are well formed with their subcortical circuits. From an evolutionary point of view the corpus callosum is another attempt to achieve unified brain function. In order to achieve this integration, 200 million neurons have been allocated and a complicated, ontogenetically late, rewiring of the existing circuitry has to be carried out. The corpus callosum is for this reason Man's biggest brain tract.

The neurobiologist R. Sperry (1964), a pupil of the famous biologist Paul Weiss, has devoted his experimental ingenuity to unravelling some of the functions of the callosal connections in Man. This work was carried out together with the brain surgeon M. S. Gazzancica in order to extend to clinical problems Sperry's knowledge gained from experiments in trained monkeys. The patients, suffering from severe epilepsy, had had all interconnections between hemispheres cut to prevent epileptic fits spreading from one side to the other. The operation did not cause personality defects or diminished intelligence. However, objects palpated by the non-dominant hand could not be named, as the non-dominant hand could not 'ask' the language-carrying hemisphere for the object's name. This failure was caused by the severance of the callosal fibres. Furthermore, important evidence could be collected that the separation of the hemispheres also leads to a separation of motor action and relevant sensations. It appears that the corpus callosum system mediates behaviour requiring both hemispheres. A verbal command cannot be executed with the non-dominant hand after callosal damage; although the dominant hemisphere understands the order, the cross-connection to the motor system of the other hemisphere is interrupted.

The basal ganglia

The composite term basal ganglia comprises neuronal material from different neural origin. The medial walls of the hemispheres form the corpus striatum and the diencephalic vesicle from the primitive brain vesicles; the globe pallidus derives from the hypothalamic portion. Thus the basal ganglia have two parts, the striatum and the pallidum. They are structurally different in the sense that the striatum has many small neurons, while the pallidum contains large branching neurons which form the main efferent element of the basal ganglia system (Figs. 7.32 and 7.33).

The corpus striatum, of uniform structure, is divided in the embryo by the downgrowing fibres of the descending cortical fibres into two parts, the caudate nucleus and the putamen. The globus pallidus or pallidum is also divided into two or more segments by white fibres (Fig. 7.32).

Clinical aspects

The importance of the basal ganglia and their connections has so far been seen more in the realm of clinical medicine than in the field of experimental neurophysiology. The clinician may be confronted with an affliction of the basal ganglia in a newborn, when a difference in the rhesus factors of the parents has caused the destruction of the infant's red blood corpuscles and jaundice. If, despite blood transfusion, the rhesus isoimmunisation leads to death, post-mortem examination shows a distinct and selective yellow stain of the basal ganglia and destruction of its neurons.

In Wilson's disease, a familial hepatolenticular degeneration, the liver is incapable of regulating copper metabolism; the disease process becomes manifest before or shortly after puberty. The inability of the body to excrete surplus copper increases the normally high copper content of the basal ganglia, causing a toxic degeneration of the neurons. The clinical signs are muscular rigidity, involuntary movements and tremor of the limbs, especially of the arms if an aimful movement is attempted.

Trembling and rigidity can also occur in older people due to vascular deficiency of the basal ganglia resulting in Parkinson's disease and excessive rigidity is present in post-encephalitic Parkinsonism. Exogenous toxic agents such as manganese can produce Parkinsonism-like signs, as can certain drugs, such as reserpine when given for a long time or in large doses to primates.

Neuropharmacological aspects. A lack of dopamine, also a precursor of noradrenaline, has been implicated in the cause of Parkinson's disease (Fig. 7.34). Treatment of these patients with dopamine as such was unsuccessful because dopamine does not cross the blood–

Fig. 7.32. Oblique horizontal section through the brain, drawn from a Weigert-stained section. This plane illustrates the full extent of the basal ganglia and the fibre topography of the internal capsule. cl. = claustrum; e.c. = external capsule; i.c. = insular cortex; n.s. = nucleus subthalamus. 1 = corpus callosum; 2 = anterior horn of lateral ventricle; 3 = head of caudate nucleus; 4 = putamen; 4a = external medullary lamina; 4b = internal medullary lamina; 5a, 5b = lateral and medial segments of globus pallidus; 6 = anterior limb of internal capsule containing thalamus–frontal, fronto-thalamic and fronto-pontine fibres; 7 = genu of internal capsule, containing descending cortico-bulbar fibres; 8 = posterior limb of internal capsule carrying descending cortico-spinal fibres, ascending thalamo-cortical fibres to sensory cortex, more posterior auditory fibres from m.g.b (= medial geniculate body (18)) and most posterior visual fibres from l.g.b. (lateral geniculate body); 9 = cavity between layers of the septum pellucidum; 10 = descending pillars of the fornix; 11 = mamillothalamic tract; 12 = nucleus ruber; 13 = central grey matter; 14 = cerebral aqueduct; 15 = posterior colliculus; 16 = bulbo-thalamic tract; 17 = inferior brachium, auditory pathway between posterior colliculus and medial geniculate body (m.g.b.); 18 = medial geniculate body; 19 = lateral geniculate body; 20 = tail of caudate nucleus; 21 = fornix (ascending pillar); 22 = hippocampus; 23 = alveus; 24 = temporal horn of lateral ventricle; 25 = visual radiation emerging from lateral geniculate body.

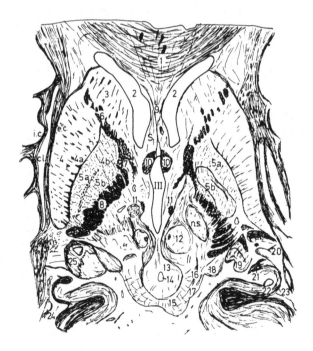

brain barrier in sufficient quantity (Silverstone & Turner, 1982), but its precursor levodopa passes readily into the brain tissue. This compound is capable of controlling rigidity but may produce side effects, including nausea, anorexia and cardiac arrhythmias.

The normal task of the basal ganglia (the extrapyramidal system)

The above brief clinical references indicate the normal functions of the basal ganglia, namely to supply a background for smooth interplay of flexors and extensors when innervated voluntarily. The supporting action of this extrapyramidal system has to be adjusted and combined with other systems, such as the cortico–pontine–cerebellar–cortical circuit, to provide the necessary muscle tone for smooth contractions. Diseases of the extrapyramidal system are characterised by rigidity and tremor, preventing voluntary movements. The burst-like onset of increased tonus in tremor makes a well-aimed movement impossible. However, it would be wrong to conclude that basal ganglia activity was the sole factor in preparation of voluntary movement. To achieve this, the cerebellum, midbrain and reticular formation are necessary components. To integrate all these units the whole extrapyramidal system needs to be integrated. One subcomponent in this system is the muscle stretch reflex, in particular the sensory portion of the muscle spindles in a given cross-striated muscle which inform the spinal cord of the degree of existing contraction and inform the motor neurons. The thin muscle fibres of the spindle itself can be set in their sensitivity by the efferent γ motor neuron (see Fig. 7.33(4)), altering the threshold of the spindle. On account of this special circuit, the motor system has a key role in regulating muscle tone (Fig. 7.33). The connections of the γ motor neurons are of decisive significance for muscle tone and the execution of the movement pattern of the voluntary motor system, for the tone or setting of the spindle regulates the tone of the whole muscle. This physiological fact can largely explain the marked motor disturbances in a

patient suffering from an extrapyramidal disease. This is aptly demonstrated if the patient attempts a movement on command and fails grotesquely. His pyramidal system is incapable of imposing its 'will' on the chaotic condition of unbalanced muscle tone. The main connections of the basal ganglia, caudate nucleus and putamen receive an input from the motor cortex, the pre-motor cortex and the thalamus. The outgoing connections of these nuclei, collectively called the corpus striatum, can be traced to the globus pallidus or pallidum. Other inputs to the striatum come from the midbrain, substantia nigra (zona reticularis; Fig. 9.18) and the red nucleus.

Fig. 7.33. Greatly simplified diagram to illustrate the influence of the basal ganglia on muscle tone.
1. Cortico-spinal pathway innervating a motor neuron (5). 2. Impulses from the basal ganglia terminate on the γ motor neuron which (4) regulates the contraction of the fusiform muscle (f.m.) of the spindle. 3. The spinal ganglion (s.g.) conveys to the α motor neuron the degree of contraction of the spindle and thus regulates the contraction of the skeletal muscle (m) via the α motor neuron 5.

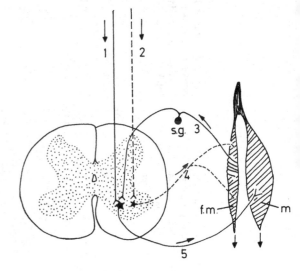

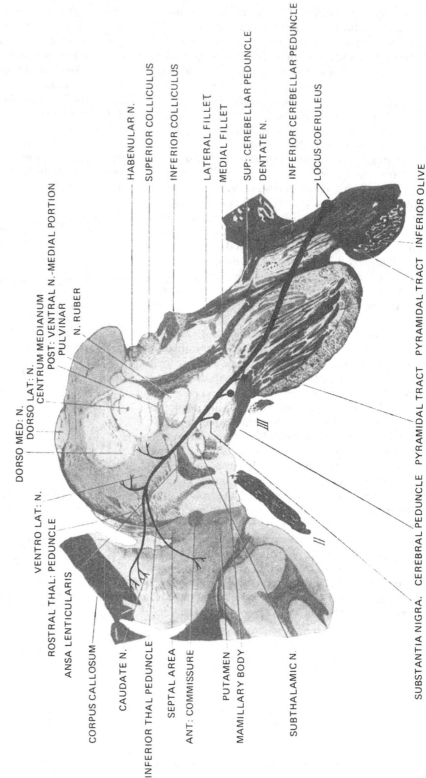

Fig. 7.34. Sagittal section through the human thalamus, caudate nucleus, putamen and caudal parts of the brainstem (Weigert stain). The black lines indicate the long ascending connections of neuronal pathways from the locus coeruleus, and other pigmented cells of the brainstem including the reticular zone of substantia nigra terminating in the thalamus, the caudate nucleus and putamen causing inhibition (the dopaminergic pathway).

CORPUS CALLOSUM

CAUDATE N.

INFERIOR THAL PEDUNCLE

SEPTAL AREA

ANT: COMMISSURE

PUTAMEN

MAMILLARY BODY

SUBTHALAMIC N.

SUBSTANTIA NIGRA.   CEREBRAL PEDUNCLE   PYRAMIDAL TRACT   PYRAMIDAL TRACT   PYRAMIDAL TRACT   INFERIOR OLIVE

VENTRO LAT: N.

ROSTRAL THAL.: PEDUNCLE

ANSA LENTICULARIS

DORSO MED: N.

DORSO LAT: N.

CENTRUM MEDIANUM

POST.: VENTRAL N.-MEDIAL PORTION

PULVINAR

N. RUBER

HABENULAR N.

SUPERIOR COLLICULUS

INFERIOR COLLICULUS

LATERAL FILLET

MEDIAL FILLET

SUP: CEREBELLAR PEDUNCLE

DENTATE N.

INFERIOR CEREBELLAR PEDUNCLE

LOCUS COERULEUS

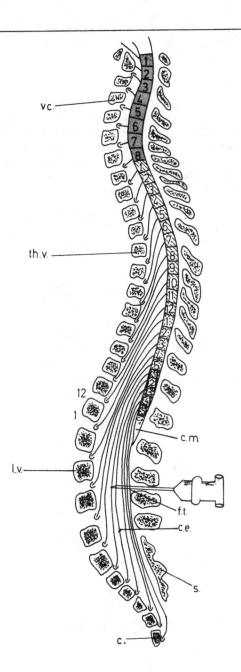

vc.

th.v.

12

1

l.v.

c.m

f.t.

c.e.

s.

c.

(a)

Fig. 8.1. (a) Diagram of a sagittal view of the vertebral column and the spinal cord showing the neural segments in relation to vertebral levels (from Glees, 1971). Note that there is a progressive caudal shift between the neural and vertebral segments. During development the cord has moved cranially and terminates between the first and second lumbar vertebrae; the exits of the spinal nerves and the location of the spinal ganglia have remained at embryonic levels, causing the formation of lengthy spinal intradural nerves, the filum terminale. Cerebrospinal fluid can be tapped without injuring the spinal cord. c. = coccyx; c.e. = cauda equina; c.m. = conus medullaris; c.v. = cervical vertebra; f.t. = filum terminale; l.v. = lumbar vertebra; s. = sacrum; th.v. = thoracic vertebra.
(b) The cutaneous distribution of sensory innervation is based on developmental neuronal segmentation (from Glees, 1971).

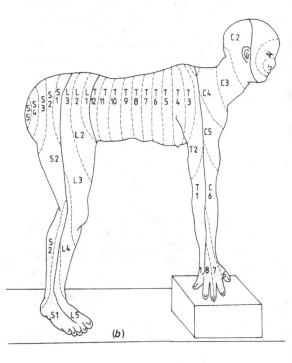

(b)

Development and general organisation

The spinal cord can be compared to a flexible white tube, the lumen of which is originally wide but narrows down considerably from its size at the neural tube stage (Fig. 2.21). The lumen is quickly filled by nerve cells and their processes. The length of the final tube is about 40–45 cm and receives considerable protection from collagenous coats and the bony vertebrae (Fig. 8.1(*a*)). In the mature state the spinal cord appears to be withdrawn cranially, terminating at the L_1–L_2 vertebrae. In the adult the lower part of the vertebral canal is filled only with nerves and is referred to as the cauda equina. The cranial withdrawal of the cord starts in the third month of pregnancy, moving the embryological spinal cord's sacral portion into the protective girdle of the lumbar vertebrae. This leaves the formerly occupied space free for a CSF chamber, which can be tapped for medical and biochemical examinations (p. 000). In addition to gaining shelter from vertebrae, the cord itself is ensheathed by the pia-mater, carrying the blood vessels, and the dura mater, a very firm tough skin; between the dura and pia loose trabeculae expands, filled with CSF, and act as a protective water cushion (Fig. 8.2). The dural sack extends down to the second sacral vertebra, while the finely drawn-out end of the conus terminalis, the filum terminale, reaches to the first coccygeal vertebra.

Special organisation

In cross-section the spinal cord reveals distinct differences between the grey substance of neurons and the white substance of myelinated fibre tracts (Fig. 8.3). The ventral aspect of the cord shows a deep cleft penetrated by blood vessels enveloped by pia-arachnoidal tissue. These blood vessels supply the grey matter of the cord much more densely than the white substance as the neurons have a higher metabolic rate in contrast to the fibres.

Regional differences

On account of the need to supply the extremities with nerves, the neural regions close to the embryological somites from which the muscles derive show distinct increases in the size of grey matter and larger spinal ganglia. This is the reason why cervical and lumbo-sacral portions of the cord show enlargements (Fig. 8.3). The spinal cord is divided into neural seg-

Fig. 8.3. The relative distribution of white matter (myelinated axons) and grey matter (neurons and non-myelinated axons) at different levels of the spinal cord.

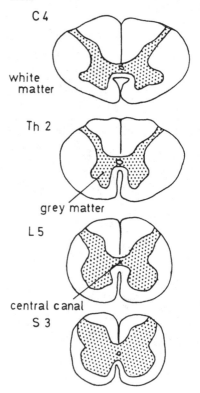

Fig. 8.2. Transverse section through a cervical vertebra illustrating the surrounding connective tissue coats. a.s. = arachnoid space; a.t. = anterior tubercle; c. = centrum; d.l. = denticulate ligament; d.m. = dura mater; d.r. = dorsal root; pg.r. = preganglionic ramus; p.t. = posterior tubercle; p.a. = pia arachnoid; s.a.p. = superior articular process; s-d.s. = sub-dural space; s.g. = sympathetic ganglion; s.p. = spinal process (bifid); sp.a. = spinal arachnoid; sp.art. = spinal artery; sp.g. = spinal ganglion; v.arc. = vertebral arch; v.art. = vertebral artery; v.pl. = vertebral plexus; v.r. = ventral root.

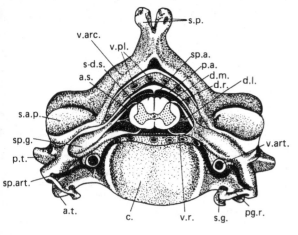

ments: cervical, thoracic, lumbar and sacral. These neural segments are not identical with the vertebral segments, due to the embryological cranial shift of the cord (Fig. 8.1(*b*)). The grey substance can be divided into a ventral half or motor portion and a dorsal half, the sensory part. A small intermediate area contains autonomic neurons for the innervation of smooth muscle for example (Figs 8.4 and 10.6).

Histology

The *motor* or ventral portion contains the large multipolar neurons, the stem cells of ventral or anterior root fibres. These fibres are joined by fine, myelinated nerve fibres from cells of the intermediate cell column (Fig. 8.4) referred to as pre-ganglionic rami as these fibres can be traced to terminate in the autonomic ganglia (Figs 8.2 and 10.6). The neurons of the *sensory* part or posterior horn receive their afferent impulses from the posterior or dorsal roots. These fibres are the central processes of spinal ganglion cells, while the peripheral processes or sensory nerve fibres pick up impulses from the skin, muscles and internal organs. The motor cells of the anterior and smaller cells of the posterior horn are embedded in a dense, interwoven plexus of nerve and glial fibres. Most of

Fig. 8.4. Diagrammatic section through the spinal cord showing, on the left, afferent nerve inputs, and, on the right, vascular channels. a.sp.a. = anterior spinal artery; p.sp.a. = posterior spinal artery; v.c. = vasa corona; 1 = muscle spindle; 2 = Vater–Paccini body; 3 = Meissner corpuscle; 4 = free nerve ending; 5 = autonomic innervation of smooth muscle; 6 = voluntary innervation of striated muscle; I = ascending fibres in posterior columns; II crossed ascending fibres of spino-thalamic tract (pain and temperature).

these fibres are small and non-myelinated but larger myelinated fibres are present. The entanglement of all these fibres appears at first sight so dense that a special term, 'neuropil', was coined, indicating that their origins and distributions were unlikely to be revealed. However, modern tracing methods have unravelled many of the sites of origin and terminations of the nerve fibres composing the neuropil. The first connections to be established were the simple systems on which the reflex areas are based (Fig. 8.5).

The white matter

Ascending fibre systems. The white substance of the cord can best be divided into fibres carrying impulses cranially and those descending caudally from brain levels. The main bulk of ascending fibres is situated in the posterior columns, which in man are specially large and important (Figs 8.6 and 8.7). These columns lie between the dorsal horns of the grey matter and are separated by a dorsal septum, opposite the ventral fissure which carries the spinal blood vessels. The receptors bringing information to the cord and some reflex connections are illustrated in Fig. 8.5. The topographical arrangements of the ascending tracts regarding their entrance at successive cord levels is shown in Fig. 8.6, indicating that fibres from the leg region are medial to those from the arm regions. These axons originating from the spinal ganglia of each neural level are widely separated at lower spinal cord levels and divided into three main divisions (Fig. 8.4). In the case of fibres carrying impulses

Fig. 8.5. Simplified diagram of interactions in a reflex arc. d.r. = dorsal root; i.n. = internuncial neuron; m. = muscle (striated); m.e.p. = motor endplate; m.f. = motor fibre; sk. = skin; s.f.sk. = sensory fibre from skin; sp.g. = spinal ganglion cell; v.r. = ventral root.

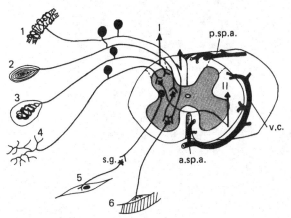

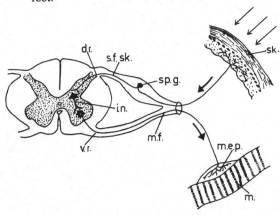

Fig. 8.6. (a) Diagram of the general distribution of descending and ascending tracts at cervical level. (b) Transverse section through the spinal cord at the level of thoracic T 11 illustrating the position of the lateral horn (LH) containing the preganglionic sympathetic column stretching from C8 to L2. The circular position of the column of Clarke (CC) or nucleus dorsalis giving rise to spino-cerebellar fibres. VH = ventral horn; DH = dorsal horn. The posterior column ranging between the dorsal horns contain the gracile tract. These fibres are processes from spinal ganglia from lumbar, sacral ganglia and lower thoracic ganglia.

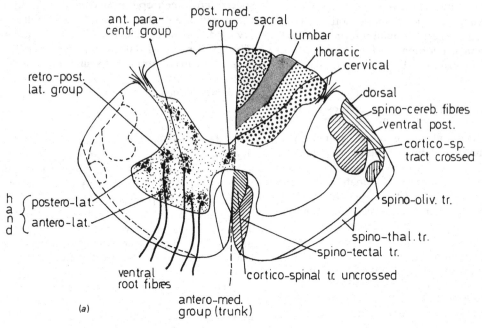

(a)

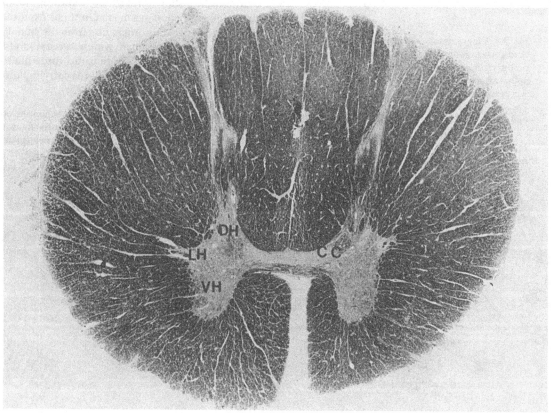

(b)

from muscle spindles, one division ascends in the posterior column, while the second division courses to anterior horn cells and is a direct reflex fibre which does not rely on internuncial cells like the fibre from a Paccinian body (Fig. 8.4). The fibres ascending in the posterior columns distribute collaterals to the neural segments while terminating in the posterior column nuclei of the lower medulla. They conduct proprioceptive impulses, such as vibrations when a tuning fork is brought into contact with a bone, recognition of the position of a particular limb in relation to the body axis, and general joint movements. Furthermore, they convey the distance between two points on the skin and recognition of numbers or simple drawings drawn on the skin, which is used in clinical testing for the examination of spinal injuries. Further ascending tracts are situated in the lateral columns, although their fibre sensity is minimal when compared to the number of posterior column fibres. The spino-thalamic tract, which mediates pain, temperature and touch, includes in its course spino-tectal fibres (Fig. 8.6), some of which cross to the opposite superior colliculus. The spino-cerebellar tracts (dorsal and ventral) supply the cerebellum with important information about the functional state of muscle via Golgi tendon organs and the position of joints, while other ascending fibres such as spino-olivary and spino-reticular fibres terminate in the lower brainstem.

The most important descending tracts. The foremost tract, the cortico-spinal or pyramidal tract, has already been dealt with in relation to the motor cortex (p. 94). Other tracts important for reflex activity are the descending vestibulo-spinal, reticulo-spinal and tecto-spinal pathways which influence muscle tone greatly. In this functional context emphasis should be placed on the interconnections, by proprio-spinal systems, from lumbar to cervical levels and vice versa; these intersegmental connections run close to the grey matter of the cord, while the long-distance ones are located more peripherally. These proprioceptive bundles or 'ground bundles' develop early in foetal time and are numerous and myelinated. Their connectivity and density vary greatly from species to species and according to way of life; Man's upright gait calls for corresponding special interspinal connections. These systems and the ones coming from supraspinal level make synaptic arrangements due to the rich influx of collaterals from numerous sources (see Kuypers (1981) and Brown (1981) for further details).

Fig. 8.7. Diagram of five different levels of the spinal cord and two levels of the medulla, illustrating the ascending course and termination of dorsal root fibres. The first medullary level shows (1) the gracile nucleus, and (2) the cuneate nucleus. The second medullary level shows (3) the medial part of the cuneate nucleus, (4) the lateral and ventral part of the cuneate nucleus, (5, 6) the vestibular nucleus and descending vestibular roots, (7) the descending root and nucleus of the trigeminal nerve. All cervical roots and the first thoracic root terminate in the cuneate nucleus, seen here in transverse section. (From Glees *et al.*, 1951.)

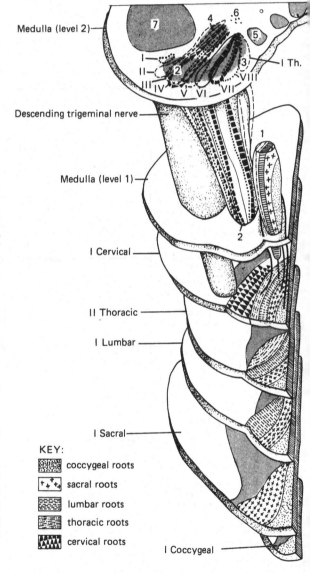

KEY:

coccygeal roots

sacral roots

lumbar roots

thoracic roots

cervical roots

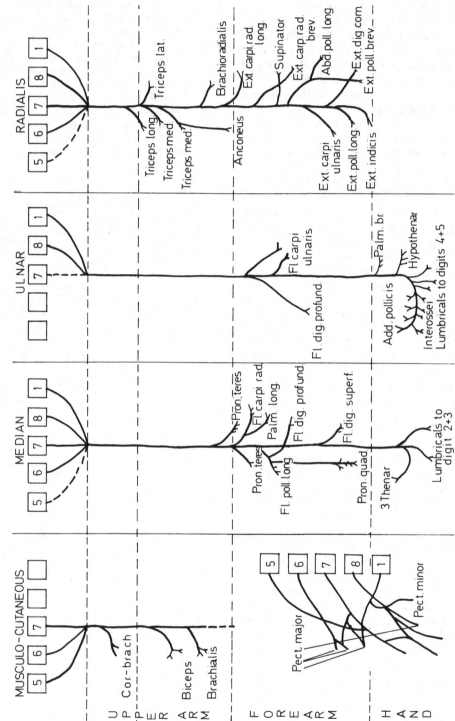

Fig. 8.8. Motor distribution to arm muscles from neuronal segments indicated by squares and segment numbers (Glees, 1971).

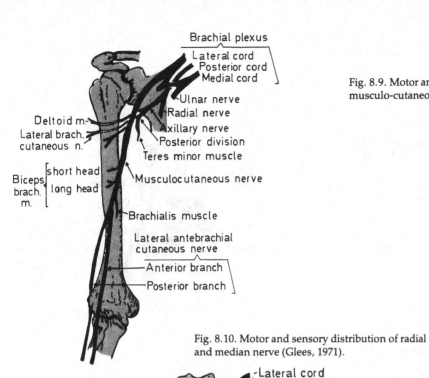

Brachial plexus
Lateral cord
Posterior cord
Medial cord

Ulnar nerve
Radial nerve
Axillary nerve
Posterior division
Teres minor muscle

Deltoid m.
Lateral brach.
cutaneous n.

Biceps
brach.
m. { short head
long head

Musculocutaneous nerve

Brachialis muscle

Lateral antebrachial
cutaneous nerve

Anterior branch
Posterior branch

Fig. 8.9. Motor and sensory distribution of the
musculo-cutaneous nerve (Glees, 1971).

Fig. 8.10. Motor and sensory distribution of radial
and median nerve (Glees, 1971).

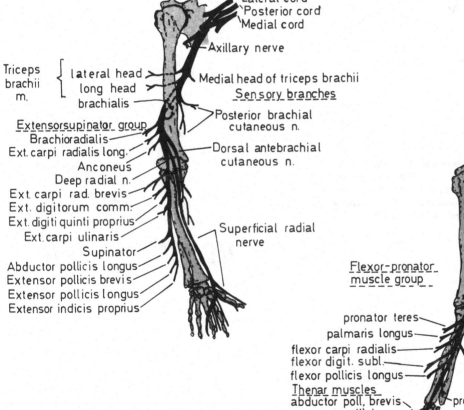

Lateral cord
Posterior cord
Medial cord

Axillary nerve

Triceps
brachii
m. { lateral head
long head
brachialis

Medial head of triceps brachii
Sensory branches

Extensorsupinator group
Brachioradialis
Ext. carpi radialis long.
Anconeus
Deep radial n.
Ext. carpi rad. brevis
Ext. digitorum comm.
Ext. digiti quinti proprius
Ext. carpi ulinaris
Supinator
Abductor pollicis longus
Extensor pollicis brevis
Extensor pollicis longus
Extensor indicis proprius

Posterior brachial
cutaneous n.

Dorsal antebrachial
cutaneous n.

Superficial radial
nerve

Lateral cord
Medial cord

Flexor-pronator
muscle group

Articular rami (2)

pronator teres
palmaris longus
flexor carpi radialis
flexor digit. subl.
flexor pollicis longus
Thenar muscles
abductor poll. brevis
opponens pollicis
flexor poll brevis
(superficial head)

Flexor digitorum
profundus
(radial portion)

pronator quadratus

Anastomosis with
ulnar nerve

First and second lumbricales

Fig. 8.11. Motor and sensory distribution of ulnar nerve (Glees, 1971).

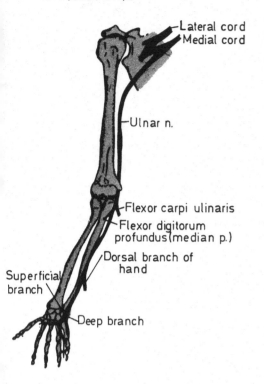

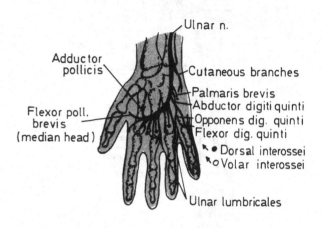

Fig. 8.12. A1, A2 sensory and motor signs in an ulnar nerve lesion. B1, B2 sensory and motor signs in a radial nerve lesion (dropped wrist). C1, C2 sensory and motor signs in a median nerve lesion (Thenar eminence muscles paralysed (Glees, 1971).

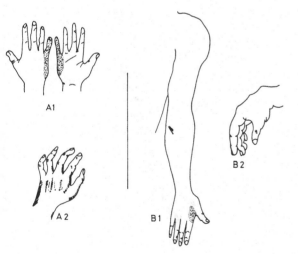

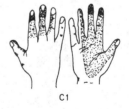

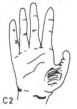

Fig. 8.13. Segmental origin and muscular branches of
sciatic, femoral and obturator nerves (Glees, 1971).

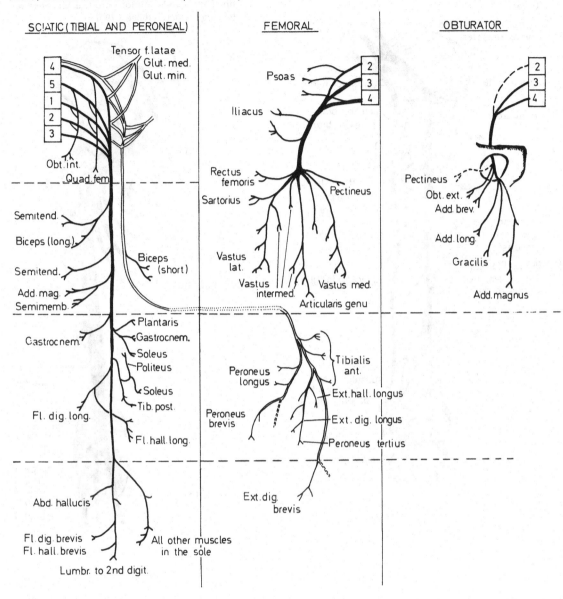

Fig. 8.14. Segmental origin and distribution of muscular branches of femoral and obturator nerves (Glees, 1971).

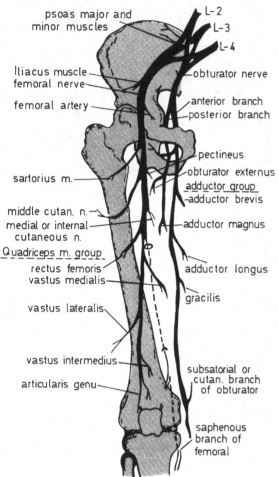

psoas major and minor muscles

L-2
L-3
L-4

Iliacus muscle
femoral nerve
obturator nerve

femoral artery
anterior branch
posterior branch

pectineus
obturator externus
adductor group
adductor brevis

sartorius m.

middle cutan. n.
medial or internal cutaneous n.
adductor magnus

Quadriceps m. group
rectus femoris
vastus medialis
adductor longus

vastus lateralis
gracilis

vastus intermedius
articularis genu
subsatorial or cutan. branch of obturator

saphenous branch of femoral

Fig. 8.15. Course and distribution of the sciatic nerve in the thigh. In this instance the nerve is divided into tibial nerve and common peroneal nerve before leaving the pelvis (Glees, 1971).

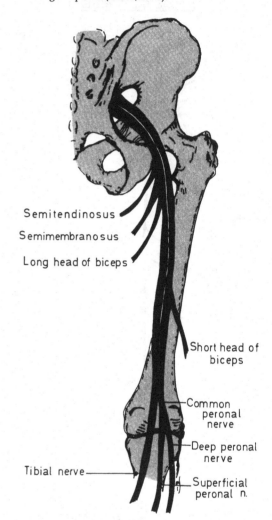

Semitendinosus
Semimembranosus
Long head of biceps

Short head of biceps

Common peronal nerve

Deep peronal nerve

Tibial nerve
Superficial peronal n.

Blood supply

The blood supply of the spinal cord has two main sources, the ventral and posterior spinal arteries. The ventral artery originates from the vertebral arteries at the level of the foramen magnum and receives regular contributions from segmental vessels further caudally. The paired posterior spinal arteries also arise from the vertebral arteries and receive segmental con-tributions from spinal arteries which reach the spinal cord through the intervertebral foramina, the exits of the spinal nerves.

The neural supply of arm and leg

These peripheral regions of innervation are illustrated in Figs 8.8–8.17.

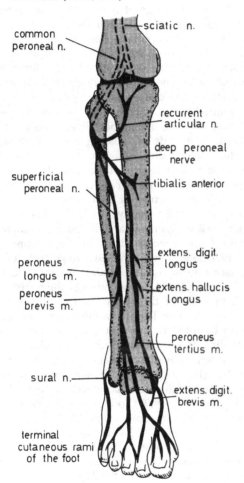

Fig. 8.16. Distribution of the peroneal nerve in the lower limb (Glees, 1971).

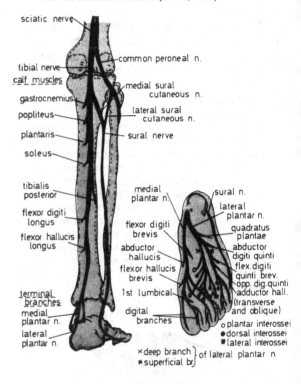

Fig. 8.17. Distribution of the tibial and peroneal nerves in the lower limb (Glees, 1971).

9
The brainstem and cerebellum

The medulla

The medulla is the lower portion of the brainstem, linking the pons and the cord, and has a conical shape (Fig. 9.1). The basic structure of the medulla is derived from the spinal cord, but this is made obscure by the crossings of two major fibre systems, the decussation of the cortico-spinal tract and the medial lemniscus or bulbothalamic tract. The cortico-spinal tract crosses it from a ventral position dorso-laterally (Fig. 9.2(*a*)) and the bulbothalamic fibres arising from the neurons of the dorsally situated gracile and cuneate nuclei cross from one side to the opposite side ventrally (Fig. 9.2(*b*)). Furthermore, a special medullary nucleus, the inferior olive, sends its axons to the opposite side by crossing the midline raphe in a dorso-lateral direction. The more fundamental embryological architecture of the medulla in relation to the spinal cord is shown in Fig. 9.3, which draws attention to the opening of the central canal into the wide space of the fourth ventricle. By this opening some neural components are shifted dorso-laterally, in particular the specialised neurons subserving hearing and balance. Fundamental components of the medulla are the motor and sensory nuclei of the cranial nerves (Figs 9.4–9.7), homologous to the ventral and dorsal neurons of the spinal cord. The pyramidal tracts, which came late in evolution and ontogeny, have to be fitted to the ventral aspect (Fig. 9.8) of the medulla (Glees, 1982). Specific medullary nuclei are the inferior olivary nuclei and the nuclei of cranial nerve VIII (Fig. 9.8), while the nuclei of the reticular system begin at the medullary level and extend into the thalamus (Fig. 9.9). To illustrate the position of the many nuclear groups, several transverse sections from the early work of Jacobsohn (1909) are reproduced as some of these nuclei have wider and more important ascending connections than believed hitherto and are summarised in the dopamine transmitter system (Fig. 7.30). To start with a simplified picture of the medulla, however, we refer to the diagram shown in Fig. 9.8. This diagram shows the motor nucleus for the tongue muscles, the hypoglossal nucleus; it illustrates the level of the vagal nucleus, the motor and sensory nerve of the foregut, and is at the level of cranial VIII nuclei, subserving hearing and equilibrium.

Fig. 9.1. Dorsal view of the lower brainstem (quadrigeminal plate, rhombencephalon) and a view of the fourth ventricle (Glees, 1961a). c.t. = cuneate tubercle; e. = epiphysis (pineal body); g.t. = gracile tubercle; i.c. = inferior colliculus of quadrigeminal plate; i.c.p. = inferior cerebellar peduncle (cut surface); i.f. = inferior fovea; l.g.b. = lateral geniculate body; m.c.p. = middle cerebellar peduncle (cut surface); m.g.b. = medial geniculate body; m.s. = median sulcus; o. = obex; s.c. = superior colliculus of quadrigeminal plate; s.c.p. = superior cerebellar peduncle (cut surface); s.f. = superior fovea; sp.c. = upper part of spinal cord; t.n. = trochlear nerve; th.p.l. = cut surface of thalamus at pulvinar level.

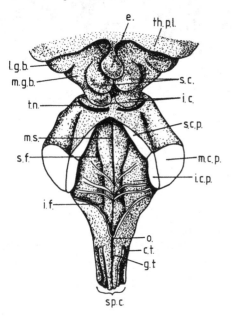

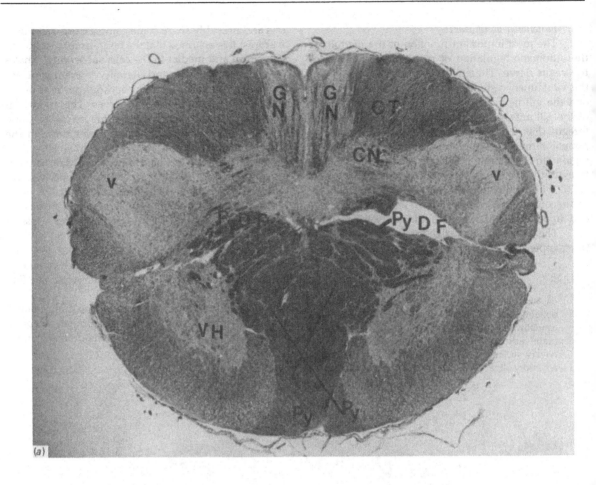

(a)

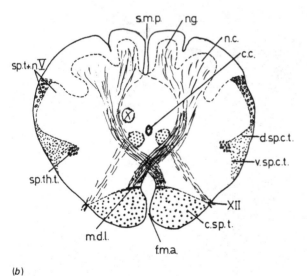

(b)

Fig. 9.2. (*a*) Lower end of medulla at the level of the crossing (X) of ipsilateral pyramidal fibres (Py) to the opposite or contralateral side (PyDF) GN = gracile nucleus; CT = cuneate tract; CN = cuneate nucleus; V = descending or spinal nucleus of the V. cranial nerve; VH = ventral horn. Gray matter and fibre tracts are clearly distinguishable. On the right side is a tear in the section.

(*b*) Diagrammatic representation of a lower medullary section at the level of medial lemniscus formation from internal arcuate fibres. s.m.p. = medial posterior sulcus; n.g. = gracile nucleus; n.c. = cuneate nucleus; c.c. = central canal; d.sp.c.t. = dorsal spino-cerebellar tract; v.sp.c.t. = ventral spino-cerebellar tract; XII = emergence of hypoglossal roots; c.sp.t. = cortico-spinal tract; f.m.a. = anterior median sulcus; m.d.l. = decussation of internal arcuate fibres, forming medial fillet; sp.th.t. = spino-thalamic tract; sp.t. + n.V = descending trigeminal fibres and spinal nucleus of V; X = vagal nucleus.

Functional significance

The most important function of the medulla is the automatic regulation of respiration, the task of the vagus nerve. The endowment of the vagus with this vital function stems from the evolution of the gills and the gill nerve supplying the area. The muscles of the gill arch, which is a functional portion of the foregut (Fig. 2.33), are supplied by the motor component of the vagus migrating caudally from the neck regions to the thorax. As the lungs bud off from the foregut, the airway is also a vagus territory (Figs 9.10–9.12). Due to this evolutionary history the medulla has become the neural integration centre for breathing and for parasympathetic gut regulation (see Fig. 10.7).

The neurons responsible for regulation of breathing appear to be part of the reticular system of neurons and probably share some common organisational features. It is assumed that the neurons for inspiration lie ventral and medial to the cells subserving exhalation, situated dorsally and laterally. Afferent impulses reach these neurons from the sensory portions of the vagus and glossopharyngeal nerves. The motor signals for contraction reach the diaphragm via the phrenic nerves and the intercostal muscles through the intercostal nerves.

Cutting the vagal nerves, which contain somatosensory, somato-motor, viscero-motor and viscero-sensory nerve fibres, causes paralysis of the vocal cords and the oesophagus and a reduction of the acid secretion of stomach glands. Furthermore, a loss of respiratory reflexes and altered cardiac activity are noticeable. Section of the vagal nerve on one side causes paralysis of one vocal cord and hoarseness. (Innervation by medullary part of nerve XI, see Fig. 9.12.)

After severing the vagus, breathing shows marked changes, as the activity of the stretch receptors in the lungs is not reaching their medullary centre.

Fig. 9.2 contd.

(c) A microscopic section (Weigert stain) cut in an oblique transverse plane (the dorsal part is more caudally than the ventral portion). Due to the slope of the section the ventral part contains the inferior olivary nucleus (ION) and the medial and the dorsal accessory olive (MAO, DAO) PyT = pyramidal tract.

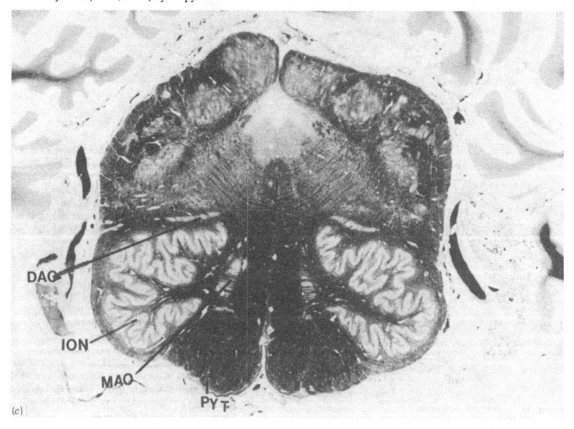

(c)

Respiration becomes slower and deeper, with frequent intervals after inspiration and expiration. Additional signals reaching the respiratory centre arise from pressure receptors in the carotid sinus and its chemoreceptors and from the aortic arch.

Cranial nerve IX, the glossopharyngeal, has close functional and topographical relations with the vagal nerve and, like it, has afferent and efferent connections (Fig. 9.11). The afferent fibres have their cell bodies in the superior petrosal ganglion close to the jugular foramen, and also in the inferior petrosal ganglion. These ganglia are responsible for afferent signals from touch, pain and temperature receptors seated in the back of the tongue, the tonsillar area and eustachian tube (Figs 9.11 and 9.16). Furthermore, the IX nerve mediates the main taste sensations from the circumvallate papillae on the back of the tongue. The afferent, incoming fibres of IX form the tractus solitarius, synapsing with the neurons close to the tract (Fig. 9.8).

Fig. 9.3. A composite diagram showing the evolutionary organisation of the rhombencephalon. On the right side is shown the distribution of cranial nerve nuclei, and on the left, the vascular supply. ASA = vertebral arteries and medial branches from spinal arteries; PSA = posterior spinal artery; PICA = posterior inferior cerebellar artery supplying lateral and dorso-lateral areas; AM = anterior medial branch.

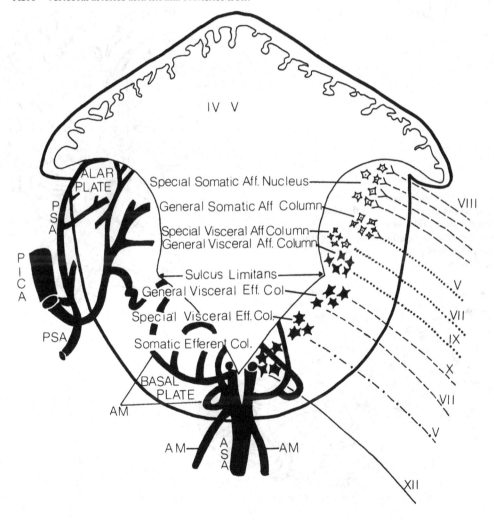

Fig. 9.4. Ventral view of the brainstem.

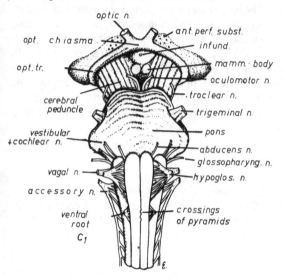

Fig. 9.5. Sagittal section through the brainstem, illustrating the location of cranial nerve nuclei and their longitudinal extent (Glees, 1971). 1, 2 = oculomotor nuclei (motor and parasympathetic); 3 = oculomotor nerve; 4 = trochlear nucleus and nerve; 5 = trigeminal motor root; 6 = trigeminal sensory root; 7 = abducens nucleus; 8 = facial nucleus; 9 = facial nerve and auditory nerve; 10 = abducens nerve; 11 = imperior salivary nucleus; 12 = nucleus ambiguous (X); 13 = glossopharyngeal nerve; 14 = hypoglossal nerve; 15 = vagal nerve; 16 = rootlets of hypoglossal nerve; 17 = descending or spinal nucleus of trigeminal nerve; 18 = accessory nerve; 19 = accessory nucleus; 20 = central canal; 21 = quadrigeminal plate; 22 = motor nucleus of cranial nerve V; 23 = internal knee of facial nerve; 24 = fourth ventricle; 25 = tractus solitarius; 26 = motor nucleus of vagus nerve; 27 = choroid plexus of fourth ventricle; 28 = hypoglossal nucleus.

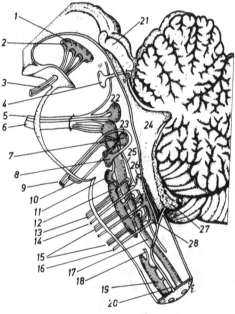

Fig. 9.6. The thalamus, the dorsal part of the diencephalon, forms the cranial end of the brainstem. This drawing shows the relative positions of thalamus, midbrain, pons, medulla and cerebellum. P.C.M. = the position of posterior column nuclei of medulla (from Glees, 1961a).

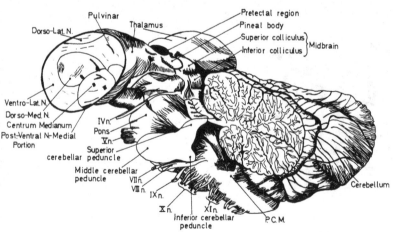

A very important afferent nerve is the carotid sinus nerve. The sinus is a small dilatation in the wall of the common carotid artery at the branching point into external and internal carotid arteries. Elevation of blood pressure is recorded by the sinus nerve and sent to the medulla, reaching the dorsal nucleus of the vagus which, in turn, informs the neurons in the atria of the heart. These neurons pass the signals on to the neighbouring autonomic neurons of the sino-auricular and atrio-ventricular nodes of the conduct-

ing system and finally produce a drop in blood pressure. In doing so, the afferent receptors and fibres of the IX nerve and the efferent fibres of X form a circuit for blood pressure regulation, a reflex, particularly important when changing posture from lying down to an upright position. This postural change forces on the heart more work in order to keep the brain well supplied with blood, otherwise a loss of consciousness results. These postural factors have to be considered when pressure-reducing drugs are prescribed which lower the blood pressure but prevent at the same time the vital compensatory autonomic neural signals for pressure regulation to the brain. This is an unpleasant side effect from such drugs as reserpine which cause orthostatic hypotonia and reduced cerebral blood flow.

Fig. 9.7. A dorsal view of the brainstem, showing the distribution of the cranial nerves (after Chusid & McDonald, 1967). 1 = superior colliculus; 2 = pulvinar; 3 = medial geniculate body; 4 = lateral geniculate body; 5 = main sensory nucleus of V; 6 = dorsal nucleus of vestibular nerve; 7 = medial nucleus of vestibular nerve; 8 = cochlear nerve; 9 = lateral vestibular nucleus; 10 = vestibular nerve; 11 = ventral cochlear nucleus; 12 = dorsal cochlear nucleus; 13 = glossopharyngeal nerve; 14 = vagal nerve; 15 = spinal vestibular nucleus; 16 = spinal tract and spinal nucleus of V; 17 = ala cinerea; 18 = oculomotor nucleus; 19 = trochlear nucleus; 20 = trochlear nerve; 21 = descending mesencephalic root of V; 22 = semilunar ganglion; 23 = sensory root of V; 24 = motor root of V; 25 = motor nucleus of V; 26 = internal knee of VII; 27 = abducens nucleus; 28 = facial nucleus; 29 = facial nerve; 30 = motor nucleus of IX and X (nucleus ambiguous); 31 = glossopharyngeal nerve; 32 = parasympathetic nucleus of X; 33 = vagal nerve; 34 = accessory nerve; 35 = hypoglossal nucleus; 36 = nucleus of ala cinerea; 37 = accessory nucleus.

Fig. 9.8. Diagram of medulla, indicating main fibre tracts and nuclei. 4v. = fourth ventricle; hyp.n. and XII = hypoglossal nucleus; n.v.d. = dorsal of vagus (viscero-motor nucleus); n.a. = nucleus ambiguous (motor nucleus of vagus); v.n, = vestibular nucleus; c.n. = cuneate nucleus; sp.n.V = spinal nucleus of trigeminus (V); d.tr.V = descending tract of V; vagal n. = vagal nerve (X); sp.th.tr. = spino thalamic tract; t.-o.t. = segmento-olivary tract; i.o.n. = inferior olivary nucleus; hyp.nerve = hypoglossal nerve; c.sp.t. = cortico-spinal tract; l.m. = medial lumniscus or fillet; n.o.a.m. = olivary nucleus, accessory and medial part; d access. olive = dorsal accessory olivary nucleus; m.r.n. = medial reticular nucleus; t.sp.-t. = spino-tectal tract; t.sp.-c.v. = spino-cerebellar tract, ventral part; t.sp.-c.d. = spino-tectal tract, dorsal part; n.t.s. = nucleus of tratus solitarius; f.l.m. = fasciculus longitudinalis medialis.

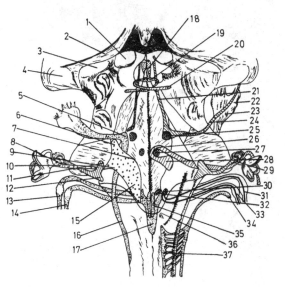

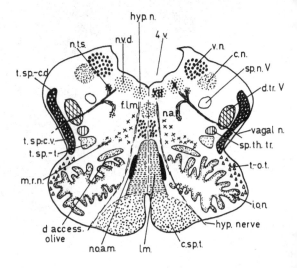

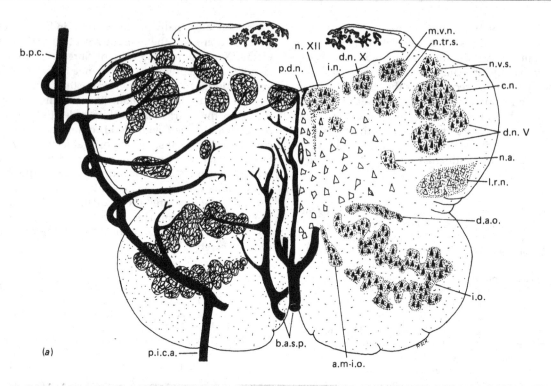

(a)

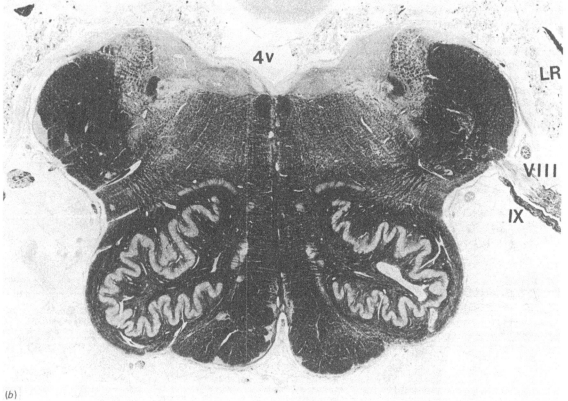

(b)

Opposite

Fig. 9.9. (*a*) A composite diagram of the medulla showing blood supply on the left and neuronal nuclear groups on the right. Note that the blood supply areas co-occur with the neuronal groupings. a.m-i.o. = accessory medio-inferior olive; b.a.s.p. = branches of anterior spinal artery; b.p.c. = branch of post. inf. cerebellar a. to cerebellum; c.n. = cuneate nucleus; d.a.o. = dorsal accessory olive; d.n.V. = descending (or spinal) nucleus of cranial nerve V; d.n.X = dorsal nucleus of the vagus nerve; i.n. = intercalate nucleus; i.o. = inferior olive; l.r.n. = lateral reticular nucleus; m.v.n. = medial vestibular nucleus; n.a. = nucleus

ambiguus; n.tr.s. = nucleus of tractus solitarius; n.v.s. = nucleus vestibularis, spinal part; n.XII = hypoglossal nucleus; p.d.n. = paramedian dorsal nucleus; p.i.c.a. = posterior inferior cerebellar artery.

(*b*) To illustrate further the complexity of the medullary fibre pattern and arrangement of nuclei shown in (*a*) which includes the vascular pattern, a myelin stained microphotograph is included. This actual picture should be studied with the keys supplied in (*a*) and the diagrams of the medulla. The level is at nerves IX, VIII and the lateral recess (LR) of the fourth ventricle (4 V).

Fig. 9.10. Peripheral distribution of the vagal nerve (NX) (after Chusid & McDonald, 1967). 1 = sensory nerve to the dura; 2 = sensory nerve to the external and auditory meatus; 3 = branch to the carotid body (afferents from the aortic body); 4 = motor branches to pharynx; 4′ = soft palate branches (sensory); 5 = sensory branches to larynx; 6 = motor branches to external laryngeal muscle; 7 = cardiac branch; 8 = recurrent laryngeal nerve, motor to vocal muscles, oesophageal branches.

Fig. 9.11. Peripheral distribution of the glossopharyngeal nerve (N.IX) (after Chusid & McDonald, 1967). 1. sensory nerve to tympanic membrane; 2. sensory nerve to carotid body (blood pressure regulation); 3, 4 = motor fibres to pharyngeal muscle; 5. sensory branches to tonsillar area; 6. taste fibres to circumvallate papillae.

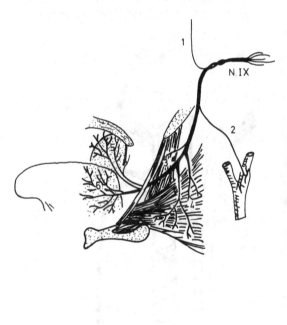

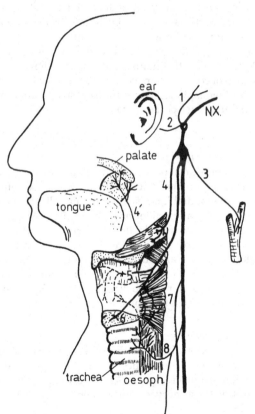

Another important reflex is mediated by the IX nerve, which is initiated by chemoreceptors. This reflex serves the recording of the chemical composition of the arterial blood and is a part of the autonomic control of respiration and circulation. The receptors are located in the carotid glomus and in the wall of the aortic arch, while pressure receptors are widely distributed in the walls of large arteries. As these receptors are built into the vascular walls they act as stretch receptors: increased blood pressure stretches the wall, stimulates these receptors to discharge and,

by this, reduces sympathetic activity and inhibits respiration. In arteriosclerosis, causing rigidity of the aortic walls, these receptors are prevented from serving their function properly.

There is one more point of clinical interest. The neurons of the respiratory centres are large and are susceptible, like all large motor neurons, to poliomyelitis, causing a further complication in an already severe disease of lower motor neurons as respiration ceases. This explains why the polio patient needs to be kept in a respirator.

The pons
Nuclei pontis
The pons, between the medulla and cerebellum, owes its name to its ridge-like appearance in ventral view (Fig. 9.13(*a*)). The main pontine bulge consists of neurons, the nuclei pontis; the arms of the bridge are the axonal processes of these cells, which terminate in the cerebellum (Fig. 9.13(*b*)). The dorsal part of the pons has the structure of the medulla and is called tegmentum (see below). The formation of a large bridge between the upper part of the medulla and the cerebellum is typical in primates, for these nuclei serve as an intermediate station between the cerebral cortex and the cerebellum. The development of pontine nuclei is in accord with the upright gait and is in particular related to the independent and skilful use of the hands and fingers, demanding a wealth of cortical connections to be relayed to the cerebellar hemisphere, while the cortico-spinal or pyramidal tract just passes through the pons (Fig. 9.13(*a*) PYT).

Tegmentum pontis
This dorsal portion of the pons provides an area of passage for the bulbo-thalamic tract, also referred to as the medial lemniscus or medial fillet. Laterally, we find the lateral fillet or auditory fillet arising from crossing cochlear nuclei fibres referred to as the trapezoid body. The spino-cerebellar fibres ascend in the inferior cerebellar peduncle, while the ventral fibres reach the anterior part of the cerebellum, ascending via the superior cerebellar peduncle by coursing dorso-laterally in the pons.

Cranial nerves
The dorsal part of the pons contains the facial nerve nucleus, the abducens, and the trigeminal and vestibular nuclei (Figs 9.14 and 9.15). The peripheral areas of these nerves can be seen in Figs 9.16, 9.17 and 9.36.

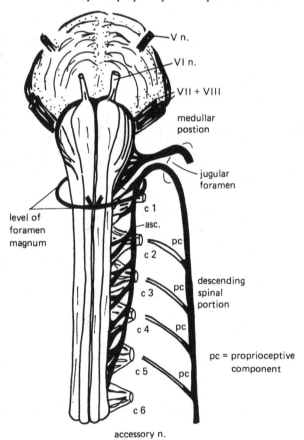

Fig. 9.12. Ventral view of cervical cord, medulla and pons, showing the composition of the accessory nerve (XI). The spinal portion ascends (asc.) through the foramen magnum, joins the medullary portion, and descends with the vagus and glossopharyngeal nerves through the jugular foramen. The medullary portion supplies the vocal muscles (via the vagus), neck muscles, trapezius and sternocleido-mastoid (after Chusid & McDonald, 1967). c1–c6 = cervical vertebrae; p.c. = proprioceptive component.

Fig. 9.13. (a) Microphotograph of a Weigert stained section through the lower pons illustrating the massive crossed connection of the pontine nuclei with the cerebellum, the middle cerebral peduncles ICP = inferior cerebellar peduncle; MCP = middle cerebellar peduncle; DN = dentate nucleus with emerging superior cerebellar peduncle; PYT = pyramidal tract; VC = vermis cerebelli; ML = medial lemniscus.
(b) The distribution of neurons at the pontine level (after Jacobsohn, 1909). abd.n. = abducens nucleus; b.-p.n. = bulbo-pontine nucleus; d.n. = dendate nucleus; d.pm.n. = dorsal paramedian nucleus; main V = main sensory nucleus of cranial nerve V; m.r.n.(a) = medial reticular nucleus (ascending part; m.r.n.(b) = medial reticular nucleus; m.ve.n. = medial vestibular nucleus; n.ang.ve. = nucleus angularis vestibularis; n.pig.tg.-c. = nucleus pigmentosus tegmento-cerebellaris; s.o. = superior olive; sp.th.t.n. = spino-thalamic tract nucleus; VII ac. = accessory facial nucleus; VII n.fac. = main facial nucleus.

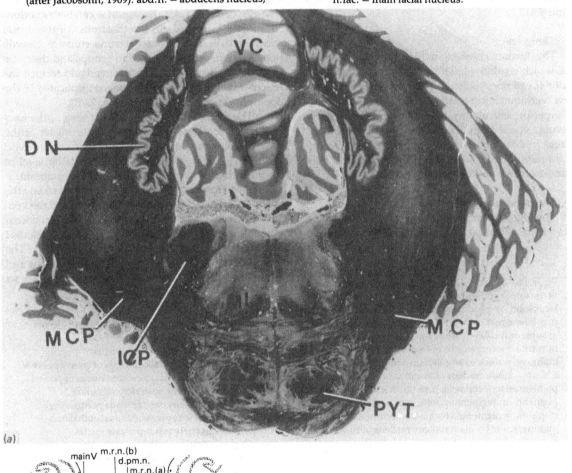

(a)

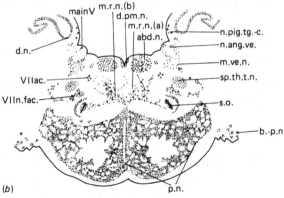

(b)

The midbrain

The midbrain is relatively large in the embryo (Fig. 2.27); but loses its dominant foetal position due to the rapidly developing cerebral cortex. Its position in the living person can now be seen in a nuclear magnetic resonance picture (see Fig. 7.4) and is illustrated in Figs 9.18 and 9.19. The midbrain is subdivided dorso-ventrally into three parts, most dorsally the tectum (or roof), the tegmentum, and ventrally the cerebral peduncles (or crura cerebri) (see Figs 7.1 and 9.1).

The tectum

The tectum consists in Man of the collicular plate, which is subdivided into anterior (superior) and inferior (posterior) colliculi. The superior colliculi in 'lower' vertebrates are often referred to as the tectum. The superior colliculi are the only part of the tectum receiving visual input and are important reflex centres. In Man the superior colliculus also serves visual reflex activity while the posterior colliculus is a reflex centre for auditory input.

The tegmentum, fibre tracts and nuclei

The tegmentum provides passage for important tracts such as the auditory lemniscus (or lateral fillet),

the spino-thalamic tract, which intermingles with lateral fillet fibres, and the spino-tectal tract. Ventral and medial lie the fibres of the bulbo-thalamic tract (or medial fillet (lemniscus)) which, further frontally, enters the posterior ventral part of the thalamus. Two very prominent nuclei are situated in the midbrain, giving cross-sections of very characteristic pattern, the nucleus ruber (red nucleus) and the substantia nigra (Figs 9.19 and 9.20). The large round area of the nucleus ruber contains relatively few large neurons but a wealth of fibres from the superior cerebellar peduncle coursing upwards to the thalamus. In the dorsal substantia nigra the compact zone contains heavily pigmented neurons arranged in groups and the more ventral area is more loosely arranged and termed the reticular zone. The reticular zone is implicated in the dopamine system illustrated in Fig. 7.30.

The fibres which penetrate the area of the nucleus ruber originate from the dendate nuclei of the cerebellum, come from a dorsal direction and descend ventrally into the midbrain, crossing at the level of the posterior (or inferior) colliculus of the midbrain.

Two further crossings are clearly marked: the dorsal tegmental decussation of Meynert and the ventral tegmental decussation of Forel. The dorsal decussation arising from cells in the superior colliculus descends as tecto-bulbar and tecto-spinal fibres. The ventral decussation is composed of rubro-bulbar and rubro-spinal fibres. One very conspicuous fibre tract

Fig. 9.14. Neuronal distribution at the dorsal portion of the upper pons, showing trigeminal nuclei (after Jacobsohn, 1906). d.n. = dendate nucleus; l.p.tg.-p. = lateral part of pigmented tegmento-pontine cell groups; m.n.cbl. = midline nuclei of cerebellum; m.n.tri. = motor nucleus of trigeminal nerve; n.ang.ve. = nucleus angularis vestibularis; n.m.fr. = motor nucleus of; n.pi.t.cbl. = nuclei pigmentosi tecti cerebelli; n.pi.t.p. = nucleus pigmentosus tegmento-pontis; p.n. = pontine nuclei; p.tg.p.m. = pigmented tegmento-pontine cells of midline; s.n.tri. = main sensory nucleus of trigeminal nerve.

Fig. 9.15. Cellular distribution at the uppermost pontine level (after Jacobsohn, 1906). iped.n. = interpeduncular nucleus; m.n.V = mesencephalic nucleus of cranial nerve V; m.pig.n.p. = medial pigmented nuclei of pons; n.p.c. = nucleus of posterior colliculus; n.pig.p. = nucleus pigmentosus ponti; n.pig. (st.pe.) = nucleus pigmentosus (subthalamo-peduncular part); p.n = pontine nuclei; r.n.p. = reticular nucleus of pons; teg.-p.n.p. = tegmento-peduncular nucleus of pons.

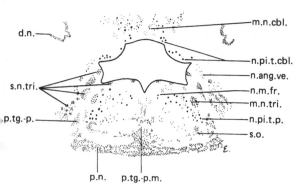

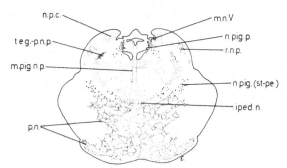

assembled at the superior collicular level is the central tegmental tract, composed of descending collicular fibres and tegmental reticular neurons. These fibres are very conspicuous in Man and terminate in the inferior olive, as shown by Glees & Zander (1950), who also discussed the relevant literature of this large midbrain connection to the cerebellum via the inferior olive. This pathway is an ancient component of the brainstem, whose highest centre is the midbrain. This is superceded by the cerebral cortex, which causes

the development of the pontine nuclei conveying its commands and information to the cerebellum but does not replace the tegmento-olivary tract as a channel between the midbrain and cerebellum. Two motor nuclei are built into the web of midbrain fibre connections: one supplies, via the trochlear nerve, the superior oblique eye muscle; the other, the oculomotor, supplies a number of eye muscles – three of the recti muscles (the superior, inferior and medial) and the elevator of the upper eye lid, the levator palpebrae

Fig. 9.16. Peripheral distribution of the trigeminal nerve (after Chusid & McDonald, 1967). The upper two branches, ophthalmic and maxillary, are entirely sensory; the lower branch, the mandibular, carries motor fibres to muscles for mastication.

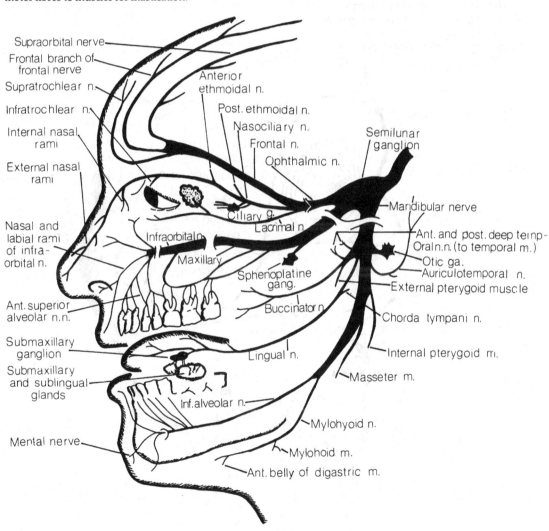

superior. The oculomotor nerve carries parasympathetic impulses to the iris of the eye, via the ciliary ganglion, in order to narrow the pupillary opening, preventing excessive light reaching the retina. The cells responsible are small neurons closely related topographically to the large motor cells for eye muscle innervation and are collectively called the Edinger–Westphal nucleus and the anterior median nucleus. These small cells are similar to the visceral motor components of the vagus at medullary level and are pre-ganglionic to the autonomic ganglion in the orbit, the ciliary ganglion.

The reticular formation of the brainstem
Organisation

The name 'reticular formation' is easily understood when looking at Figs 9.21–9.24 which show the large neurons of the reticular system spreading out among the ascending and descending fibres, supplying numerous synaptic contacts. The smaller and larger neurons are independent of the neurons supplying cranial nerves or of well-defined nuclear formations such as the inferior olive (Fig. 9.2(*c*)). Brodal (1957) was able to separate the reticular system in a greater number of nuclei stretching from the medulla

Fig. 9.17. Peripheral distribution of the facial nerve, mainly motor to muscles of facial expression (after Chusid & McDonald, 1967). Note nervous intermedius (from the superior salivary nucleus) which is pre-ganglionic to the parasympathetic ganglia of the head. The sympathetic nerve supply originates in the superior cervical ganglion.

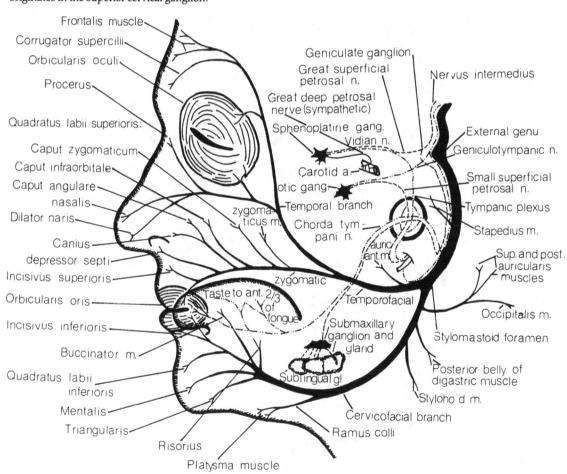

Fig. 9.18. Oblique transverse section through midbrain and upper pons. CG = central grey; PC = posterior colliculus; LL = termination of lateral limniscus; S = spino thalamic tract; ML = medial lemniscus; DSCP = decussation of superior cerebellar peduncle (from dentate nucleus); SCA = superior cerebellar artery; TN = trochlear nerve (IV) and vessels; TP = deep and transverse pontine fibres cut longitudinally while pontine and cortical spinal fibres are cut transversally.

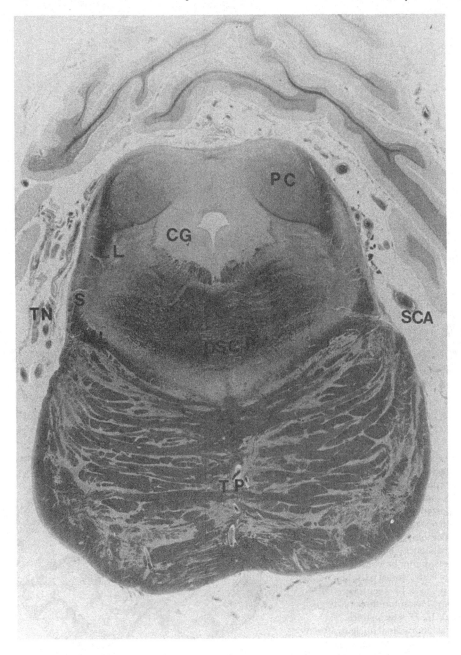

Fig. 9.19. Transverse section through level of superior colliculus of midbrain (Weigert stain). SC = superior colliculus; CG = central grey; S = Sylvian acquaduct; III N = oculomotor nuclei; III = oculomotor nerve

entering the interpeduncular fossa; SN = substantia nigra composed of a compact zone (CZ) and a reticular zone (RZ); R = nucleus ruber; MGB = medial geniculate body; CP = cerebral peduncle.

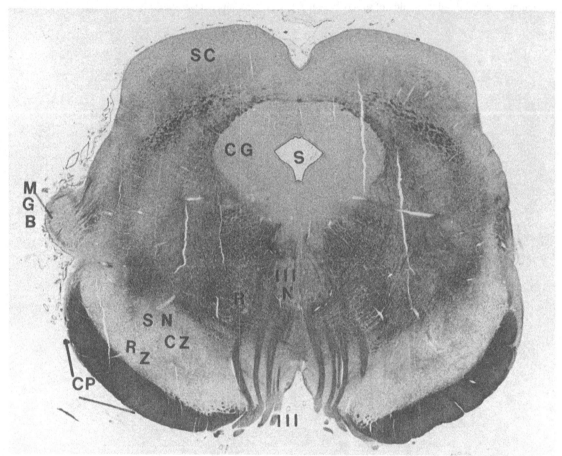

Fig. 9.20. Area of transition between the midbrain and the thalamus. 1 = pineal gland (epiphysis); 2 = pretectal area; 3 = commissure between superior colliculi; 4 = part of posterior commissure; 5 = central grey area; 6 = position of oculomotor nuclei; 7 = emergence of oculomotor nerve; 8 = medial nucleus of pulvinar thalami; 9 = lateral nucleus of pulvinar thalami; 10 = superior brachium; 11 = medial geniculate body, dorsal part; 12 = medial geniculate body, medial part; 13 = ventral part of medial geniculate body; 14 = spino-thalamic tract; 15 = medial lemniscus; 16, 17 = tectal nuclei; 18 = position of medial longitudinal nucleus; 19 = red nucleus (nucleus ruber); 20, 21, 22 = position of substantia nigra and subdivisions; 23 = fronto-pontine tract; 24 = cortico-spinal tract; 25 = parieto-temporo-pontine tract; 23, 24, 25 = collective cerebral peduncle.

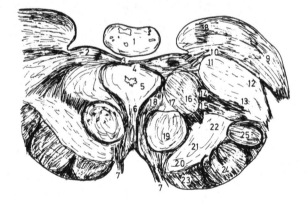

Fig. 9.21. Neuronal distribution at the superior collicular level of the midbrain (after Jacobsohn, 1909). c.g.s. = central grey substance; d.teg. = dorsal tegmental cells; l.p.n. = lateral peripeduncular nucleus; m.g.b. = medial geniculate body; mes.n.V. = mesencephalic nucleus of cranial nerve V; m.tec. = medial cell groups of tectum; n.r. = nucleus ruber; oc.n. = oculomotor nucleus; pig.n.p. = pigmented neurons of nucleus subthalamo-peduncularis; ret.f. = reticular formation; s.n. = subsantia nigra; st.gr. = stratum granulosum; st.lem. = stratum lemnisci; st.o. = stratum opticum; tg.-ped.n. = tegmento-peduncular nucleus.

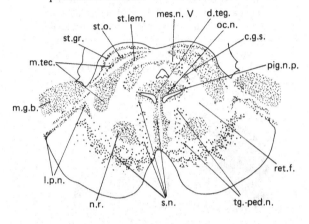

Fig. 9.22. A general diagram of the ascending reticular system. 1 = reticular formation (r.f.) in thalamus; 2 = reticular nuclei in midbrain 3 = r.f. in pons; 4 = position of parvicellular nucleus of r.f.; 5 = reticular nuclei at upper medulla; 6 = paramedial r.f. of medulla; 7 = lateral r.f. The thick black line (r.s.) represents the whole ascending reticular system.

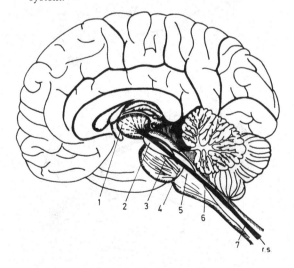

Fig. 9.23. A detailed diagram of the ascending reticular system (reticular formation, R.F.), based on the concepts of Magoun and co-workers. Dots represent the neurons of the R.F. spread around the midline of the raphe, reaching from the brainstem into the thalamus. The system receives continuous contributions from the ascending medial lemniscus (proprioceptive) which terminates in the posterior ventral nucleus of the thalamus (P.V.N.). The lateral lemniscus (L.L.), carrying auditory impulses, distributes afferents to the R.F. Due to the multiple input from all afferent sources, the R.F. is continuously activated and in turn alerts the cerebral cortex. A.C. = auditory cortex; I.C. = inferior colliculus; M.G.B. = medial geniculate body; M.L. = medial lemniscus; S.C. = sensory cortex; Sci.N. = sciatic nerve; TH. = thalamus; VIII = cranial nerve VIII – auditory division.

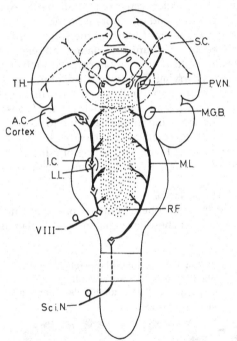

up to the thalamus and hypothalamus. The neurons send their axons in either an ascending or a descending direction and, by extensive collateralisation, influence cranial nerve nuclei and relay centres. The position of reticular nuclei is shown diagrammatically in Fig. 9.9(*a*).

The medullary reticular neurons project on to the cerebellum and the spinal cord.

Functional considerations

Neurophysiological investigations, in particular the early observations by Magoun and his co-workers (see Glees, 1961a), have shown that the neurons of the reticular system receive impulses from all afferent fibres, in particular from the lateral and medial lemniscus, and trigeminal, vestibular and spino-thalamic fibres. The reticular system or formation (RF) exercises both facilitating and inhibitory influences on the cerebral cortex, the brainstem and the spinal cord. It has therefore an important modulating influence on the cortex in an unspecific way in contrast to the specific pathways carrying specific sensory information. The alerting influence of the RF on cerebral function leads to cortical awareness and regulates state of consciousness. The inhibiting influence of the RF is related to sleep. Both these effects can clearly be seen in EEG recordings, and brainstem injuries or tumours involving the RF can lead to profound unconsciousness.

The thalamus

Each hemisphere contains one thalamus, the dorsal part of the diencephalon. The thalamus has

Fig. 9.24. Drawing of the large reticular cells embedded in the mass of ascending and descending fibres. These cells monitor impulses and regulate our state of consciousness.

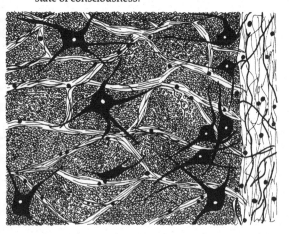

the size and form of a hen's egg with its axis situated horizontally. Anatomically the thalamus is divided into two main portions, a medial and a lateral, subdivided by a layer of myelinated (white) fibres called the lamina medullaris interna. The medially situated

Fig. 9.25. Topological relations of thalamic nuclei to the cerebral cortex (areas of projection) (after Netter, 1953). (A) Lateral view of left hemisphere.
c.s. = central sulcus. (B) Thalamic nuclei.
a.n. = anterior nuclear group; a.v.n. = anterior ventral nucleus; d.l.n. = dorso-lateral nucleus; d.m.n. = dorso-medial nucleus; l.g.b. = lateral geniculate body; m.g.b. = medial geniculate body; m.i. = massa intermedia; p.-l.n. = posterio-lateral nucleus; pulv. = pulvinar; v.l.n. = ventro-lateral nucleus; v.p.n. = ventral posterior nucleus (lateral part). (C) Medial view of right hemisphere.
t.p. = temporal pole. Cortical areas in white receive no direct thalamic projections.

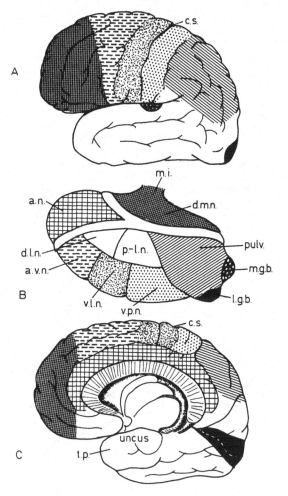

Fig. 9.26. (*a*) Photograph and explanatory diagram of thalamic nuclei. 1 = caudate nucleus; 2 = dorso-lateral nucleus; CC = corpus callosum; F = fornix; 3 = third ventricle; 4 = internal capsule; 5 = hippocampal area; 6 = lateral geniculate body (or nucleus); 7 = medial geniculate body (or nucleus); 8 = lateral nuclei of thalamus; 9 = ventral posterior nucleus, medial part; 10 = dorso-medial nucleus; I = insula.

(*b*) Frontal section through the cerebral hemispheres, low power micro-photograph Weigert stain. (Explanations as in (*a*).)

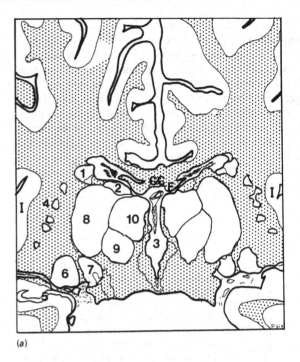

(*a*)

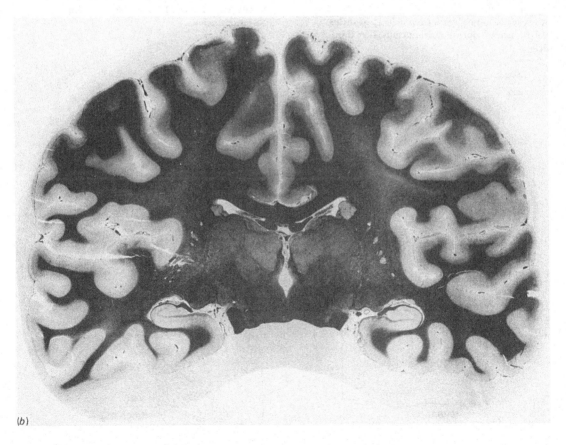

(*b*)

nuclei are divided into a dorsal, the dorso-medial, nucleus and a central median nucleus (or centrum medianum), plus some smaller nuclei close to the midline. The left and right thalamus enclose between them the third ventricular cavity. Laterally the thalami are separated from the fibres of the internal capsule by the external medullary lamina; between this lamina and the internal capsule are the neurons of the thalamic reticular nucleus. Figure 9.25 shows diagrammatically the thalamic nuclei and Fig. 9.26 shows a transverse section of the thalamus, both diagrammatically and an actual microphotograph.

Nuclei

Lateral nuclei. The most posterior lateral nucleus is the postero-lateral ventral nucleus, which receives afferent fibres from the posterior column nuclei, the medial lemniscus (or bulbo-thalamic tract), the spino-thalamic fibres and the fibres from the trigeminal fillet (Fig. 9.27(*a*)). In turn, the nucleus transmits its impulses to the sensory cortex or post-central gyrus (Fig. 9.27(*b*)). The ventral lateral nucleus receives signals from the cerebellum, arriving via the superior brachium, and from the red nucleus, transmitting its activity to the motor cortex or the pre-central gyrus.

Fig. 9.27. (*a*) Terminations of the large ascending tracts to the thalamus can be traced using the classical method of Marchi (Glees, 1961a). The medial lemniscus (m.l.) and spino-thalamic tracts (sp.th.tr.) terminate in the shaded areas – the lateral and medial portions of the posterior ventral nucleus.
c.i. = capsula interna; c.m.n. = median nucleus;
c.n. = caudate nucleus; d.l.n. = dorso-lateral nucleus;
d.m.n. = dorso-medial nucleus;
d.s.c.p. = decussating superior cerebellar peduncles;
p.d.l.n. = posterior dorso-lateral nucleus; III = third ventricle.

(*b*) Tracing cortical connections. When ablated, thalamic projection neurons in the shaded area (sensory cortex) undergo chromatolysis and can be recognized. The injected horseradish peroxidase (H.R.P.) is taken up by cortical neurons allowing the tracing of efferent cortical pathways. c. = cortex; c.c. = corpus callosum; deg.c.th.f. = degenerating cortico-thalamic fibres; retrogr.deg. = retrograde Nissel degeneration; Th. = thalamus; v.p.n. = ventral posterior nucleus.

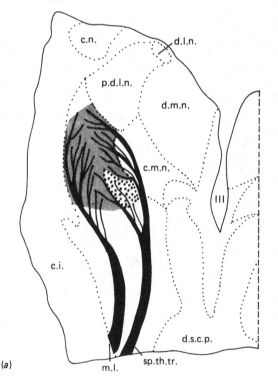

(*a*)

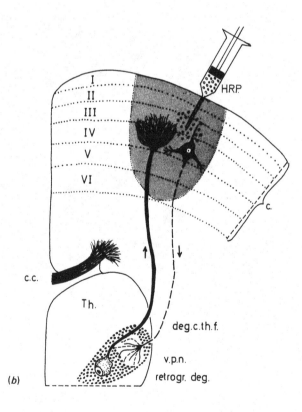

(*b*)

The dorso-lateral and posterior lateral nuclei send their information to the parietal cortex (Area 5). A further nucleus of the lateral group is the anterior ventral nucleus, which receives input from the basal ganglia.

Posterior nuclei. The nuclei of the pulvinar thalami and the lateral and medial geniculate bodies are components of the posterior thalamic area. The pulvinar nuclei have connections with the parietal and temporal cortex. The medial geniculate receives *auditory*

impulses via the lateral fillet or lemniscus and the inferior brachium, a connecting link between posterior colliculus and medial geniculate, which in turn projects onto the central receiving station, the transverse gyrus of Heschl of the temporal lobe (see Fig. 12.5). The lateral geniculate receives *retinal* input and is dealt with in Chapter 13 on vision and visual pathways.

Medial nuclei. Two main nuclei are referred to: the dorso-medial nucleus' projection to the pre-frontal lobe, receiving an input from there; and the centre median nucleus, connected with the basal ganglia.

Anterior nuclei. The anterior nucleus is seen macroscopically as a dorso-frontal protrusion and is subdivided microscopically into three portions – medial, dorsal and ventral. The anterior nucleus (Fig. 9.28) (or, better, the anterior nuclear group) receives input from the mamillary body, via the fornix, and projects

Fig. 9.28 Diagram of thalamic nuclei and neighbouring structures. ACA = anterior cerebral arteries; AN = anterior nucleus; CC = corpus callosum; CI = capsula interna; CN = caudate nucleus; DM = dorso-medial nucleus; F = fornix; GC = gyrus cinguli; GL PAL = globus pallidus; IML = internal medullary lamina; LA = lateral and anterior nuclear groups; V = ventricle. Arrows point to the choroid plexi of the third and lateral ventricles.

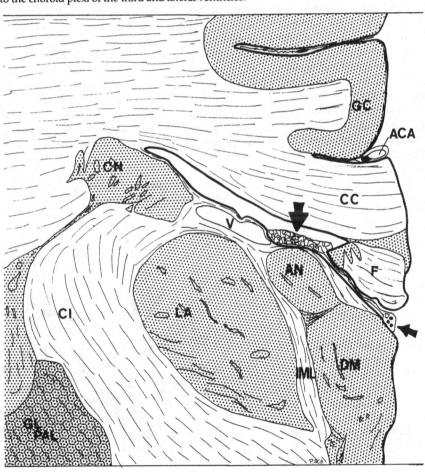

onto the cingular gyrus, above the corpus callosum (Fig. 9.25) which is a part of the limbic system of Mac-Lean (see below).

The limbic system

The limbic system owes its name to the French neurologist Broca who, in 1878, attempted to separate functionally the medial portions of the hemisphere from the lateral and dorsal aspects by giving it the name of the limbic lobe. The American neurobiologist MacLean (1954) used many ingenious experimental designs to explore the limbic lobe, which he called the visceral brain and endowed with psychosomatic functions. His concepts were further elaborated by Ploog & MacLean (1963).

The anterior nuclear group of the thalamus interconnects two parts of the limbic system, the hypothalamus (mamillary body), the evolutionarily oldest part of the diencephalon, and the cingular gyrus, a part of the neocortex (see Fig. 7.27). Included in the limbic system are the hippocampus–fornix, the amygdaloid nuclei, olfactory areas, hypothalamus and the mamillo-thalamic tract (Fig. 7.27). These widely spread anatomical structures appear to neuro-physiologists to house a number of functional circuits ranging from emotional behaviour to psychosomatic diseases. I was present, however, when the late brain surgeon Sir Hugh Cairns stimulated, under local scalp anaesthesia, the gyrus cinguli in a fully conscious man without eliciting any of the supposed functions, thus questioning whether the gyrus cinguli was indeed the centre for emotional behaviour.

Functional considerations

At first sight the thalamus appears to be a relay station for external sensory input onto the cerebral cortex. For some thalamic nuclei (lateral and some posterior) this appears to be convincing and they are called relay or projection nuclei, and the relevant cortices referred to as projection areas. However, these projection nuclei receive other inputs as well as input from the cerebral cortex.

Other thalamic nuclei, such as the dorso-medial, seem to receive no 'outside' information and can be called 'associational' in function, projecting onto the pre-frontal lobe, making this part of the cerebral cortex an association area. This connection has received special attention through the neurosurgical intervention of leucotomy and is dealt with on pp. 95–6. Furthermore, the connections between basal ganglia and the thalamus have been cut by neurosurgeons using

stereotactic instrumentation to locate these connecting fibres. This approach was carried out in the past to alleviate Parkinsonism but progress in neurobiochemistry (see p. 108) has made surgical intervention obsolete.

The cerebellum
Morphology and general function

The cerebellum (Figs 7.6 and 9.29) has an entirely different structure from the cerebrum and a separate cranial cavity, the posterior fossa, sharing this with the brainstem. Its weight is only a tenth of that of the cerebrum, about 120 g. The internal structure is grossly simplified and comprises three layers (Fig. 9.30). Its main function is the evaluation of data controlling motor performance. It is generally assumed that the cerebellum does not take part in mental activity or contribute to the state of consciousness. However, Glees & James (1957) observed a microcephalic, amentia patient whose brain weight was 870 g; the most obvious histopathology was the complete absence of Purkinje cells in the cerebellum, while sensory and motor pathways and the cerebral cortex appeared normal. The patient suffered from profound hypotonia, a functional state explainable by the lack of Purkinje neurons. We assumed that this abnormality could also have contributed to the state of amentia and stupor, for the low brain weight as such could not have been the sole course for this mental condition. The efferent cerebellar pathways affect the reticular formation's activity, reducing its alerting function.

Fig. 9.29. Sagittal section through the cerebellum showing the general division into white (myelinated fibres, w.) and grey (neurons and dendrites, g.) cortical matter (from Glees, 1971).

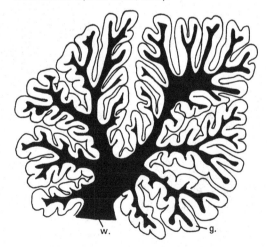

Evolutionary and functional aspects

Cerebellar and vestibular function are clearly associated from early in development and there is evidence that the medullary vestibular area 'dispatches' embryonic neurons from the rhombic lip to lay the foundation for the Purkinje cells, which form the archi- and palaeocerebellum, serving vestibular information and spinal impulses. This evolutionarily older part appears first in ontogeny and is eventually joined by the neocerebellum, forming the large cerebellar hemispheres. This latter development is related to the primates' acquisition of upright gait and independently moveable upper extremities. Due to these changes in posture the neocerebellum becomes a computer-like aid to the cerebral motor cortex commands.

Fibre connections

The three large connecting pathways of the cerebellum are called peduncles or stalks. The lower or inferior peduncle carries spinal, vestibular, reticular and olivary pathways. The middle peduncle is the pontine brachium (see p. 131) and the upper peduncle or superior brachium is the main efferent channel of the cerebellum.

Histology and ultrastructure

Only knowledge of the detailed histological structure allows understanding of cerebellar connec-

tivity and synaptology. The key element is the large flask-like cell of Purkinje (Fig. 3.1). These cells are arranged in rows in a systematic fashion, their large and numerous dendritic branches stretching towards the surface, their axons emerging opposite the dendrites towards the white or fibrous matter (Figs 9.30–9.33). The Purkinje cell has no direct access to 'outside' information; all stimuli reach the receptive membranes from inside the CNS and via a number of synapses. The afferent fibres are called climbing fibres, basket fibres and tangential or parallel fibres, according to their histological appearances (Fig. 9.32). The climbing fibres wind like branches of ivy around the dendrites of the Purkinje neurons. The basket fibres have their basket-like arrangement around the cell body (Fig. 9.31). The parallel fibres are axons of the neurons situated in the granular layer below the layer of Purkinje neurons (Fig. 9.32). These cells receive

Fig. 9.31. A simplified wiring diagram of the cerebellum (from Glees, 1971). The mossy fibres of spino-cerebellar, vestibular pontine origin (m.f.) terminate in the granular layer, synapsing with granular neurons (g) whose axons ascend to the molecular layer, seen in a lateral view (l.v.) which shows the Purkinje cells. The ascending climbing fibres (a.f.) synapse with the dendrites of Purkinje cells shown in a ventral view (v.v.). The cell bodies of Purkinje neurons (P) receive synapses from basket cells (b.c.). Ascending fibres to the Purkinje cells supply collaterals (c.f.m.) to the dendate nuclei (d.n.). These collaterals act as emergency circuits in diseases involving the Purkinje cells.

Fig. 9.30. Section through a cerebellar lobule stained with Glees' silver technique, showing the principal divisions into layers (from Glees, 1971).

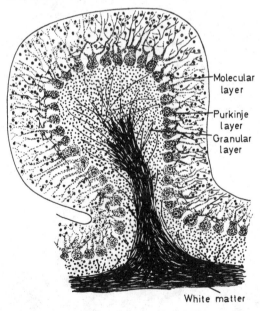

Molecular layer

Purkinje layer

Granular layer

White matter

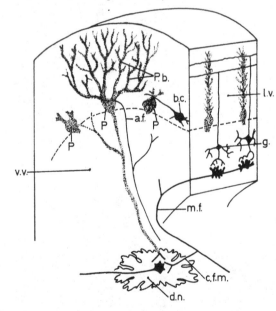

Fig. 9.32. (*a*) Cerebellar layers under higher power
(Glees, silver impregnation) illustrating the close
contacts between climbing fibres and Purkinje
dendrites (marked by arrows) and the basket contacts
with the cell bodies (b.c.) (Glees, 1971).
GL = granular layer; PCL = Purkinje cell layer;
ML = molecular layer. The black dots in the ML are
the nuclei neuroglia cells.
(*b*) High power microphotograph of a Purkinje cell
(Glees preparation). From the cell body large
branching dendrites emerge in intimate contact with
climbing fibres. Dendrites and climbing fibres are
'immersed' into the molecular layer which is the
synaptic substratum. To the right of the Purkinje cells
is the granular layer whose synaptic relationships
could only be revealed by electronmicroscopy (see
Fig. 9.33).

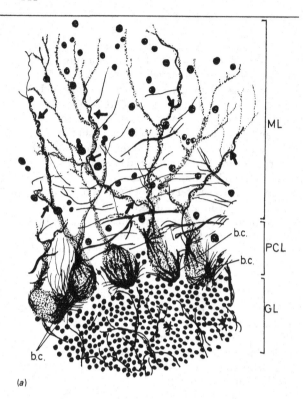

(*a*)

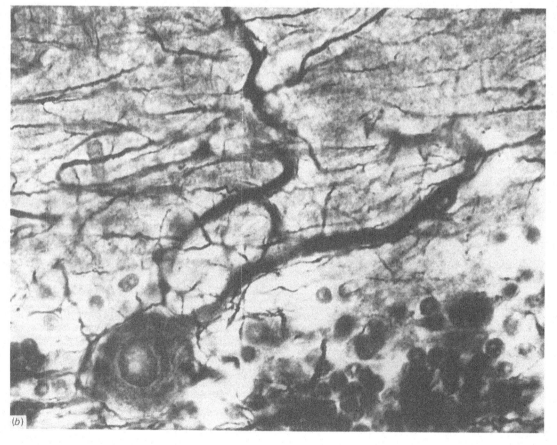

(*b*)

input from a number of sources from spinal, vestibular and pontine levels, terminating as mossy fibres and synapsing with the short dendrites of the granular neurons in an interdigitating manner. These synaptic complexes are called glomeruli (Fig. 9.34). The granular neurons send their axons into the molecular layer, forming synapses with the dendritic spines of Purkinje cells and with the basket cells. The exception from the type of mossy terminations in the granular layer are the climbing fibres. According to Szentágothai (Szentágothai & Rajkovits, 1959) these fibres originate in the inferior olive, have extensive synapses with the smooth stems and are excitatory for the Purkinje neuron (Eccles, 1968). The synapses from mossy and climbing fibres are shown diagrammatically and based on ultrastructural studies of a number of authors in Fig. 9.34.

Quantitative data

The total cortical surface area of the strongly folded cerebellum is about 1000 cm^2, while the cerebral cortex occupies an area of 2500 cm^2. It has been estimated that there are 500 million granular cells and 14 million Purkinje neurons. The high number of granular cells can be explained by the fact that the cerebellum is most of the time activated by motor tasks and

that the granular cells face these tasks in rotation. The relatively low number of Purkinje neurons indicates a marked convergence and confluence of impulses on Purkinje cells, further condensed when their axons converge on the roof nuclei, e.g. the dendate nuclei of the cerebellum, where they exercise inhibitions (Fig. 9.31).

Exteroceptive impulses

Apart from the influx of proprioceptive impulses from muscles, joints and other sources, exteroceptive stimuli from vision and hearing also reach the cerebellum, as can be seen in physiological experiments, but these impulses serve no apparent function.

Disturbances of cerebellar function

The cortico–pontine–cerebellar circuits serve discrete integration of aimful movements, and in cere-

Fig. 9.34. Cerebellar circuitry at the electron microscope level. Arrows indicate the directions of conduction of impulses (from Glees, 1971).
a.g. = axons of granule cells; these synapse with Golgi thorns in axo-dendritic synapses (a-d.s.). AP = axon of Purkinje cell. b.c. = basket cell of larger synapse on Purkinje cell body (axo-somatic synapse). c.G. = stellate Golgi cell which contributes to synapses in the granular layer (s.G.). cl.f. = climbing fibre. cl.f.s. = multiple synapses from climbing fibre on smooth stem of Purkinje dendrite. d. = dendrite of granule cell. f.p.1, f.p.2 = parallel fibres. m.f. = termination of mossy fibres on dendrites of granule cells. P.1, P.2, P.3 = Purkinje cells. s.v. = synaptic vesicles.

Fig. 9.33. A Purkinje cell as seen after Golgi impregnation. The Golgi thorns are the 'spines' seen with the election microscope (sps) (from Glees, 1971).

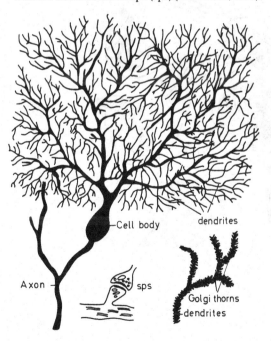

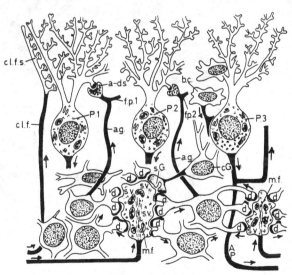

bellar dysfunction tremor and dysmetria are apparent. The Purkinje cells can be compared to computer elements, evaluating data and sending the results via the superior peduncular cable to the lateral nucleus of the thalamus to be forwarded to the sensory-motor cortex. In this way the cerebellum mediates between the cerebral cortex and the motor neurons of the spinal cord. Cerebellar dysfunctions can result in inability to execute aimful movements correctly, dysmetria, or the failure to perform quick alternating supination and pronation (rotatory movements), adiadochokinesia. Extracerebellar compensation can largely cover up these deficiencies, but closure of the eyes, depriving the patient of visual control, quickly shows up the cerebellar dysfunction in the so-called finger–nose

test. With vision allowed, the test is performed fairly well; without vision, gross misplacements occur, i.e. the patient cannot touch the end of his nose with a finger from an arms-outstretched position. Often, large lesions caused by tumours or surgical ablation show surprisingly few clinical signs and as long as the cerebellar bypass is intact (Fig. 9.31) some cerebellar function is maintained. This compensation appears to be carried out by the roof nuclei and the dendate nucleus. Furthermore, connections between the cerebral cortex and the reticular formation of the brainstem can take over some cerebellar function.

For general revision and overview we conclude Chapter 9 with Fig. 9.35.

Fig. 9.35. Ventral view of the human brain showing the peripheral distributions of the cranial nerves (after Netter, 1953).

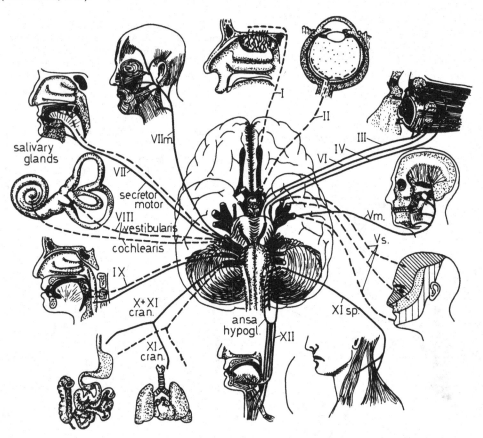

10
The hypothalamus and the autonomic nervous system

The hypothalamus
Structure

The central switchboard is composed of the hypothalamus and its endocrine outlet, the pituitary gland. The hypothalamus is a relatively small funnel-shaped pouch of the ventral part of the diencephalon and lies on the basal surface of the brain (Figs 10.1 and 10.2). A stalk connects the hypothalamus with the pituitary gland, which consists of two different parts or lobes, often called hypophysis in contrast to the epiphysis – a dorsal pouch of the diencephalon.

The stalk connects with the posterior lobe and is thus an outgrowth from the hypothalamus. The posterior lobe is for this reason referred to as the neurohypophysis and the anterior lobe, developing in ontogeny from the roof of the oral cavity, is glandular in structure and also called the adenohypophysis. The two lobes in primates are closely approximated with an intermediate zone between, but in some vertebrates, such as the elephant, they are separated. The glandular or anterior part has a number of differently granulated cells, which also stain differently. Histology discriminates five cell types: (1) undifferentiated stem cells; (2) α cells; (3) β cells; (4) γ cells; and (5) δ cells (Fig. 10.1).

Immunohistochemistry shows that alpha-cells secrete growth hormone and prolactin, beta-cells adreno-cortico-trophic hormone and thyrotrophic hormone, and the delta-cells secrete gonadotrophic hormones (Martin *et al.*, 1977; Bhatnagar, 1983).

The stalk itself carries pathways and also fibres which transport neurosecretory granules (Figs 10.3 and 10.4). These granules are taken up by the capillaries of the posterior lobe. In the hypothalamic nuclei (Figs 10.4 and 10.5) we encounter a clear double neuronal function, to produce action potentials and neurosecretory granules. Most hypothalamic neurons are relatively small, apart from the supraoptic nucleus

Fig. 10.1. Functional and topographical relations between the hypothalamus and the hypophysis (pituitary gland) seen in a lateral view (from Glees, 1971). a.c. = anterior commissure; a.l. = anterior lobe; c.α = alpha cells (eosinophils, acidophils); c.β = beta cells (basophils); c.γ = gamma cells (chromophobe cells, replacement cells); c.δ = delta cells; f. = fornix; i. = infundibular stalk; l.t. = lamina terminalis; m.b. = mamillary body; m.i. = massa intermedia; o.ch. = optic chiasma; p.l. = posterior lobe (neurohypophysis); pv.n. = parvicellular nucleus; r.c. = rete capillare; so.n. = supraoptic nucleus; v.2 = afferent and efferent vessels transporting neurosecretion; v.3 = vessels to neurosecretory nuclei.

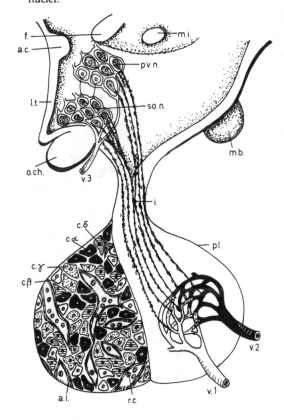

(Fig. 10.5) and are well supplied with dense capillary nets, for the hypothalamus records blood temperature and its composition and regulates via the posterior lobe of the pituitary water metabolism and urine secretion. Close functional relations exist between the hypothalamus and the pituitary gland, brought about via neurosecretory fibres and venous vessels communicating with the blood vessels of the anterior lobe (portal-hypophyseal vessels) (Fig. 10.3). The anterior lobe of the pituitary discharges its secretions into the blood in which they reach their target areas the endocrine glands (Fig. 10.4), e.g. the thyroid, suprarenal, and the gonads. On this basis, the hypothalamus and anterior pituitary regulate the sexual cycle in women. The activity of the anterior lobe is itself influenced by the feedback from the endocrines via the vascular channels, stopping if necessary the stimulating hormones from the pituitary. In the interchange between central and peripheral places of hormone production many disturbances in orderly production may ensue,

not only in the anterior lobe or peripherally in the gonads but also in the hypothalamus itself. Disturbances in metabolism or sexual function show the close interdependence of all the structures and their functions involved.

The study of evolution has shown that the hypothalamus is a relatively large and constant part of the forebrain which regulates, together with the pituitary, the whole inner milieu of the body, the functions of all endocrines, the composition of body fluids and the regulation of temperature in warm-blooded animals. The hypothalamus is well qualified for these functions, for it can send messages or transmitters by neurosecretion and by pulse-like action potentials of ordinary nerve impulses.

Fibre connections

The most important connecting fibre tract is a longitudinally running pathway, arising in the basal olfactory centres coursing through the hypothalamus and the midbrain. This pathway consists of a chain of neurons, many of which terminate on their fronto-basal route and are replaced by new cells; collectively this pathway is referred to as the medial forebrain

Fig. 10.2. Topography and structure of the pituitary gland in Man. cav.sin. = cavernous venous sinus; int.car.a. = internal carotid artery; III, IV, V, VI = cranial nerves.

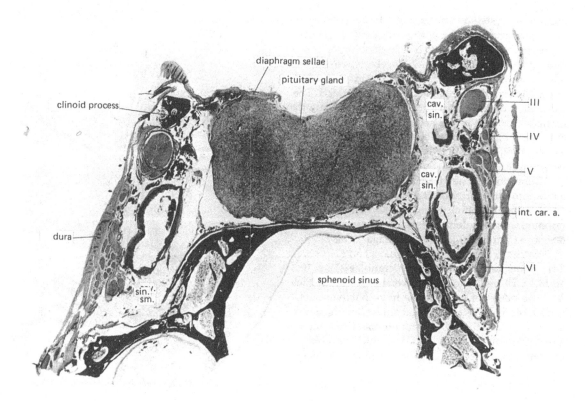

bundle. Fibre connections can be traced from the hypothalamus into the dorso-medial thalamic nucleus, the periventricular system of fibres, which contains fibres from and to the midbrain. The strong connection of the medial part of the mamillary body with the anterior thalamic nuclei has already been mentioned.

Cortico-hypothalamic connections

The ventro-medial nucleus has cortical connections with the temporal lobe and the frontal lobe, in particular the orbital cortex, which receives additional fibres from the lateral hypothalamic, supraoptic and paraventricular nuclei.

Connections of the neurohypophysis

These connections pass through the stalk of the posterior lobe (or neurohypophysis), the embryological outgrowth from the hypothalamus. The neurons of this connection compose the paraventricular and supraoptic nuclei. Axons from neurons of the infundibular nucleus terminate on the vessels of the hypophyseal stalk to deliver neurosecretion for the anterior lobe. The myelinated connections of the hypothalamus to the posterior lobe are

Fig. 10.3. Diagrammatic representation of neurosecretory mechanism, after O. Scharrer, the discoverer of neurosecretion. The posterior lobe (Post.l.) of the pituitary gland receives direct neurosecretory granule-carrying fibres. The anterior lobe receives neurosecretion indirectly via vascular loops (see arrow). O.ch. = optic chiasma.

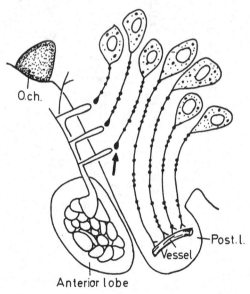

Fig. 10.4. Diagram of neurosecretory pathways (after Bargmann, 1968). The neurons of the neurosecretory centre are stimulated via synapses (s.s., described by Oksche). The axons of the neurosecretory cells transport the secretory granules to stores from which the granules reach the vascular bed. Larger amounts of granules are called Herring bodies (H.b.) Neurosecretions are carried by the blood to target organs which report back to the centre and effect hormonal regulation. endo. = endocrine organs.

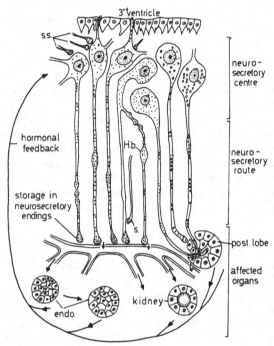

Fig. 10.5. The most important hypothalamic nuclei seen in sagittal section. These nuclei are arbitarily divided into an anterior group at the level of the optic chiasma, a medial group and a posterior group in relation to the mamillary body or corpus mamillare.

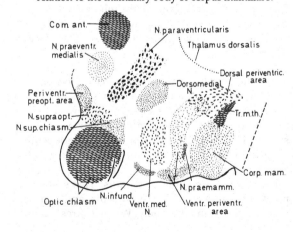

special in the sense that although they are impulse-conducting, they also transport the secretory granules to the capillary walls of the neurohypophysis (Fig. 10.1).

Functional aspects

The essential function of the hypothalamus is to ensure a well-balanced regulation of metabolism by means of nervous and vascular connections with the pituitary.

Descending and ascending connections with the autonomic nervous system are finely tuned to assure a balanced motor outlet for the various metabolic demands of the body in emotional stress. This metabolic activity embraces the neurosecretory nuclei and the neurohypophysis (posterior lobe) to regulate water metabolism; disturbance leads to diabetes insipidus, characterised by uncontrollable thirst and massive output of dilute urine. Other hypothalamic disease processes or malfunctions are adiposity and anorexia nervosa; in children adiposity can be combined with genital dystrophy. Skull trauma, involving direct injury to basal parts of the brain, can cause conditions similar to those described below.

Malfunction of the pituitary

Excessive secretion of thyrotrophic hormone can produce a thyrotoxicosis and exophthalmus. Cerebral gigantism is a disease of retarded children. Acromegaly, which appears fully in adults, is caused by a tumour in the pituitary (eosinophilic adenoma) which causes increased bone formation in the tips of the feet and hands, in the skull bones and in the tip of the chin. Additionally, diabetes mellitus can occur.

Cushing's syndrome. Regarding the cause of this disease, it is assumed that proliferations of β-cells (Fig. 10.1) cause a hyperplasia of the suprarenal glands and thus a profound imbalance of the mineral metabolism, glycosuria, hypertension, increase of hair growth and skin abnormalities. Adiposity causes the face to become round, 'moon-shaped'.

The peripheral autonomic nervous system

Apart from the central nervous system (CNS), conducting our conscious and voluntary activities, another neural system is present in our bodies. This system is relatively autonomous and independent from the CNS. It regulates the autonomic (involuntary) functions of the gut and circulation and many aspects of the urogenital apparatus. This system has many built-in feedback mechanisms and normally works securely and discretely. When in stressful situations, however, our 'embarrassment' is only too obvious – we blush, cry, are frightened, our heart rate goes up and cold sweat appears. Sudden anxieties can lead to diarrhoea or micturition. These disturbances illustrate that the normally present self-regulation has broken down and its 'sympathy' with external events is only too apparent.

Distribution and arrangement

In order to understand this normally well hidden system, a division into sympathetic and parasympathetic systems is informative (Figs 10.6–10.8). Both divisions control the smooth muscles of blood vessels, the gut, the glands and the genital organs. The sympathetic system is directed from special neurons situated in the cord or close to the cord, the sympathetic chain, and clusters of sympathetic neurons, the peripheral sympathetic ganglia. Their interconnections are shown in Fig. 10.6 together with their divisions in pre- and post-ganglionic fibres.

The parasympathetic system has its pre-ganglionic cells of origin in the brainstem and in the sacral

Fig. 10.6. Wiring diagram of the sympathetic nervous system (from Glees, 1971). C.p.p. = cardiopulmonary plexus; G.sp.n. = greater splanchnic nerve; L.sp.n. = lesser splanchnic nerve; I.M.G. = inferior mesenteric ganglion; S.M.G. = superior mesenteric ganglion.

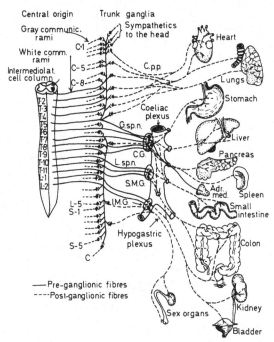

portion of the spinal cord. The axons of the post-ganglionic cells on the whole have only a short course within the intestine and abdominal organs.

Functions of the autonomic system

The sympathetic division regulates those body reactions expressing fear and aggression. These reactions give both attacker and defender a better chance of survival by increasing blood pressure, releasing more glucose for muscle work, and dilating pupils to frighten the opponent. These reactions can be well studied in fighting cats. This heightened sympathetic reaction is a mass reaction and spreads over the whole body. The neurotransmitter released in these reactions is noradrenaline and this is the reason for calling the sympathetic reaction 'adrenergic', but this definition appears too simple, for Burn (1967) proved that adrenergic nerve endings secrete acetylcholine initially. The double function of sympathetic endings is supported by electron microscope studies showing that certain synaptic endings contain vesicles with a dense core (probably adrenergic), as well as clear vesicles.

The Swiss physiologist and Nobel prize winner Hess, an authority on the autonomic nervous system, called the hypothalamic area responsible for directing sympathetic activity the ergotrophic zone and the area responsible for parasympathetic activity the tropho-troph–endophylactic zone. Hess (1954) saw the tasks of these zones as follows. The parasympathetic zone had the task of reducing and relaxing autonomic body functions and in this sense was antisympathetic. For this concept sleep would be the most important aspect of parasympathetic tone, a state of lowered blood pressure, reduced respiration and narrow pupils to keep out arousing light stimuli. The transmitter of the parasympathetic system is acetylcholine and the parasympathetic system is referred to as cholinergic. The term autonomic should not be taken too literally as some dependence on the CNS exists, although in normal unstressed life we expect our internal organs to work smoothly without penetration into consciousness (e.g. circulation, digestion and genital functions). A hypothalamic malfunction can, however, produce angina pectoris, bronchial asthma, diabetes mellitus and hypertension. Regulation of body temperature is easily interfered with by hypothalamic injury, in particular the protection of the body against heat. The structures responsible for the regulation are not strictly separated topographically, but we can assume that the hypothalamic neurons responsible for defence against heat loss are in the sympathetic zone, as heat preservation is achieved by contraction of peripheral vessels; this and heat production are tasks of the sympathetic system. However, heat production can proceed within certain limits without the hypothalamus.

Control of appetite. Injury to the ventro-medial hypothalamic nucleus in experimental animals causes an increased urge for feeding and a consequent increase in body weight. If this lesion is made in cats, not only

Fig. 10.7. Diagram of the origin and distribution of the parasympathetic system (from Glees, 1971).
C.p.p. = cardio-pulmonary plexus; D.m.n.X = dorsal motor nucleus of vagus; O.p. = oesophageal plexus; S3, S4 = pre-ganglionic sacral origin of parasympathetic nerve supply.

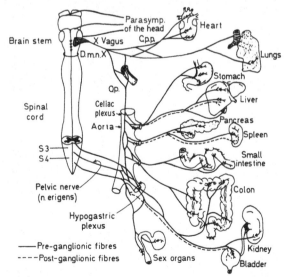

Fig. 10.8. Peripheral distribution of the autonomic nervous system illustrated by the innervation of the intestine (after Chusid & McDonald, 1967).

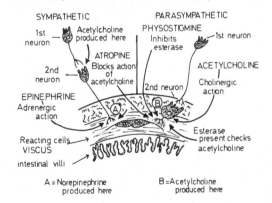

is appetite but also aggression is heightened. A small lesion lateral to the ventro-medial nucleus causes loss of appetite and cachexia. In Man hypothalamic tumours can produce disturbance of appetite control, such as satiation, leading to adiposity or marked weight loss.

Reactions to stress. Sensory impulses arriving from sense organs are primarily directed to CNS relay stations, but the cerebral cortex passes on the information to the autonomic centres for emotional evaluation, illustrating the interdependence of the cerebral cortex and the autonomic system. Under many conditions of modern life, this dependency leads to uncontrollable stress reactions; mismanagement in the autonomic sphere and strong excitements can cause diarrhoea and circulatory failure. These worries or excitements don't necessarily need to be acute, they can be present in the 'mind' only and still cause unwanted stress reactions by exceeding the person's tolerance. Observations on young drivers in London traffic reveal increases in heart rate of 100% and many people show abnormalities in their electrocardiograms in traffic stress, while bus drivers can show an increase in blood pressure and a risk of apoplexy (Taggert & Gibbons, 1967). The branch of medicine researching into the overlap of cerebral awareness and autonomic reactions has led to a new speciality – that of psychosomatic medicine. The important relationship of the central autonomic connections to psychosomatic medicine and clinical pathology with special reference to CNS control centres has been emphasised by Glees & Hasan (1976b) in a handbook on the autonomic nervous system.

11
Olfaction and taste

Olfaction
Introduction

The ability to smell, a highly sensitive modality even in Man, is of great significance for our social life, both physiologically and psychologically. From a biochemical point of view olfaction is related to taste and both are chemical senses. Many animals are guided almost exclusively by the sense of smell in periods of sexual activity, and dogs and cats appear almost blind and deaf to other stimuli when 'on heat'. A surprisingly small amount of substance is required for detection by olfactory receptors.

To characterise the strong effect odours have on behaviour a specific term 'pheromone', was introduced by Karlson & Lüscher (1959) in their work on insects searching for a mate and guided by odour. Pheromones are olfactorily active substances which, when smelled, trigger a specific behavioural pattern in neuroendocrine mechanisms in a similar way to hormones. These pheromones may cause profound changes in endocrine secretory systems or may simply attract the opposite sex, in which case they are referred to as primer pheromones (Keverne, 1983).

The sense of smell in Man is highly efficient, in spite of the fact that the area in the nose housing the receptors is very small (Figs 9.35 and 11.1) and the greater part of our nasal mucosa serves to warm the inhaled air. The olfactory cells in Man occupy a relatively small area in the upper part of the nose and nasal septum and, for this reason, odiferous substances transported by air and inhaled do not reach this upper nasal portion (Fig. 9.35) directly but by diffusion inside the nose. This is why we sniff the air in order to reach the receptors. It also explains the interval before we smell, the long time it takes before we have 'lost' the smell, and why we cannot smell if the nose is blocked. Furthermore, we *adapt* quickly to a specific smell, but new substances are noted quickly.

Receptors

The olfactory receptor is a combination of nerve cell and sensory cell, a unit construction of ancient evolutionary history and, presumably, highly successful since it has not been replaced. The receptive pole when viewed with a high-power microscope, looks like a daisy; the flower leaves are mobile fine extensions from a club-like terminal swelling of the receptive pole (Figs 11.1 and 11.2).

The surface ultrastructure of the olfactory epithelium has been clearly illustrated by Porter & Bonneville (1965). It is composed mainly of receptor cell ciliated terminals and microvilli. Glees & Spoerri (1978) observed that the surface of olfactory receptors possesses, in addition to the previously described extremely long cilia, several branched or unbranched cytoplasmic protrusions similar to microvilli. Extending from the tips and from the distal portions of the

Fig. 11.1. The olfactory mucosa is composed of supporting cells (s.c.) and the actual olfactory cells (o.c.). Each olfactory cell is a combination of a sensory cell with a receptive pole (r.p.) and a transmitting pole (t.p.) emitting a fine non-medullated axon (from Glees, 1971). b.c. = basal cells (replacement cells); sub.ep.l. = subepithelial layer; v. = vessels.

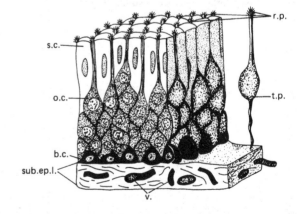

shafts of these elevations into the neighbouring portions of the extracellular space are numerous very delicate lace-like filaments. The filaments diminish in length and number towards the base of the processes. While these fur-like filaments attached to separate cytoplasmic protrusions have not been reported previously in connection with olfactory cells, Yamada (1955) in his classical paper on the gall bladder epithelium noted similar delicate extracellular adornments radiating from microvillous projections and called them antennulae microvillares. Similarly, Choi (1963) observed on the outer surface of the microvilli of the urinary bladder a pile or nap of filaments. Such a network of filaments is in actuality an extracellular coat, rich in polysaccharides and known as the surface coat (Fawcett, 1969). Many types of cells possess such a polysaccharide-rich coat, which, however, cannot always be distinguished with the electron microscope. Several functions have been attributed to the surface coat (Brandt, 1962; Bennett, 1963), some of which may be applicable to the filamentous structures seen on the microvilli of the olfactory epithelium. It is known

that a surface coat may exercise a filtration action and thus influence the concentration of substances in the immediate vicinity of the plasma membrane. Binding sites may selectively bind certain ions such as Ca^{2+} or K^+ and render them available for uptake into the cell by pinocytosis and other mechanisms. For the olfactory receptor these fine hair-like filaments may act as a receptive surface, while the cilia may be responsible for motility only, as their microtubular structure suggests. Glees & Spoerri assume that the numerous microvillous processes covered by very fine spines should be considered as receptive structures leading to membrane depolarisation.

The cell body is small and almost filled by the nucleus, while the basal pole is continuous with the axon, forming with many others bundles of non-myelinated olfactory nerve fibres. These olfactory nerve fibres (many millions) pass through the holes of the cribriform plate and synapse with the glomeruli – the dendritic expansions of mitral cells (Figs 11.3 and 11.4) of the olfactory bulb lying closely applied to the cribriform plate. The axons of the mitral cells,

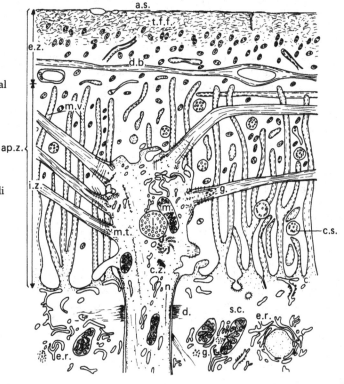

Fig. 11.2. Drawing from an electron micrograph of the upper part of an olfactory cell, the sensory (receptive) pole, showing the emergence of sensory hairs. Most distal branches are embedded in a terminal fluid film (after Andres, 1969). ap.z. = apical zone; a.s. = air space; c. = cysterne; c.z. = central zone; transverse section through cilium; d. = desmosomes; d.b. = distal branches; e.r. = endoplasmic reticulum budding from outer nuclear membrane; e.z. = external zone; g. = glycogen granules; i.z. = internal zone; l. = lysomes; m. = mitochondrion; mt. = microtubules of sensory hairs; mv. = microvilli of supporting cells; s.c. = supporting cell; t.f.f. = terminal fluid film.

having received up to 20000 fibres, convey via the olfactory tract the impulses to the basal olfactory centres below the frontal lobes.

The first receiving and distributing station is the olfactory bulb, from where the medial and lateral olfactory roots pass to the anterior olfactory nucleus, the pre-pyriform cortex, olfactory tubercle, the medial nucleus of the amygdaloid complex and to the entorhinal cortex. The hippocampal cortex – usually considered also to receive olfactory input – has apparently no direct olfactory connection, but by being a part of the limbic system receives olfactory input indirectly in conjunction with emotional and instinctive behaviour. Furthermore, the hippocampus receives other sensory input, e.g. visual, auditory and tactile.

Evolutionary significance of olfaction

It is of general interest that the olfactory bulb is, from the evolutionary point of view, a part of the forebrain and its main sensory input. This should in itself be a sufficient reason to provide olfactory input also to the 'improved version' of the forebrain, the telencephalon, deriving from the cortical plate (Fig. 2.32). However, this step has not taken place;

although olfactory input remained an important external signal, it contributed nothing to neocortical telencephalic input. The main reason must be that the sense of smell contributed nothing to topographical insight of the external world, in contrast to the precision of vision, and is informative both day and night. Although an animal is directed to the source of a smell, its diffuse way of being conducted by wind or water current does not permit a definite external parameter. It is characteristic that animals with a strong sense of smell proceed with their nose 'glued' to the ground, while vision encourages upright gait, gaining a bigger action radius.

The neurons engaged in the elaboration of smell are, however, capable of supplying highly specialised

Fig. 11.3. Wiring diagram of primary olfactory connections. Arrows indicate the directions of impulse conduction (after Ramón y Cajal, 1928).
A = bipolar olfactory cells; B = lateral olfactory tract; C = olfactory part of anterior commissure.

Fig. 11.4. Section through the olfactory bulb of a young cat. (Golgi stain, after Ramón y Cajal, 1928.) The afferent olfactory terminations and dendrites of mitral cells are drawn separately, while in reality these neural branches form intimate synaptic contacts and the mitral dendrites and olfactory terminations together make up an olfactory glomerulus.
A = glomerular layer; B = outer plexiform layer; C = mitral cell layer; D = inner plexiform layer; E = granular layer and fibre layer; 1, 2 = glomerular part of olfactory terminations; 3 = dendritic part of mitral terminals; 4 = brush-like cells; 5 = mitral cells; 6 = branches of mitral cell axon (inner granular layer); 7 = axon of a brush-like cell; 8 = recurrent collateral of a mitral cell axon; 9 = granule cells.

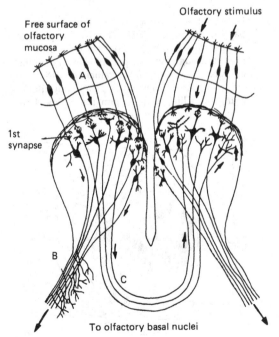

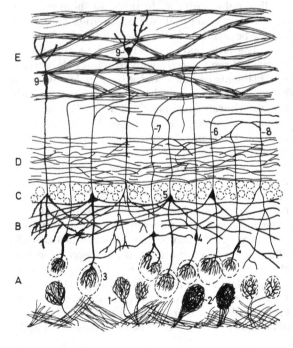

information of the external world and information is stored on olfaction of events far back. In fact, certain childhood events are recalled by smells only. All this should remind the reader that the relatively simple neuronal chains occurring in the olfactory pathways have great significance for our mental life in spite of the fact that none of the olfactory centres has the refined structure of the neocortex.

Psychologists and some industrial enterprises have attempted to classify smells into four fundamental qualities – musk, sour, burnt, and sweaty – and some modern perfumes are said to combine all four of them. Other classifications include mercaptan and the smell of violets. However, the judgement on olfactory properties depends on personality, sex and the phase of a sexual cycle, when sensitivity is either enhanced or a particular quality rejected. The failure to smell anything at all is associated with a cold or a destruction of the receptors due to long periods in extremely dry air. Increased sensitivity occurs in drug-induced states, while misjudgements of odoriferous substances are typical for schizophrenics or hysterical persons. Olfactory hallucinations are said to occur with tumours of the base of the brain.

Taste

The sense of taste is, like smell, chemically mediated. The substance has to be dissolved in the mucous fluid of the oral cavity to be carried to the taste buds. The separation of the senses of taste and smell is rather artificial. In principle, both are very similar if not identical, for odoriferous substances have to be dissolved in the nasal fluid.

The taste buds (Fig. 11.5) are an assembly of specialised sensory cells, with an apical pole carrying fine filaments or hairs, and a basal pole enveloped by nerve terminals, which not only convey the taste sensation but also maintain the 'integrity' of the receptor (if a taste nerve, e.g. the glossopharyngeal, is cut, the taste buds atrophy and regenerate when nerve fibres return (Guth, 1957, 1958)).

It is not only the glossopharyngeal nerve (IX) that contributes to the innervation of taste but also branches of cranial nerves VII and X (Fig. 9.35). Four basic taste qualities have been put forward: acid, salt, bitter and sweet. Unfortunately, or fortunately in view of dietary considerations, these qualities have no definite relation to chemical structure – sugar and saccharin both taste sweet but are chemically unrelated. The problem arises as to whether the taste is being sensed by chemical reaction with the receptor membrane of the taste hairs or whether the configuration of the molecule is decisive. The taste buds have special

distributions and locations on the tongue's surface. Bitter receptors are situated in the posterior third of the tongue, sweet taste in the tip, and salt and sour in between. The most conspicuous taste receptors, the circumvallate papillae, are located between the anterior two-thirds and the posterior third of the tongue.

Regarding taste sensation, the most important message it seems to convey is whether a given tasted substance is good and nourishing or harmful and therefore metabolically not advisable to eat. The desire for particular food or spicing may be a sign of the lack of a special substance. Some people find even small salt concentrations repulsive, while others seem to need large quantities, depending on the kidney's ability to retain salt. Surprising too is the change in taste and consequently in diet during pregnancy, when a woman may demand in large quantities certain foods usually found objectionable.

The nerve supply from the taste buds reaches the brain in the case of VII via the geniculate ganglion and chorda tympani, in the case of IX from the circumvallate papillae via the petrosal ganglion, in the case of X via a vagal ganglion. These fibres are collected for central distribution in the tractus solitarius and are received by the nucleus tractus solitarius (Figs 9.8 and 9.9). From this medullary nucleus taste information is sent up to the arcuate nucleus of the thalamus and to the primary sensory cortex in the depth of the Sylvian fissure.

Fig. 11.5. Section through a taste bud (circumvillate papilla) (from Glees, 1971). The taste receptors are elongated cells with apical sensory hairs which project through the taste pore (gustatory opening, g.o.). Nerve supply is from cranial nerve IX.
c.n.f. = cutaneous nerve fibre penetrating epithelial lining; l.e. = lingual epithelium; n.f. = nerve fibre of IX nerve; rep.c. = replacement cell.

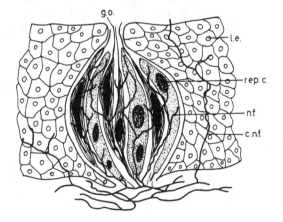

12
The auditory system

Structure and developmental origin

The auditory apparatus is composed of three separate and distinct divisions. First, the outer ear and auditory meatus, which are both ectodermal in origin; these lead to the tympanic membrane or eardrum. The middle ear, the second division, develops chiefly from the first pharyngeal pouch, as does the Eustachian tube, the passage which joins the pharynx to the middle ear. The lateral wall of the middle ear is formed by the tympanic membrane, and the medial wall contains two apertures, the fenestra ovalis and the fenestra rotunda, each also covered by a membrane. Within this second division are the three auditory ossicles – malleus (hammer), incus (anvil) and stapes (stirrup) – formed from the cartilages of the first and second pharyngeal arches. The process of the malleus (the 'handle') is fixed to the tympanic membrane and the head fits into the joint cavity of the incus. The incus has two processes, one fixed to the posterior wall of the inner ear and the other, a longer process, which articulates with the process of the stapes. The base of the stapes enlarges and forms a plate which is inserted into the fenestra ovalis, covering the entire membrane. The ossicles with their processes, therefore, together constitute a mechanical connection between the outer and the inner ear (Fig. 12.1).

Fig. 12.2. Longitudinal section through the mesencephalon and rhombencephalon of a 5 mm embryo to show the developing inner ear (from Glees, 1961a). *M* = mesencephalon; *mes* = mesoderm; *O* = otic vesicle; *Rh* = rhombencephalon; *IV* = fourth ventricle.

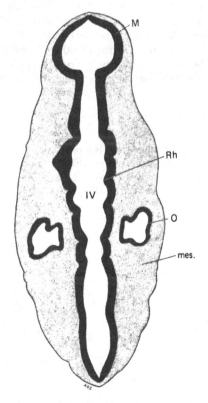

Fig. 12.1. Overview of the auditory and vestibular receptors (from Glees, 1971). 1 = auricle; 2 = cartilages in outer meatus; 3 = outer auditory meatus; 4 = bony part of meatus; 5 = tympanic membrane; 6 = bony capsule of middle ear; 7 = malleus; 8 = incus; 9 = stapes; 10 = semicircular canal; 11 = vestibular nerve; 12 = auditory nerve; 13 = cochlea; 14 = eustachian tube.

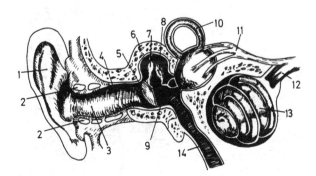

The receiving station

The final anatomical division of the auditory apparatus, the inner ear, consists of cochlea, semicircular canals, utricle and saccule, of which only the cochlea is primarily concerned with the *reception of auditory impulses*. This develops from the auditory placode, an ectodermal thickening, the otocyst (Fig. 12.2), which grows down into the underlying mesoderm near the rhombencephalon and there forms the cochlear duct, a spiral hollow tube of cells which by then has lost all connection with ectoderm (Fig. 12.3). In the lateral wall of the duct is the area vasculosa, the source of the endolymph with which the duct is filled (as are the utricle, saccule and semicircular canals). Two other ducts containing perilymph develop from mesenchyme, and they follow the same spiral course on either side of the cochlear duct, on the dorsal side the scala vestibuli, on the ventral side the scala tympani (Fig. 12.3). They join each other at the apex and at the base both lead to the middle ear, the scala tympani separated from it by the membrane of the fenestra ovalis, the scala vestibuli by the membrane of the fenestra rotunda. The dorsal wall of the fully developed cochlear duct, known as Reissner's membrane, is extremely thin, but the ventral wall, the basilar membrane, is somewhat thicker and from it a number of sensory cells protrude into the duct (Figs 12.4 and 12.5). This layer of cells spirals up the cochlear duct, in Man its total length is 33.5 mm and it contains anything from 15 000 to 24 000 cells. The cells themselves are of two types, though both types have a number of filaments which stick out from the receptor pole of the cell and are the reason for

the name 'hair cell' for sensory cells of the inner ear (Fig. 12.5). By far the greater number of them (12 000–20 000) have round nuclei and as many as a hundred filaments each (Wüstenfeldt, 1957), these are the outer hair cells, that is, those which are furthest from the cochlear nerve and they are arranged in parallel columns of approximately 3400 cells, the number of columns dropping from four to three from the base to the apex of the duct. The inner hair cells, with oval nuclei and both fewer and shorter filaments, are contained in a single column. Both types of hair cell are cylindrical in shape with the nucleus near the basal end, which in the outer hair cells is rounded and in the inner cells an irregular shape. The end of the hair within the cell is thinner than the protruding part, which has a protoplasmic sheath enveloping the filament. The region of the cell between the nucleus and the upper cuticle contains a number of mitochondria and – in the outer hair cells only – a larger structure known as the Hensen body, which seems to alter its shape when the cells are exposed to intense sounds (Engström & Wersäll, 1958); below the nucleus are a number of small round granules.

The hair cells are sandwiched between the basilar membrane and a further membrane, the tectorial membrane (Fig. 12.6), a gel-like structure similar to the membranes that cover the sensory cells of the semicircular canals. The light microscope shows the tectorial membrane to be fibrillated, and it has been suggested that the tectorial fibrils join the filaments of the hair cells; but with the electron microscope no

Fig. 12.3. The cochlea of a three month human embryo, cut at different levels (from Glees, 1961a). The outline of the duct is shown black to indicate its origin from the otic vesicle (see Fig. 12.2). The scala vestibuli and scala tympani are well developed. *g* = spiral ganglion.

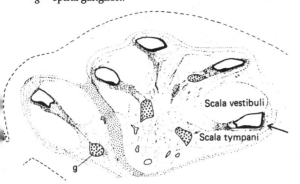

Fig. 12.4. Larger scale diagram of the portion of the cochlear duct indicated by the arrow in Fig. 12.3 (from Glees, 1961a). The developing organ of Corti is very clearly seen. Note the thickening of the wall and the appearance of the tectorial membrane (*M.t.*); the upper wall remains thin. *R.m.* = Reissner's membrane.

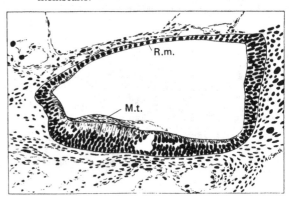

sign of fibrils can be seen, which makes this method of junction between sensory cell and membrane less likely (Engström & Wersäll, 1958). It is, however, assumed that the hairs are embedded in, or at least in contact with, the tectorial membrane. This cannot,

of course, be easily established in the living animal, and the fixation and dehydration necessary for histological preparation may grossly distort the actual relationship between hairs and membrane because of the gel-like consistency of the membrane. However,

Fig. 12.5. Diagram (after Retzius, 1884) of a section through the organ of Corti. (*a*) The basal turn. (*b*) The apical turn. Note the difference in width between the two turns of the cochlear duct. Fibres of the spiral ligament (*L*) continue into the basilar membrane (*M*). *m.t.* = tectorial membrane; *n.f.* = nerve fibres.

(*c*) Diagram (after Ramón y Cajal, 1952) of the developing cochlea of the mouse showing nerve fibres (*n.f.*) supplying three outer hair cells (*O.hc.*) and one inner hair cell (*I.hc.*). *G.* = vessel; *M.b.* = basilar membrane; *M.t.* = tectorial membrane.

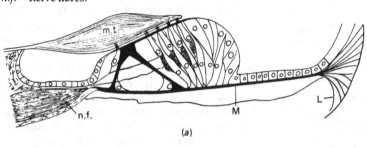

(*a*)

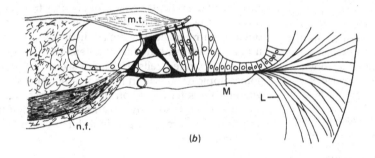

(*b*)

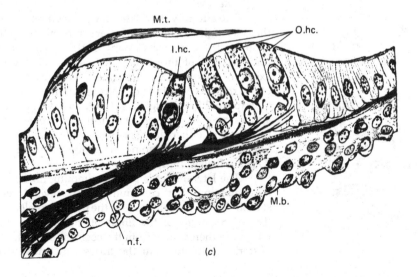

(*c*)

instantaneous freezing of the cochlea in liquid air and the use of phase contrast, a procedure which avoids dehydration and staining, has shown that the sensory hairs are firmly attached to the tectorial membrane (de Vries, 1949).

The basilar membrane, tectorial membrane and the sensory hair cells, together with a number of supporting (Deiters) cells, form the organ of Corti (Fig. 12.6), the mechanism for transforming the sound waves into electrical activity which ultimately reaches the brain, the connection being made initially by the peripheral processes of cells of the spiral ganglion which terminate round the basal pole of the hair cells. These processes start with a myelin sheath but this disappears as they approach the hair cells. At this point the fibres run through a groove in the Deiters cells, which in this respect correspond to the Schwann cells surrounding the peripheral nerve fibres. The Deiters cells are packed close around the basal end of the hair cells, leaving only small gaps through which the fibres can reach the sensory cells. A number of fibres end under or around each hair cell in large terminal swellings (Fig. 12.6) which, like all true synaptic terminal swellings, contain a large number of mitochondria. Although the nerve endings make contact with the thin plasma membrane of the hair cell, they do not fuse with it, for their own plasma membrane maintains its integrity. The spiral ganglion cells lie in the modiolus, the central bony column round which the cochlear duct spirals, and they probably derive from the neural crest. The central processes of these cells terminate on the dorsal and ventral cochlear nuclei in the medulla, which develop from the rhomboencephalon (Fig. 12.6). The most important fibre influx to the dorsal nucleus is naturally from the cochlear nerve, but other afferent fibres also terminate there from the reticular system or possibly from higher levels of the CNS. The dorsal nucleus is laminated but the ventral nucleus, which is distinctly subdivided into a postero-ventral and an antero-ventral portion, contains scattered cells, but there seems to be some somatotopic organisation in the manner in which the afferent fibres terminate on the cells of each nucleus and the neurons sensitive to auditory stimuli of high and low pitch are arranged in a dorso-ventral plane (Rose *et al.*, 1959).

The lateral fillet

The auditory impulses, having been relayed by the cells of the cochlear nuclei, are transmitted by the axons of these neurons. Many of these cross at the midline, and of those that cross some (chiefly the axons from the dorsal nucleus) are relayed by the cells of the trapezoid body and the connection is resumed by trapezoid fibres (Fig. 12.10). All, however, crossed and uncrossed, relayed and unrelayed, eventually form part of either the ipsilateral or the contralateral fillet, where they join spino-thalamic and other fibres (Glees & Bailey, 1951).

The lateral fillet is peculiar among fibre tracts in containing, but continuing past, several relay stations before it finally ends in the posterior colliculus (Fig. 12.6). Some of the fibres of the fillet are thus relayed in their course from the cochlear nuclei to the posterior colliculus, but the fibres which take over

Fig. 12.6. Diagram of the auditory pathway (from Glees, 1961a). A – The pathway and its terminations. The cochlear nerve (c.n.) enters the medulla terminating in the dorsal cochlear nucleus (d.c.n.) and ventral cochlear nucleus (v.c.n.). These nuclei send their axons across the midline, collectively called the trapezoid body. Some fibres terminate in the superior olivary nucleus (s.o.), others in the nucleus of the lateral lemniscus (n.l.l.). Cranially, lateral lemniscus fibres terminate in the inferior colliculus (i.c.) or the opposite inferior colliculus. Via the inferior brachium (i.br. linking the inferior colliculus with the medial geniculate body), the rest of the lateral lemniscus fibres terminate in the medial geniculate body (m.g.b.), whose neurons send out the auditory radiation (aud.r.), and the auditory cortex (aud.c.). B – The receptor units = organ of Corti. i.h.c. = internal hair cell; D.s.c. = Deiters supporting cell; e.h.c. = external hair cell; m.t. = membrana tectoria. C – Cross-section through the cochlea. c.d. = cochlear duct; sp.g. = ganglionic spiral; sc.v. = scala vestibuli; sc.t. = scala tympani. D – Position of the auditory cortex in the human brain.

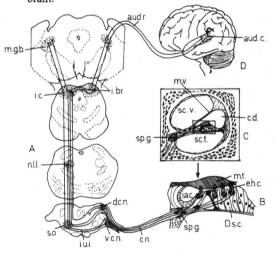

transmission continue along the same tract. The extent of this intermediate relay differs in different species. The cat, for instance, has not only very numerous nerve cells in the trapezoid body but a superior olive equal in size to the inferior olive, where the relay of fibres in the lateral fillet is extensive; in man the superior olive is very poorly developed. At the upper pontine level there is again a relay station, the nucleus of the lateral fillet. The lateral fillet ends at the posterior colliculus, and here is another point of decussation, the connection with the medial geniculate body being completed by the brachium inferior (Fig. 12.6). Although some auditory impulses may reach the posterior colliculus without being relayed, it is unlikely that any auditory fibres run direct to the medial geniculate body; in Marchi preparations there is no sign of degeneration, which suggests a connection to the medial fillet when the trapezoid body has been severed (Glees, 1944).

Medial geniculate body and auditory cortex

The medial geniculate body lies between the midbrain and the thalamus, dorso-lateral to and close by the cerebral peduncle, and it is the final relay station for both contralateral and ipsilateral auditory impulses before they reach the auditory cortex. This is its most important afferent connection, and fibres from the medial geniculate body (known as the auditory radiation (Fig. 12.6) of Flechsig) pass through the posterior limb of the internal capsule behind and beneath the basal ganglia to reach the auditory cortex, which is a small portion of the temporal lobe. In lower mammals it is on the surface of the brain, in monkeys it is buried in the Sylvian fissure, and the human auditory cortex (the gyrus transversalis of Heschl) runs transversely from the superior temporal gyrus to the insula, which is in the depths of the vertebral cortex (Fig. 12.6). The primary auditory cortex in Man is, in Brodmann's terms, Area 41; the neighbouring region, Area 42, is thought to be an association area for auditory impulses. Area 41 is composed of very small nerve cells, particularly layer IV which is a thick granular layer, and this is the reason for its third name of 'coniocortex'.

The cochlea is projected on to the auditory cortex in frequency bands and is thus represented several times. An early neurophysiological finding of this multiple representation is shown in Fig. 12.7. It is from a dog's temporal lobe where the auditory cortex is fully exposed to the surface, while in primates and Man it is hidden in the depth of the Sylvian fissure.

The auditory cortex of different animals can be located by neurophysiological means; the simplest technique is the click response giving a short auditory stimulus and leading the evoked potential from the surface of the cortex. More refined microelectrode recording and stimulating with pure tones have revealed a very detailed mode of sound projections, but the older method of evoked potentials still has its value in clinical testing, as it can be done from the scalp of patients without causing any injury. In a similar way the evoked potential method is used for other sensory input to the cerebral cortex such as after optic stimulation, tactile or simple peripheral nerve stimulation (see Fig. 7.20).

The most important auditory for Man is of course the human language and much time in early infancy is devoted for learning this means of communication. The pattern of the language can be studied with the help of an oscilloscope which shows a complex pattern of periodic and aperiodic waves. The aperiodic part is caused by consonants, while noise too gives an aperiodic and irregular sound pattern.

The capacity for hearing is measured by using an audiometer, producing pure tones of different frequencies, whose volume can be finely adjusted. It is the rule that older persons, particularly men, have a *deafness* for high pitch, essentially for understanding of language; this is probably due to wear and tear of cochlear receptor cells and is referred to as nerve deafness in contrast to conduction deafness caused

Fig. 12.7. Projection areas of auditory impulses of varying frequencies (Hz) in the cerebral cortex of the dog (from Glees, 1971). c.g. = coronary gyrus; c.s. = cruciate sulcus (motor area); e.g. = ecto-Sylvian gyrus; o.g. = orbital gyrus; P.L. = pyriform lobe and olfactory tract; S.f. = Sylvian fissure; S.g. = Sylvian gyrus; s.g. = sigmoid gyrus; s.s. = supra-Sylvian gyrus.

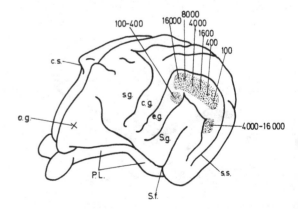

by blockage in the outer or middle ear. In addition the sound energy can be measured; the lowest degree of intensity which we can hear is $2 \times 10^{-9} N/m^2$. Sound is measured in decibels (dB): a whisper is usually 20 dB, normal speech 50–70 dB, and thunder 110 dB, while a low-passing jet reaches 120 dB, a painful and excessive noise. The source of a sound is localised using the difference in the time the sound reaches the left and right ears and the ensuing phase differences. Turning the head can help sound location. This fact becomes painfully clear when with progressing age one side receives sound less well and the person cannot locate the whereabouts of a caller.

Equilibrium: the vestibular organ

The significance of the sense of equilibrium (or balance) has been made abundantly clear to everyone by space science and the state of weightlessness. The relevant sensory apparatus is stimulated by gravity in relation to the prevailing gravitational field. This means that the acceleration is perceived intensely when leaving the earth's gravitational field. The subsequent loss when outside this force and coming back

to earth, readjustment to these previously lost sensory messages recorded again by the disused vestibular apparatus is most difficult and takes considerable time. Orientation in space without vision and movements such as upright gait (posture) are dependent upon vestibular information, and the hook-up of auxilliary structures to this information service is very considerable.

The sensors are situated in the dilatations of the semicircular canals – the ampullae, utricle and saccules. The three semicircular canals are orientated in the parameters of three-dimensional space and their sensory parts are supplied by the divisions of the vestibular ganglia (Fig. 12.8). The sensory cells in these five units are mechanoreceptors and, like the auditory receptors, have a series of sterociliae and kinociliae, which are embedded in a gel-like substance (Fig. 12.9). The kinociliae seen ultrastructurally consist of a ring of nine filaments with two centrally placed filaments. These sensory cells are mounted on an elevation of the epithelial covering of the internal surface of an ampulla, called a crista, while the ciliae and the covering gel are called the cupula. The cupula responds

Fig. 12.8. A diagrammatic representation of the vestibular receptor, consisting of three semicircular canals, superior, lateral (horizontal) and posterior. The receptive units are located in dilatations referred to as ampullae. Further receptors are present in the utriculus and sacculus (from Glees, 1971).
1 = superior semicircular canal; 2 = lateral semicircular canal; 3 = ampulla; 4 = vestibular ganglia; 5 = superior portion; 6 = inferior part; 6a = vestibular nerve branches; 7 = cochlear nerve; 8 = spiral ganglion cells; 9 = cochlear duct (stretches out); 10 = macula (location of sense organs); 11 = ampulla; 12 = posterior semicircular canal; 13 = endolymphatic sac; 14 = utricle; 15 = saccule.

Fig. 12.9. Diagram of the vestibular receptors, serving rotatory acceleration which arise from the crisa ampullaris (from Glees, 1971). c.a. = cupula ampullaris; e.c.s. = epithelial cells covering semicircular canals; m.n.f. = myelinated nerve fibres from vestibular ganglion which receive and conduct impulses from the sensory cells; s.c. = sensory cells; s.h. = sensory hairs.

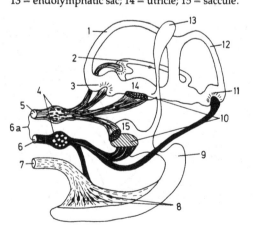

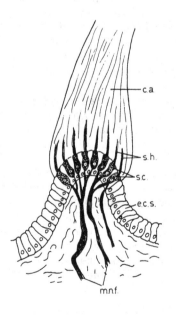

by bending to acceleration, steady rotation and deceleration which cause movements of the fluid inside the canals. The transducing of mechanical distortion energy into electrical impulses is done by the sensory cells in conjunction with the terminations of the vestibular nerve fibres at the base of the sensory or hair cell. The vestibular sensory cells discharge while at rest, thus providing a background discharge for future mechanically caused stimulation, which means any change in the body position in relation to the gravitational forces will find alert sensory cells.

On account of its mechanoreceptors the vestibular organ is eminently suited to regulating muscle tone. Indeed the whole of the switchboard arrangement for vestibular input serves muscle adjustments in relation to gravity, achieving appropriate posture when accelerating or decelerating forces act. In astronauts, when gravitational force is excluded from muscle tone, not only are vestibular influences limited or put out of action but other mechanoreceptors in the joints are disturbed. The tonus-enhancing influence of vestibular impulses is normally expressed in extensor muscle tone, for the extensors are responsible for man's upright gait and by this overcome gravity. The vestibular neurons for this task are located in the caudal part of the brainstem, the lateral vestibular nucleus

and its descending spinal tract (Fig. 12.10). The other vestibular nuclei send their information to the cerebellum, the vestibulocerebellar tract; further contributions enter the medial longitudinal fasciculus for brainstem and spinal cord neurons (Fig. 12.11). These vestibular impulses coordinate neck and head movements with eye movements and trunk turning. The dominant influence of vestibular impulses on eye movements is clearly demonstrated when a subject seated in a rotary chair fixes an object. When the chair rotates the subject at first keeps looking in a direction opposite to the rotation until he loses the object; the eyes then jerk back and follow the direction of rotation to regain object fixation. This is called nystagmus. If such eye-rolling occurs in a non-experimental setting it is a sign of disease. Nystagmus is referred to as left or right to denote the direction of eye movement following head turning.

Finally, some reference to evolution must be made for the reader will wonder why hearing and

Fig. 12.11. Connections of the vestibular nuclei with eye muscle nuclei ascending via the medial longitudinal bundle (7), in a horizontal view. The cerebellum has been removed and the floor of the fourth ventricle lies open (from Glees, 1971). 1 = superior vestibular nucleus; 2 = lateral vestibular nucleus; 3 = vestibular root fibres and ganglion; 4 = interstitial vestibular nucleus; 5 = inferior vestibular nucleus; 6 = medial vestibular nucleus; 7 = medial longitudinal bundle; 8 = vestibular spinal tract in transverse section; 9 = secondary vestibulo-cerebellar fibres; 10 = middle cerebellar peduncle; 11 = abducens nucleus; 12 = trochlear nucleus; 13 = oculomotor nucleus; 14 = thalamus.

Fig. 12.10. Diagram of transverse section through the pons, showing terminations of vestibular afferent fibres (from Glees, 1971). 1 = dendate nucleus; 2 = ascending vestibular fibres to cerebellum (juxta-restiform body); 3 = inferior cerebellar peduncle; 4 = middle cerebellar peduncle; 5 = vestibular ganglion; 6 = spinal tract of V; 7 = cortico-spinal tract; 8 = medial lemniscus; 9 = lateral lemniscus; 10 = position of superior olive; 11 = medial vestibular nucleus; 12 = lateral vestibular nucleus; 13 = superior vestibular nucleus; 14 = vermis cerebelli; 15 = fastigial nucleus.

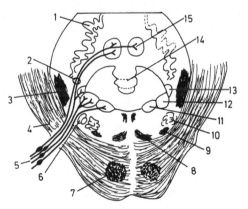

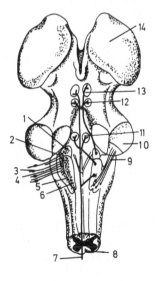

equilibrium sensation are developmentally closely associated and appear as a unit construction from the otocyst or auditory vesicle (Fig. 12.2). The vestibular organ appears first in evolution, while the organ for hearing, the cochlea, is first a small appendix, as 'hearing' in water is to say the least very limited and pressure differences are only those occurring and transmitted in a fluid medium. The perilymph and endolymph take over mechanical pressure oscillation at the level of the oval window. This has to be seen from an evolutionary point of view as the appropriate mode for aquatic animals emerging onto land to change to air conduction. Similarly, cochlear function to start with is similar to that of the vestibular system, i.e. it is coupled with muscular activity. Human babies still respond to sound waves with head and arm movements and beat music is more effective on muscles than on cortical centres.

13
Vision and visual pathways

The eye is Man's most important sense organ and visual input accounts for almost 40% of all incoming fibres to the CNS from the outside world. Light receptors range from dermal receptors or pigment spots, enabling at least a sensitivity to light, to the enormous variety of eye constructions in insects and vertebrates (Duke-Elder, 1958). Light sensitivity ranges from simple awareness of dark and light to using light as an image producer of outside events. One could compare this range with that between a simple light meter and a camera with a built-in image analyser. The detailed construction of the optic apparatus shows great variety in comparative histology: some animals can change the focal distance considerably, while we can only change the shape of the lens by accommodation due to the action of the ciliary muscle. Those mammals living in water, e.g. dolphins, whales and seals, have a further disadvantage as the light intensity decreases

rapidly under water and at a depth of 40 m it is only 1% of the white light incident on the surface. Those dolphins living and hunting at this depth have an atrophic visual sense like other deep-sea animals and have to rely on other mechanisms, e.g. echolocation, for hunting. The evolution of the eye is one of the most exciting chapters in biology and the vast comparative information collected by Duke-Elder (1958) should be consulted. A similarly valuable reference containing most excellent illustrations by Polyak (1957) is highly recommended. In vertebrates, photosensitive cells derive from the neural tube at the level of the diencephalic portions (Fig. 13.1). In fact, the brain turns its cells towards the light and organises the reception of light and the transmission of the elicited energy sequences.

Light is an ideal medium for gaining information quickly as the speed of light is unsurpassed; this property is made use of in fibre optics. The wavelengths for light reception in the human eye are 400–700 nm (Fig. 13.2). The energy of these electromagnetic waves can be expressed in quanta and is perceived by the receptors of the eye.

The photosensitive cell is a typical example of bipolar differentiation. One pole shows elaborate membranous layer differentiation for light reception while the other pole transmits the signal onto a neuron (Fig. 5.7). The whole eye is an elaboration on this basic

Fig. 13.1. Development of the retina from the optic vesicle of the forebrain (from Glees, 1961a).
(a) Emergence of the optic vesicle (opt.v.). l.pl. = lens placode; Th = thalamus. (b) Invagination of the optic vesicle. c = cornea; l.v. = lens vesicle; opt.st. = optic stalk. (c) Differentiation of the inner wall of the vesicle into layer of ganglion cells (stippled) and a layer of sensory cells (shaded). The outer wall forms the pigment layer (p.l.). (The surrounding vascular layer and connective tissue coat are not shown.)
f.w. = forebrain wall; l = lens.

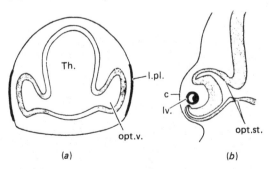

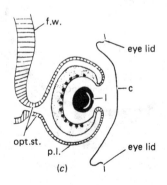

Fig. 13.2. The visible light range occupies only a small part of the total spectrum of electromagnetic radiation (from Glees, 1971).

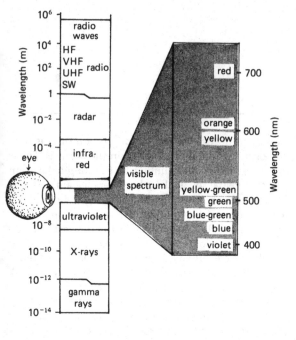

construction of a photosensitive element and a long-distance transmitter, the neuron. Making a technical comparison with a camera, we find the sensory receptor cell is comparable to a photographic plate or film, the camera body is the casing of the retina, and the optic lens and curved cornea show the most important elements of the composite camera lens. The muscles attached to the eyeball keep the eye in a particular position and turn the globe: they are camera stand and movers at the same time.

The retina, however, the assemblage of neurons and photosensitive cells, has the capability of receiving, 'digitalising' and processing the information received by the photosensitive cells. The optic nerve is actually no primitive nerve but a brain tract carrying information of a higher order than would be possible from sensory cells alone.

Fine structure of the retina

The future retina, derived from the embryonic brain wall, divides into several layers; from its innermost layer the photosensitive receptors develop. This in itself is a disadvantage, because the light has to penetrate several cell layers before striking the receptors (Figs 13.3–13.6). In order to achieve maximal resolution a special retinal portion develops, the fovea, arising from the fact that all those cells not engaged in photoreception are pushed to the periphery, allowing the sensory elements more direct light contact (Figs 13.7 and 13.8). The ability of the retina to perceive light was not realised until the neoclassical

Fig. 13.3. Horizontal section through the left eye (from Glees, 1961a). V.A. = visual axis.

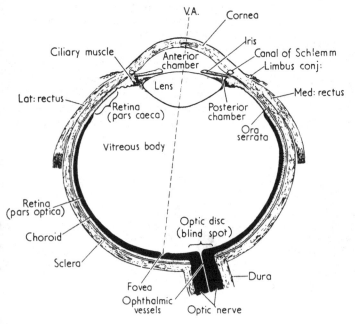

Fig. 13.4. Section through the retina of a rhesus monkey (from Glees, 1961a). On the left can be seen the blind spot (B.S.) where the optic nerve leaves the retina and the layers of the retina are interrupted. The fovea centralis (F.C.) to the right of the section can be seen in Fig. 13.7. B.V. = blood vessels; C = choroid; I = interneurons; O = optic fibres; R = receptor layer; S = sclera.

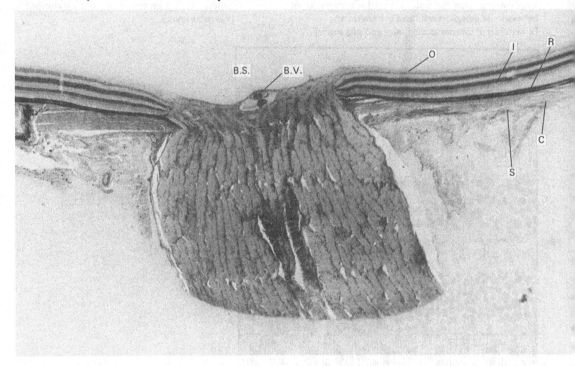

Fig. 13.5. The structure of the retina (from Glees, 1961a). ax = axon; c = cone; d = dendrite; G = layer of ganglion cells; I = layer of interneurons; i.n. = interretinal neuron; O = optic fibres; P = layer of pigment cells; r = rod; R = layer of receptor cells; s.l. = synaptic layers.

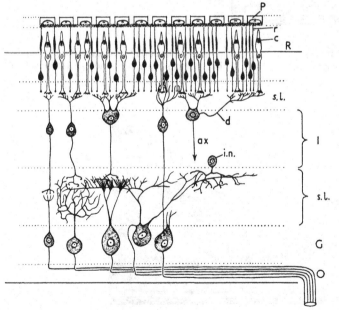

Fig. 13.6. Enlarged diagram of the layers of the retina seen in Fig. 13.4. (500×) (from Glees, 1961a).
I. = nerve fibres forming the optic nerve, plus supporting glia fibres; II = the layer of ganglion cells whose axons form the optic nerve; III = synaptic layer between the ganglion cells and interneurons; IV = nuclei of interneurons (pale) and glia nuclei (dark); V = synaptic layer between rods and cones and interneurons; VI = glia nuclei (dark) and nuclei of rods and cones (pale); VIIa = inner members of rods and cones; VIIb = outer members of rods and cones; VIII = pigment cell layer; IX = choroid (vascular layer).

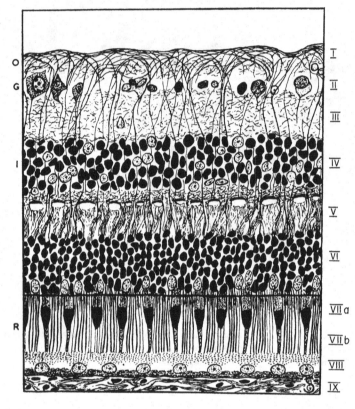

Fig. 13.7. Drawing from a photomicrograph of the fovea (200×) (from Glees, 1961a). The layers of ganglion cells and interneurons are to the sides so that light can reach the cones in the fovea direct.

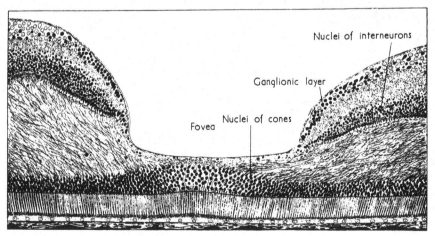

period, by the astronomer Kepler (1571–1630). In 1625 Schreiner removed the posterior coats from an ox eye and showed for the first time, in an early period of experimental biology, that the lens and the cornea produced a reduced and inverted picture of the outside world.

Retinal receptors

Receptors can be subdivided into rods and cones according to their shape. The rods are highly sensitive to light and allow monochromatic vision at low light levels, e.g. in moonlight. The cones respond to different light frequencies and allow colour vision, but they need strong illumination for stimulation. Cones are concentrated in the central part of the retina, especially in the fovea, which is the area of highest resolution. The fovea in Man has a diameter of only 0.1 mm and contains about 2000 cones (Fig. 13.9). The total number of receptors in the human retina amounts to 130 million. Gregory (1966), in his fascinating book on eye and brain, wrote that the total number of cones reached the number of people living in the greater New York area and that the total number of rods approached the total population of North America. This number of rods and cones are assembled on a retina with the area of a postage stamp.

The receptive pole (the outer segment) of the photosensitive cell is essentially a shelf-like system of membranes which are connected by a connecting stalk to the body of the receptor cell (Figs 13.8 and 13.10). Detailed electron microscope studies have revealed that the arrangement of the membranes in rod and cone receptors is different: the cone outer segment consists of a single membrane folded back and forth, forming a concertina-like structure that encloses the intracellular space, while the membrane layers in the rod outer segment are joined together in pairs and form flattened sacs that are called discs (Young, 1978). The stack of discs is enclosed by the

Fig. 13.8. A simplified diagram of the vertebrate retina based on electron microscope studies, emphasising the organizational arrangement of the Müller cells as the main glial component and showing scattered astrocytes (from Glees, 1971). (After Karchin *et al.*, 1986.) g.c.l. = ganglionic cell layer; l.b.c. = layer of bipolar cells; opt.f.l. = optic fibre layer; p.c.l. = pigment cell layer; r.l. = receptor layer; Sl = first synaptic layer; S2 = second synaptic layer; t.exp.M. = terminal expansion of Müller cells, fusing with the basement membrane.

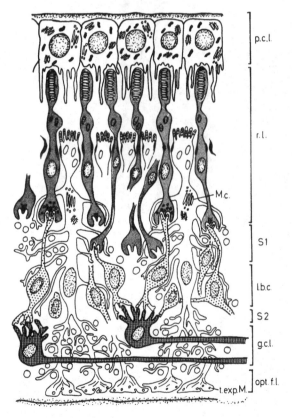

Fig. 13.9. Horizontal sections through the retina of a baboon, showing various levels of the outer members of rods and cones in transverse section. 1. Through the centre of the fovea which contains only cones. 2. 0.5 mm from the centre of the fovea. 3. 1.5 mm from the centre of the fovea. 4. 3 mm from the centre of the fovea. Note that the number of rods increases towards the periphery. (Sections kindly supplied by the late Mr E. H. Leach.)

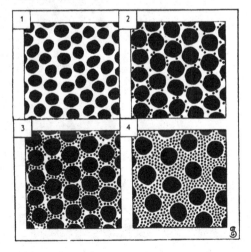

outer cell membrane, and so the outer segment is divided into two kinds of enclosed volume, the intra-disc space and the interdisc space (Fig. 13.10). (In the rhesus monkey, a rod cell contains about 900 discs.)

The photoreceptive proteins, the visual pigments, are embedded in the membranes. The inner segment of the photoreceptive cells contains a large number of mitochondria for the high metabolic demands of the cell (Fig. 13.11). The membrane segments are continuously shed at the distal end and regenerated at the proximal end. Shed membrane segments are slowly degraded by the pigment epithelium (Young, 1978). The rate of disc replacement is very rapid: in the rhesus monkey a new disc is formed every 20 min, and the whole outer segment is replaced every 12 days.

Fig. 13.10. Electron micrograph of the outer light-receptive section of a photoreceptor.

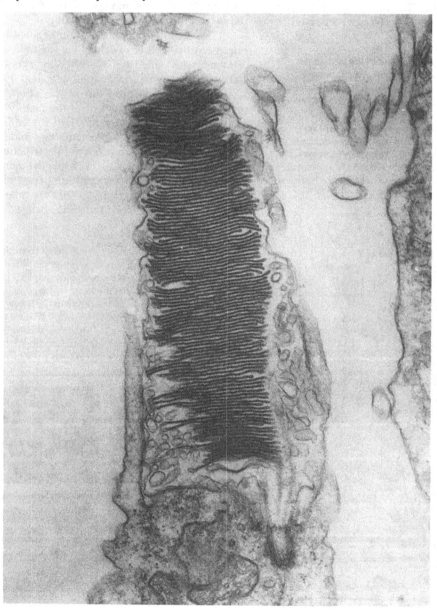

The basal pole of the receptor contains a neuro-transmitter in vesicular structures, many of which are arranged around ribbon-like microtubular structures (Spoerri & Glees, 1977). The neurotransmitter of the photosensitive cell is unknown, but aspartate has been implicated (Thomas & Redburn, 1979).

It is generally accepted that the photoreceptors are modified neurons. The view taken here assumes that the receptors derive from the stem cells of the neural tube. These stem cells may differentiate into neurons, photoreceptive cells or the supporting cells. This view is illustrated in Fig. 13.11 and is supported by electron microscope observations that the receptors develop from ependymal cells. The inner and outer segments of a receptor are connected by a stem containing microfibrils. It may well be that these fibrillary structures are capable of contraction, pulling the outer segment away from the shelter of the pigment cells or extending it into the pigmented shelter in response to variation in light intensity.

Biochemistry of vision

The biochemistry of vision is a fast-growing field, and only a brief summary is attempted here.

Light absorption by the visual pigment causes a change in its chemical structure. The major com-ponent of the visual pigment is a protein molecule of molecular weight about 40000. This protein is asso-ciated with a polyene molecule called retinal. Photon absorption by the visual pigment causes the isomerisa-tion of 11-*trans*-retinal to 11-*cis*-retinal (Wald, 1968). 11-*cis*-retinal cannot bind to the protein, and the com-plex dissociates.

The light-activated visual pigment then diffuses to interact with the protein transducin: one activated visual pigment molecule can activate many transducin molecules. Transducin activation involves the dis-placement of bound GDP (guanosine diphosphate) from transducin by GTP (guanosine triphosphate). The transducin–GTP complex then fragments: the γ- and β-subunits dissociate from the GTP-α-subunit complex. This complex then binds to a cyclic 3',5'-guanosine monophosphate (cGMP) phospho-diesterase to activate the enzyme, and the level of intracellular cGMP falls (Lamb, 1986).

It has been shown that the decrease in cGMP levels precedes the decrease in the 'dark current' in the photoreceptor cells (Cote *et al.*, 1984), and that light causes a cGMP level decrease within 10 ms of the stimulus (Stryer, 1986). This cascade enables the original signal to be greatly amplified: one photon can cause the hydrolysis of 10^5 cGMP molecules (Stryer, 1986). The presence of a multiple-step cascade also means that the transduction process can be regulated at various points in the cascade. It is also interesting to note that this cascade bears great resemblance to the enzymic cascade responsible for the activation of adenylate cyclase by certain hormones and neuro-transmitters.

The rod cells are only capable of monochromatic vision. Colour vision is only possible with cones because the three types of cone cells present in the human retina have different sensitivities to light of different wavelengths. This arises from the different kinds of pigments in different cone cells. An excellent review on colour vision has been written by Mollon (1982).

The visual world

The threshold of vision depends on the type of receptor activated. For scotopic vision, that is, monochromatic vision in very dim light, only the rods are activated, since rods have a lower threshold than cones. In strong light, the cone cells are activated and colour vision is possible. The visible electromagnetic spectrum for vision is a comparatively narrow band (400–700 nm), and each type of receptor is maximally activated at a characteristic wavelength.

The fact that it has proved to be possible, in

Fig. 13.11. Cellular differentiation of retinal cells from a common matrix cell. (After Meller, 1968.)
a.p. = axonic pole; d. = desmosome; d.p. = dendritic pole; e.r. = endoplasmic reticulum; g.c. = ganglion cell; m. = mitochondrion; m.c. = matrix cell; M.c. = Müller cell; m.e. = mitochondria in 'mitochondrial bag'; n. = nucleus; p. = receptor pedicle; R = photoreceptor; rib. = ribosomes; r.p. = receptor pole; s.p. = synaptic pole.

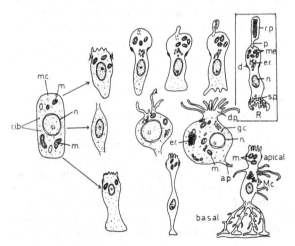

favourable conditions, to see an ordinary lighted candle at a distance of 27 km (Pirenne, 1948) is evidence of the low threshold of scotopic vision; the faintest star discernible from the earth has a brilliance of a mere 10^{-14} times that of the sun. The receptors which respond to these low intensities of light lie 20 degrees away from the centre of the fovea. Indeed the fovea, although it has the sharpest focus, is virtually blind to faint lights for it contains only cones, and an attempt to focus the eye on a faint star only has the result of banishing it from sight.

It is the amount of light energy to reach the receptor within the first millisecond that counts (Hecht *et al.*, 1942); there will be a summation of the stimulation effect for 0.1 s but not thereafter. Within this limit, therefore, a light stimulus of a certain intensity lasting 0.03 s will have the same effect as one 100 times stronger lasting 0.0003 s (Pirenne, 1948).

The intensity of the light stimulus may be expressed in physical terms as the number of particles or quanta of energy produced by the source of light. It was Planck's quantum theory of light which first focused attention on the importance of the energy particles produced by the source of light rather than on the wavelength which carries the particles from that source to the eye. Some of this energy will, of course, be absorbed by the cornea before it reaches the retina and as little as 10% of the energy which strikes the cornea may penetrate to the retinal receptors (Marriott *et al.*, 1959). The lowest estimation of the number of quanta that this 10% must contain to produce a sensation of light is five, though probably more are required. Less will no doubt produce some effect on the rod but not necessarily reach the threshold for vision (Baumgardt, 1952). The fact that the visual receptors are more sensitive to shorter wavelengths is explained by the greater number of quanta carried by shorter wavelengths, and the necessary five quanta then reach the rods in less time.

Pirenne (1953, 1956) assumed that one quantum would affect one molecule of the photosensitive substance (rhodopsin) contained in the rods, and that to reach the threshold of vision about ten separate quanta must attack molecules in a number of rods. The effect of summation might then be achieved by a build-up of the chemical reaction within a rod, or it might be neurophysiological and concern the convergence of a number of rods on one ganglion cell, a possibility which will be explored in more detail later in this chapter.

The commonly expressed opinion that light sensitivity is related to the amount of light energy which reaches the receptors of the eye is certainly valid, but the calculation of the exact threshold of the receptors in terms of numbers of quanta is not such a simple matter. A purely biophysical analysis of receptor function can be of great importance if related to a rigid experimental setting or confined to very simple systems, but the capacity of any living material to adapt to constantly changing conditions brings with it a continuous variation in the level of excitation, particularly in the more complex nervous systems of mammals, and this can only undermine the significance of any absolute estimation of receptor thresholds. The threshold of visual receptors, like that of auditory receptors, may also be influenced by central connections from the cortex. The retina is in itself an extremely labile system which can be triggered off by factors other than light: a rise in temperature causes a condition of heightened sensitivity which may require the addition of only one quantum of energy to produce light sensation. Johannes Müller, the eminent nineteenth-century German physiologist, made a special study of extraneous factors which have this effect (see Ebbecke, 1951): the sensation of light produced by pressure on a dark-adapted eye, and the coloured patterns seen when the eyes are shut, which are probably the result of spontaneous discharges initiated by the kinetic energy of the blood in the capillary bed of the retina. The ganglion cells of the retina are known to discharge spontaneously even in complete darkness, an activity which varies in degree from one region of the retina to another but is constant except when depressed by anaesthetic drugs such as barbituric acid. This suggests that the neuronal components of the retina can also be activated in the absence of light stimuli (Kuffler, 1952).

The task of the eye is obviously more than that of an exposure meter, telling day from night. The main task is the recognition of objects in space, their motion and their exact location, and further the awareness of colour. The three-dimensional distribution of objects in space (the depth in space) is a further improvement in seeing the world. The combination of the world of touch and hearing with the world of vision is a highly complex early experience in childhood and deserves a separate evaluation which has recently been made by Robinson & Petersen (1985).

The visual pathway (optic nerve and tract)

The axons of the ganglion cells of the retina are the fibres of the optic tract, which forms the first lap of the visual pathway. At the optic chiasma some of the fibres decussate, and the number of fibres which do so will vary according to the species. In animals with panoramic vision, whole eyes being placed on either side of the head must work independently and decussation appears to be complete. The number of uncrossed fibres increases with the increase in overlap of the two fields of vision and with the development of binocular (stereoscopic) vision. Thus the rabbit is believed to have few uncrossed fibres, in the cat about one third of the total number cross, and in Man and monkey about half cross. The pathway has been extensively studied using HRP degeneration techniques in the cat. (Wässle, 1982, 1984; Karchin *et al.*, 1986).

The retinal cells of the cat project to the lateral geniculate body and to the superior colliculus; 30% of all retinal cells project to both relay stations (e.g. all large α cells of the retina). Small densely arborising β cells project to the lateral geniculate but 10% of the cells send collaterals to the superior colliculus. All γ cells send their axons to the superior colliculus and half of the cells also to the lateral geniculate (Wässle, 1984).

In Man and animals with any degree of stereoscopic vision an object on the left is recorded on the right half of each retina and projected onto the visual cortex of the right hemisphere. It is the fibres from the right or nasal half of the left retina which must decussate before they reach the cortex to converge with those from the corresponding half of the right retina. The reverse procedure occurs with objects on the right. Thus, it is the fibres from the nasal half of both retinae which cross at the optic chiasma, those from the temporal half are the uncrossed fibres. The division between the nasal and temporal portions runs through the middle of the fovea.

This arrangement admirably suits the relaying of impulses initiated by the mirror reception of the visual image in the retina and the integration of the two visual images, which in animals with stereoscopic vision will be approximately the same. The complete optic decussation in animals with panoramic vision has never been satisfactorily explained and seems to have no very obvious reason.

The lateral geniculate body

One of the interesting features of the lateral geniculate body is the manner in which the optic fibres terminate there after the point of decussation in the optic chiasma. The lateral geniculate body consists of a number of layers of cells, and the anatomical evidence is that the crossed and uncrossed fibres terminate separately in different layers. The transneuronal degeneration which follows the cutting of optic fibres is indirect proof of this, for the layer of post-synaptic geniculate cells which is affected depends on the

crossed or uncrossed route of the optic fibres (Minkowski, 1913). An examination of terminal degeneration in the monkey gives a more exact picture of the synaptic connections in the lateral geniculate body (Glees, 1940, 1958a,b; Glees & Le Gros Clark, 1941; Glees, 1961b; Beresford, 1963; Glees *et al.*, 1966a; Glees *et al.*, 1966b; Glees & Neuhoff, 1967; Campos-Ortega *et al.*, 1968; Hubel & Wiesel, 1977).

The visual cortex

In the cat, rabbit and monkey the visual cortex (or striate cortex, so-called because of its histological structure) lies on the surface of the brain. In the monkey it covers a vast area of the dorsal, lateral, and medial surface of the occipital lobe, but in man it is comparatively small – limited to the medial surface with only a small extension towards the posterior tip of the lobe – and partly hidden in the calcarine fissure, the earliest fissure to develop in the human foetus. A comparison of the surface area of the visual cortex and the size of the retina shows that the 'enlargement' of the image will be considerable. Polyak (1957) puts the ratio at 1:7 (retina $350\,mm^2$, visual cortex $2613\,mm^2$). Illuminating an area of the monkey's fovea (0.005 mm radius) Talbot & Marshall (1941) recorded potential changes in the visual cortex over a region with a radius of 0.5 mm, i.e. an area 10 000 times the size. Stimulation of the half fovea projecting onto one hemisphere affects an area 6 mm in radius near the lunate sulcus of the visual cortex. The study of occipital lobe injuries sustained in World War I indicated that the human fovea projects to the posterior extremities of the visual cortex. The remainder of the visual cortex is connected with the peripheral regions of the retina, which are comparatively larger than the fovea, and therefore the enlargement is bound to be on a lesser scale. In this way the visual cortex receives a detailed spatial projection from the retina, in particular from the fovea. The lateral geniculate cells send their axons to pyramidal cells of layer IV of the visual cortex (Figs 13.2 and 13.13). These cells project in turn onto cells of layer III. The primary receiving cells in layer IV are referred to by neurophysiologists as S cells (simple cells) and react maximally to lines of contrast and illuminated beams in a particular orientation briefly illuminated or moved slowly in the visual field. Their receptive fields are small and very small in the foveal Area 17, assuring by this a high degree of visual resolution and sensitivity to colour. Area 17 contains complex cells (C cells) which have large receptive fields mainly in layer V on account of greater afferent convergence. All C cells react in all regions of their receptive fields with a short ON and OFF activity according to Creutzfeldt (1983) who should be consulted for further details.

The neurons responsible for visual orientation are located in strategic cell columns (orientated columns) arranged vertically in relation to the cortical surface. The primary visual cortex receives the input from both retinal halves, still separated at geniculate body level and kept separate in layer IV. This can be proved by injecting radioactive leucine into the retina which is transported by the visual pathway to the corresponding layers of the geniculate body and from here transneuronally to separate small regions of layer IV, producing a very characteristic picture of alternate markings. As mentioned above, the S cells receive input from one eye only, but 50% of the C cells are influenced by both eyes.

The cells situated in layers III and V are excited by both eyes but to a varying degree. Depending on the degree of firing by the ipsi- and contralateral eyes, a number of ocular dominance cell columns can be discriminated. The distribution of binocular and monocular neurons responsible for ocular dominance of cells and cell columns can be studied not only by neurophysiological but also by morphological methods and was shown admirably by LeVay *et al.* (1975). Hubel & Wiesel (1979) have drawn attention to the importance of normal vision soon after birth to achieve a normal and well arranged visual cortex. It appears that the number and the arrangement of effective synapses depend on early and normal usage. If this is delayed, irreparable damage is done to orientation in space and power of resolution. Early training, certainly where motor skill is involved, produces its best results when started in infancy, perhaps explaining the existance of child prodigies in music or chess when supervised by a strict taskmaster very early on in life.

The peristriate cortices

Having discussed the primary visual cortex, Area 17, the cortical areas surrounding this primary

Fig. 13.12. The visual pathway in relation to the visual fields and to the more important clinical signs of lesions (from Glees, 1961a). The fovea of the eyes converge on the common fixation point (f.p.) and the visual fields can be divided into a left binocular and monocular field of vision, and a right binocular and monocular field. The optic nerves, carrying the signals from these fields, decussate partially in the chiasma in such a way that the optic tracts are composed of corresponding or homonymous visual field fibres emerging in the left eye from the medial retinal half and from the right eye in the lateral retinal half. Each optic tract terminates in the lateral geniculate body of its side and by a medial division, drawn in black, in the pretectal region. This region is connected with midbrain neurons (Edinger Westphal nucleus) serving pupillary reflexes via the ciliary ganglion (c.g.) a parasympathetic ganglion whose postganglionic fibres (p.g.) innervate the constrictor pupillae muscle. The lateral geniculate body sends its axons (collectively called the optic radiation), passing close by the ventricle (v), to the primary visual cortex (area 17). Lesions: I. severance of one optic nerve causes blindness in the relevant eye; II. chiasmatic destruction causes bitemporal blindness or hemianopia; III. right homonymous hemianopia; IV. optic radiation injury, right homonymous hemianopia, no pupillary change. ch. = chiasma; c.p. = cerebral peduncle; F. = fovea; L.G.B. = lateral geniculate body; M.G.B. = medial geniculate body; o.n. = oculomotor nerve; P. = pulvinar; P.B. = pineal body; pt.a. = pretectal area; r.n. = red nucleus; v. = ventricle; v.c. = visual cortex; v.r. = visual radiation.

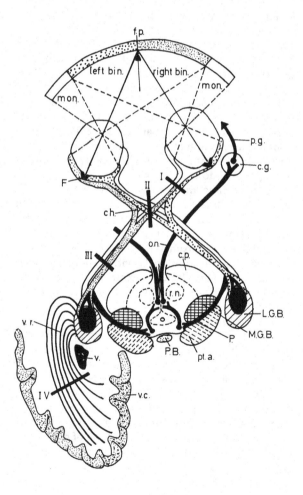

striate area have to be considered. Although Area 17 is the primary visual centre or V1, Area 18 (V2) and Area 19 (V3) also contribute to visual awareness. In V2 a complete visual field is represented, while V3 receives visual inputs. V2 and V3 get their information from the primary visual cortex (V1) and have no direct connection with the lateral geniculate body, which receives a return input from Area 17 (Beresford, 1963). The peristriate cortical areas can be termed 'associative' in relation to Area 17, receiving associative connections from Area 17 and having interconnections among themselves. Similarly, temporal lobe Areas 20, 21 and 22 take part in visual processing of information, not in reference to retinal fields or coordinates but in a higher order of visually related activity.

Clinical considerations

The connection between the two hemispheres via the corpus callosum seems to have a real value in visual coordination, the first definite indication of the true function of the corpus callosum. This has been shown very strikingly by the results of a series of experiments undertaken by Sperry, Stamm & Miner (1956). By cutting the optic chiasma in cats they destroyed all the crossed fibres so that each hemisphere received impulses from one eye only. The cats were then trained to perform various visual tests with one eye masked and therefore with one hemisphere inactive. When they were presented with the same problems with the other eye covered, their performance in the test was equally good, which can only be explained on the assumption that what had been learned could be transferred across the brain by some established link. That this link is the corpus callosum they further proved by destroying the corpus callosum as well as the optic chiasma, which had the effect of making each eye and hemisphere entirely independent, and what was learned with one could not be

Fig. 13.13. A simplified diagram of the basic cortical visual pathway, indicating the general synaptic stations. a = photoreceptor; b = bipolar cell; c = ganglion cell; d = large cell of lateral geniculate body (l.g.b.); e = cortical cell, layer IV; h = illuminated rod, moving in visual field, triggering those cells which record movement; s.1 = special ribbon-like synapses; s.2 = synapse between bipolar cell and ganglion cell; s.3 = retinal synapses in l.g.b.; s.4 = synapses of terminating fibre from l.g.b.; f = synapses of non-visual origin; g. = glomerular synapses. 1 = depolarising potential of the receptor; 2 = action potential bursts in optic nerve; 3 = evolved visual potential; 4 = EEG potentials, eyes-closed rhythm when interrupted; 5 = action potentials from cortical cells when triggered by visual stimuli. d.p. = dendritic process; o.n. = optic nerve; v.c. = visual cortex (monkey).

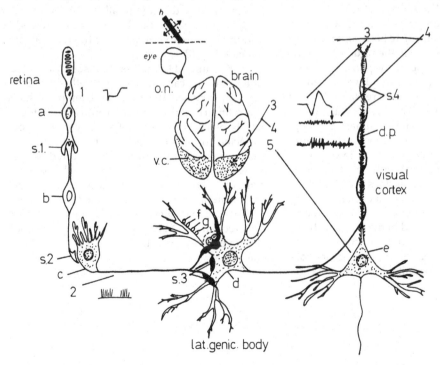

lat.genic. body

practised with the other. Much the same results were obtained by Downer (1959) in the monkey. Destruction of both the corpus callosum and the optic chiasma meant that movements initiated by one motor cortex could be visually guided only by the ipsilateral eye, although of course the limb controlled by that motor cortex would be the contralateral one.

Some parts of the corpus callosum appear to be more vital to this coordinating function than others, as Myers (1956b, 1959) discovered by destroying not the whole structure but either the anterior or posterior regions. The link between the visual cortices of each hemisphere was damaged by any interference with the corpus callosum, most seriously when the posterior half was destroyed.

Provided the corpus callosum remained intact, removal of the visual cortex in the hemisphere which the cats had been using in their one-eyed training did not abolish all their ability to perform tests on subsequent occasions with the hitherto untrained eye, although the more complicated tests proved beyond their capacity (Myers & Sperry, 1958).

Interocular transfer in experiments of this kind seems to require a previous normal use of binocular vision, as Chow & Nissen (1955) found when they tested six infant chimpanzees. These animals, kept in the dark from the age of 10 days except for periods of training one eye, showed little ability to perform the test with the untrained eye, although they learned the test more quickly with that eye.

In birds, reptiles and amphibians, who have only a very small lateral geniculate body and no visual cortex, the main visual centre is the optic lobe of the midbrain, where there is a point-for-point projection of the retina (Gaze, 1958). With the development of the cortex in mammals an ever-increasing share of the control of conscious visual function is taken over by the visual cortex, but in some mammals (cat, dog, rabbit) the superior colliculus or tectum opticum, which corresponds to the optic lobe in lower vertebrates, has not lost this function entirely. To remove the occipital lobe in these animals does not blind them totally, for with renewed training after operation they can again estimate degrees of illumination and recognise familiar objects. In Man and in the monkey, however, the superior colliculus is only concerned in the reflex visual pathway and has no significance for conscious vision, loss of the occipital lobes means complete and permanent blindness (Bürgi, 1957).

The various effects which bilateral removal of the occipital lobes has on the monkey's behaviour have been studied in great detail by Klüver (1942) with a variety of tests. A monkey blinded in this way at first crashes about in its cage but it soon manages to rely on touch, smell, and hearing to live a superficially normal existence in familiar surroundings. A strong light may evoke some sort of startle reaction but this is less likely to be due to the projection of rod vision via the superior colliculus than to the transmission of retinal impulses to the reticular formation. The monkey may close its eyes in response to a strong light and the pupils will contact (both reflex responses); on the other hand, a sudden movement close to its eyes does not make it blink, for it is presumably unaware that any such movement has taken place. Finally, the fact that Klüver found that his animals did not seem to notice any difference between the lighted and dark compartments of their cages suggests that the influence of vision on their behaviour was nonexistent.

The removal of one occipital lobe or a lesion in the optic tract above the level of the optic decussation will, of course, affect the sight of both eyes. The resulting half-blindness is called 'homonymous hemianopia', for the side of the retina put out of action is the same in both eyes. A tumour of the hypophysis, on the other hand, causes heteronymous, binasal, hemianopia by destroying all the fibres which cross in the optic chiasma but leaving the uncrossed fibres and thus the temporal halves of the retina unaffected (consult Fig. 13.12).

Bitemporal blindness is caused by an aneurysm of the internal carotid artery on both sides. Since the division between the nasal and temporal halves of the retina runs through the centre of the fovea, the effects of hemianopia is of whatever sort would be expected to extend over half the fovea (Fig. 13.12). Instances have, however, been reported of complete foveal vision even when one occipital lobe is entirely removed. Attempts have been made to explain this by a bilateral representation of the fovea on the visual cortex, but the effects of such operations as hemispherectomy in Man do not give any evidence that the fovea is less drastically attacked than the rest of the retina.

14
Touch, pain and proprioception

Touch (pressure) receptors

The human hand is especially well provided with touch receptors. For this reason the hand is the most direct information gatherer from the outside world that the brain has at its disposal. One might argue whether vision is more important but watching a blind person 'reading' Braille with his finger tips one must agree that touch can compensate. The tips of our fingers contain specialised nerve endings, the touch corpuscles of Meissner and Merkel mediating exploratory touch. Meissner's corpuscles appear to be encapsulated unmyelinated branches of several nerve fibres (Fig. 14.1) positioned close to the surface (Fig. 14.2) while Merkel's bodies or discs are situated more deeply and in very intimate contact with large epithelial cells.

Skin hairs are highly sensitive receptors, for around their roots a complex basket of nerve fibres can be found (Fig. 14.3) registering movements of the hair, while the hairshaft acts as an amplifier. Many animals use their hairs, such as whiskers, as highly sensitive indicators of air movements or to measure the size of an opening to see if they can pass through; some of these sensory hairs are surrounded by a blood sinus at their base, and thus suspended in fluid to be more sensitive. The connective tissue of the skin contains very refined sensory corpuscles, the Vater–Paccini laminar corpuscles (Fig. 14.4). They respond to pressure changes and vibrations and also occur in retroperitoneal spaces and in the mesentery. In this location they mediate intra-abdominal pressure changes and changes in intestinal blood pressure.

Fig. 14.1. A Meissner corpuscle, after Glees silver impregnation, showing the malpighian layer of the epidermis (m.l.). One to three nerve fibres (n.f.) can form a Meissner corpuscle which has a capsule (c.) formed by Schwann and neurial cells.

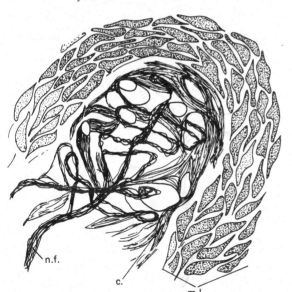

Fig. 14.2. Finger pad skin from a 3-year-old child after Glees silver impregnation. A = Meissner corpuscle; B = discs of Merkel; C = free nerve (pain, temperature); f.n.e. = free nerve ending; Str.c. = stratum corneum; Str.l. = stratum lucidum; Str.m. = stratum malpighii.

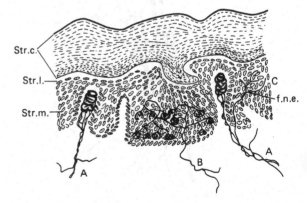

Pain and temperature

It is generally assumed that pain is subserved by free nerve endings – 'free' because they have no ensheathing cells such as Meissner or Merkel corpuscles (Fig. 14.5). Head and Rivers, two eminent Cambridge physiologists of the last century, called the perception of such an uncomplicated sensation as pain 'protopathic', to contrast it with the 'epicritic' perception of the more highly developed encapsulated receptors which have properties of greater discrimination. This division was based on Head's observation of the sensory disturbances causes by the deliberate section of a cutaneous nerve in his own arm. Pain was the first sensation to return after regeneration of the nerve, and it persisted when the sense of touch returned later. The idea later proved to be ill-founded, but the work of Head and Rivers did break new ground and acted as a spur to further research.

The free nerve endings may react directly to the stimulus, or the damage to the tissue may set up some chemical stimulus which involves the response of some bioelectrical mechanism (Breig, 1953). Most experiments on pain sensation have been based on a human subject's response to needle pricks. By recording the degree of muscle contraction caused by

cutaneous pain, Breig (1953, 1955) gained some more objective results which enabled him to study the summation of pain impulses and to make a comparison of pain sensation with other types of sensation. He recorded the contraction which occurred when a painful stimulus was drawn across an area of skin in a

Fig. 14.4. A Vater–Paccini laminar body, mediating pressure and tension. Such bodies are present in the subcutis of the palm of the hand and the sole of the foot and in the abdominal cavity. i.c. = inner core (area of nerve terminals); m. = myelinated nerve fibre.

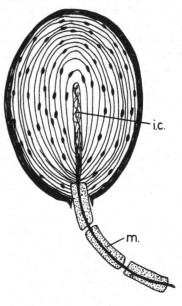

Fig. 14.3. Innervation of a hair. b. = bulbous part of hair; c. = corium; e. = epidermis; e.p. = erector pili muscle; h. = hair shaft; n.f. = nerve fibre; r.sh = root sheath; s.c. = subcutis; s.g. = sebaceous gland.

Fig. 14.5. Free nerve ending. m.sh. = myelin sheath; n.R. = node of Ranvier.

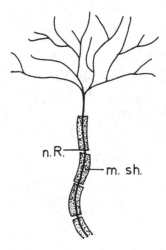

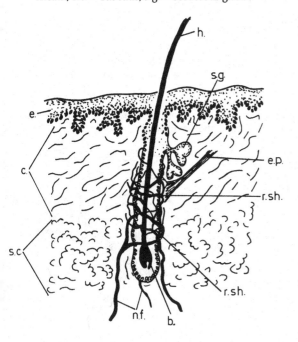

straight line, and he found that the contractions increased as the area stimulated was lengthened. (An example of a cutaneo-muscular reflex involved is the cremateric reflex when stimulation of the medial surface of the thigh results in an upward movement of the testis.)

The most puzzling feature of receptor function lies in the sensitivity to warmth and cold, or, more precisely, whether there are specific temperature receptors and, if so, what they are. The examination of 'warm' and 'cold' spots in the skin seemed a likely way of finding out but the results were soon found to be unpromising. Donaldson (1885) found no specific endings in the cold and warm spots in sections of his own arm and leg, nor could Goldscheider (1886) discover any special endings. Dallenbach (1927) examined the warm spots of his arm and then cut them out (this he did without anaesthetic in order not to damage the histological structure), but even methylene blue stain, usually specific for demonstrating end organs, failed to show any structures which might be special temperature receptors; haematoxylin and eosin, which stains most organised structures, also failed in this respect (Pendleton, 1928).

It was the discovery of the Krause and Ruffini endings and their possible connections with temperature which was responsible for a general change of opinion which held sway until recently. Studies on corneal sensitivity suggested that Krause or Ruffini endings were temperature receptors (Strugnold & Karbe, 1925). The fact that the nipple, for instance, is very sensitive to cold and that many Krause endings are to be found there has been taken as proof of their function as cold receptors; a close connection between the distribution of warm spots and that of Ruffini endings in the prepuce was found by Bazett, McGlone, Williams and Lufkin (Bazett *et al.*, 1932; Bazett, 1941). Weddell reported in 1941 the observation of a group of Krause end bulbs below a cold spot under the arm but has since changed his views, for the actual existence of Krause end bulbs is doubtful – it is possible for an oblique or cross-section through a Meissner corpuscle to be mistaken for a Krause end bulb, and more modern neurohistological methods suggest that they are no more than artifacts (Weddell *et al.*, 1955; Oppenheimer *et al.*, 1958).

Since temperature receptors respond primarily to changes in body temperature, or rather skin temperature, it would be reasonable to look for them near blood vessels or within the vascular wall, as temperature is maintained chiefly by the vascular system. In 1886 Goldscheider expressed his view that the blood vessels might themselves record temperature changes, and von Frey (1895, in Weddell *et al.*, 1955), when testing the sensitivity of the conjunctiva – which unlike the cornea is vascularised – found that the position of cold spots seemed to have a definite relationship to blood vessels.

Nafe (1934) studied the sensations produced by warm and cold stimuli; whereas ordinary physical thermometers record degrees of heat unrelated to any normal level, skin sensitivity to temperature has a starting point or baseline at about 32.5–33.5 °C, which is the average normal temperature of human skin. Temperatures above this are recorded as increased warmth and those below as increased cold. Up to 45 °C the sensation is one of warmth, above this degree the sensation becomes a mixture of heat and pressure, and around 52 °C this is followed by pain. At temperatures below 32 °C we start to feel cool and then progressively colder, at about 12 °C the sensation is pressure and pain, and at lower temperatures pain. The sensation produced by extreme cold and extreme heat, or by extreme variation from the normal, are therefore qualitatively similar. This suggests that cold and warmth are recorded by the same mechanism. Nafe concludes that the mechanism is the vascular system, believing vasoconstriction to be the process essential for the arousal of cold and vasodilation to be the process essential for warmth. But his views of thermal perception have not remained uncriticised; Jenkins (1938) summarised the evidence against them, particularly the fact inherent in Kastorf's observation that warmth stimuli applied at intervals of 0.1 s were perceived as single stimuli (Kastorf, 1920): Jenkins regarded it as improbable that the smooth musculature of the vessel wall could react so rapidly. (For the reply to this criticism see Nafe, 1938.)

Thermal sensation in Man has been studied for some considerable time, one of the early theorists on this subject being Weber (1834, in Weddell *et al.*, 1955). He considered that our sensitivity to warmth and cold was a single sense and quotes the common experience that if one hand is adapted to warm water and the other to cold, water of skin temperature will thereafter feel warm to the cold hand and cold to the warm hand.

Animal experiments with the possibility of more physiological procedures and more objective results began only when electrodes came into use and were in fact made possible by the work of E. D. Adrian & Zotterman (see Adrian, 1928). Zotterman and his colleagues in Sweden concentrated on the study of thermal sensation (see Hensel & Zotterman, 1951), stimulating the tongue of the cat with a punctate thermode and recording from fine strands of the lingual nerve. Their views were at variance with Nafe's,

Fig. 14.6. Simplified diagram of the central portion of a muscle spindle which in this instance is supplied by two thick sensory nerve fibres winding around two muscle fibres. The thicker fibre shows a nuclear bag surrounded by a nerve fibre of group I afferent fibres; the thinner fibre receives a branch of the Ia fibre and another thin fibre of group II. The motor supplies of the spindle muscle fibres are located distally from the central area drawn here.

c. = capsule; m. = myelinated nerves; p.t. = primary termination; s.p. = secondary portion.

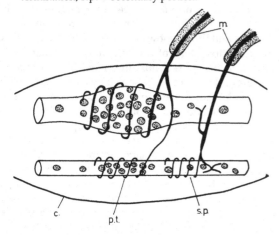

although they did not discuss his in detail, possibly due to the difficulty of comparing results achieved in such widely different settings. The main point of difference is whether there are separate receptors for warmth and for cold. Hensel & Zotterman maintained that there were not only separate types of receptor but that the afferent fibres of warmth receptors were of larger calibre than those of cold receptors. The two receptors, however, have much in common, e.g. both have a steady discharge rate at temperatures between 20 and 40 °C. Recordings made from single cold fibres showed the response of cold receptors to intracutaneous temperature gradients. At a constant temperature the discharge rate of a cold fibre was approximately 10 impulses per second, rising to approximately 140 with rapid cooling; if the new temperature was maintained the frequency dropped again to the original 10 per second. A warmth receptor reacts in the same way, the frequency rising from the steady discharge rate with increases of temperature. However, a warm stimulus applied to a cold receptor will decrease the rate of discharge, as will a cold stimulus applied to a warmth receptor (dependent on the rate of change and the height of the rise in temperature). This is some indication of the probability of separate receptors for cold and warmth. Bernhard & Granit

Fig. 14.7. A dissected muscle spindle (after Bridgemann, 1962, personal gift).

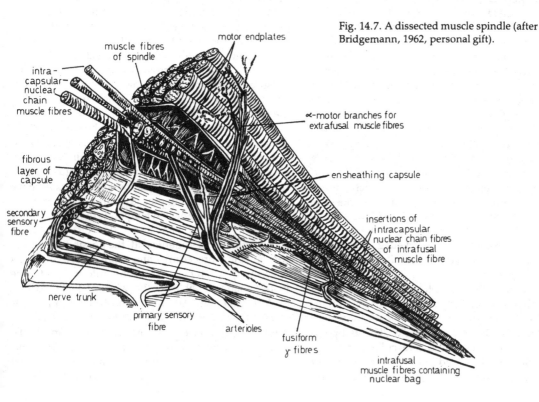

Fig. 14.8. Receptor connections with the sensory cortex (sc) seen in a basic diagram. The left part of the diagram illustrates from below the medulla seen from above, a frontal section of the thalamus and a frontal section of the sensory cerebral cortex areas 3,1,2 of Brodmann (see Fig. 7.13). The right part shows receptors in the skin, superficial and deep and joint receptors. The afferent signals reach in the case of the arm via the posterior roots the posterior column nucleus of Burdach or cuneate nucleus, whose axons cross the midline and ascent as medial lemniscusar fillet, terminating in the posterior vental nucleus of the thalamus. From there the afferent thalamic fibres reach the sensory cortex via the internal capsule. sc = sensory cortex; cc = corpus callosum; m.l. = medial lemniscus or bulbo-thalamic tract; m.p.c. = medial posterior column tract (Goll); l.p.c. = lateral posterior column tract (Burdach); c sp.g. = cervical spinal ganglion; sh.j. = shoulder joint; V.P. = Vater-Pacinian body; sk = skin; h = hair innervation; d.m.n. = dorso-medial nucleus; p.l.n. = posterior lateral nucleus; p.v.n. posterior ventral nucleus; c.m. = centrum medianum; s.c.p. = superior cerebellar peduncle; i.c. = internal capsule; B.n. = nucleus of Burdach or cuneate nucleus; 1–6 = layers of cerebral cortex.

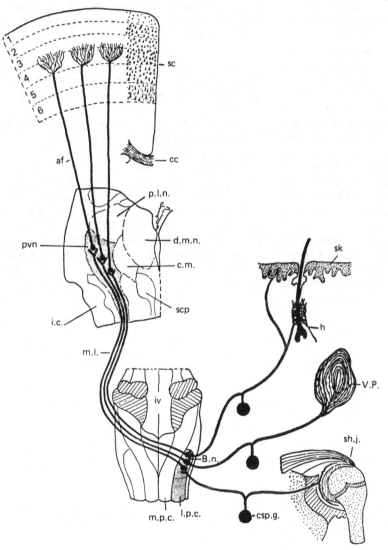

(1945), on the other hand, found that both cold and warmth produced changes in the potential in the same mammalian nerve, but, certainly in Man, the sensation produced by the stimulation of a cold receptor will be one of cold, though the stimulus may be warm, and similarly a warmth receptor always produces the sensation of warmth. This is the phenomenon of paradoxical sensation. Cold objects often feel heavier than warm ones: Hensel & Zotterman (1951) have recorded large spikes in the same nerve, initiated by rapid cooling and by pressure. The response to cooling by these mechanoreceptive fibres disappears after some time while the cold receptors maintain their discharge.

The evidence for specific receptors for warmth and cold is too weak to be accepted as conclusive, nor indeed is it established that there are any receptors which are exclusively concerned with temperature perception, for differences in temperature are felt in sections of skin in which our present methods show no specific endings. There is, however, a likelihood that the free nerve endings, so far discussed in connection with pain, are also concerned with temperature (see Ranson, 1911). The fact that extremes of temperature are felt as pain would supply a connection between two apparently unconnected sensations, and the vascular wall, together with the free nerve endings, may be sufficient to form an efficient receptor apparatus for temperature as well as for pain. A recent review by Breipohl (1986) should be consulted, dealing with the molecular aspects of temperature transduction. This review considers a concept of membrane oscillation, the basis for a dynamic response of cold-sensitive thermoreceptors and the role of Ca^{2+} for the sensation of heat.

Muscle and joint receptors

Striated (voluntary) muscles harbour sense organs built in parallel with the muscle fibres and recording the degree of muscle stretch. On account of their general shape these sensors have been called muscle spindles (Fig. 14.6). The spindle is a kind of bag containing thin muscle fibres which are fixed at either end; the state of contraction, or 'tone', is regulated by fine motor fibres. Larger sensory fibres wind around these thin muscle fibres (Figs 14.6 and 14.7). These sensory fibres report to relevant spinal cord levels the degree of stretch of the spindle if the main muscle is elongated and thereby help to regulate the stretch reflex. The muscle fibres of the spindle are contracted or relaxed by their own motor innervation, which means that the spindle can be adjusted to meet the desired degree of the main muscle contraction, regulating posture.

The connecting pathways from Pacinian bodies and muscle spindles reach the sensory cortex and the cerebellum and provide an accurate background for movements or the position of limb components in relation to the joints involved. In this way we ascertain the position of our limbs in space or in relation to the body axis. As said before skin sensations are exteroceptive, while those from joints and muscles are proprioceptive and the infomation from the intestine is called enteroceptive. A summary of the connections in reference to the upper extremity is illustrated in Fig. 14.8.

REFERENCES

Adrian, E. D. (1928). *The Basis of Sensation*. London: Christophers.

Aidley, D. J. (1978). *The Physiology of Excitable Cells*. Cambridge: Cambridge University Press.

Akert, K. (1963). *Das limbische System und seine funktionelle Bedeutung. Relaxation und Sedation des menschlichen Uterus* (2nd Symposium). Bern: Karger.

Altman, J. (1969a). Autoradiographic and histological studies of postnatal neurogenesis (Part 3). *J. comp. Neurol.*, **136**, 269.

Altman, J. (1969b). Autoradiographic and histological studies of postnatal neurogenesis (Part 4). *J. comp. Neurol.*, **137**, 433.

Altman, J. & Das, G. D. (1964). Postnatal origin of microneurons in the rat brain. *Nature*, **207**, 953.

Altman, J. & Das, G. D. (1965). Autoradiographic and histological evidence of postnatal hippocampal neurogenesis in rats. *J. comp. Neurol.*, **124**, 319.

Andres, K. H. (1969). Der olfaktorische Saum der Katze, *Z. Zellforsch.*, **96**, 250.

Andy, O. J. (1964). Quantitative comparisons of brain structures from insectivores to primates. *Amer. Zool.*, **4**, 59.

Ariens-Kappers, C. U. (1920). *Die vergleichende Anatomie des Nervensystems der Wirbeltiere und des Menschen*. Haarlem: De Erren F. Bohn.

Ariens-Kappers, C. U., Huber, G. C. & Crosby, E. (1936). *The Comparative Anatomy of the Nervous System of Vertebrates including Man*. New York: Hafner.

Auerbach, L. (1898a). Nervenendigungen in den Centralorganen. *Neurol. Zentbl.*, **10**(17), 445.

Auerbach, L. (1898b). *Neurol. Zentbl.*, p. 734.

Barbara, D. A. (1960). *Psychological and Psychiatric Aspects of Speech and Hearing*. Springfield (Ill.): Charles Thomas.

Bargmann, W. (1968). Neurohypophysis: structure and function. In *Handbuch der experimentellen Pharmakologie*, vol. 23: *Neurohypophysial Hormones and Similar Polypeptides*, ed. B. Berde, pp. 1–39. Berlin: Springer.

Bauer, K. F. (1948). Uber die zwischenzellige Organisation des Nervengewebes. *Z. Anat. Entw.*, **114**, 53.

Baumgardt, E. (1952). Sehmechanismus and Quantenstruktur des Lichtes. *Naturwiss.*, **39**, 388.

Bazett, H. G. (1941). Temperature sense in man. In *Temperature, its Measurement and Control in Science and Industry*, p. 489. New York: Reinhold.

Bazett, H. G., McGlone, B., Williams, H. G. & Lufkin, H. M. (1932). Sensation: depth, distribution and probable identification in the prepuce of sensory and organs concerned in sensations of temperature and touch, thermometric conductility. *Archs. Neurol. Psychiat., Chicago*, **27**, 489.

Bennett, H. S. (1963). Morphological aspects of extracellular polysaccharides. *J. Histochem. Cytochem.*, **2**, 14.

Beresford, W. A. (1963). The Anatomical Connections of the Visual Cortex. D.Phil. (Oxon.) thesis.

Berger, H. (1929). Uber das Elektroencephalogramm des Menschen I. *Arch. Psychiat.*, **87**, 527.

Bernhard, C. G. & Granit, R. (1945). Nerve as model temperature and organ. *J. gen. Physiol.*, **29**, 257.

Bernstein, B. (1902). Untersuchungen zur Thermodynamik der bioelektrischen Strome. *Pflügers Arch. ges. Physiol.*, **92**, 521.

Berry, W. B. N. (1968). *Growth of a Pre-historic Time Scale.* San Francisco: W. H. Freeman.

Berry, M. (1974). Development in the cerebral neocortex of the rat. In *Aspects of Neurogenesis*, ed. G. Gottlieb. New York.

Betz, W. (1874). Anatomischer Nachweis zweier Gehirncentra. *Centbl. med. Wiss.*, **12**, 578.

Betz, W. (1881). Uber die feinere Struktur der Grosshirnrinde des Menschen, *Centbl. med. Wiss.*, **19**, 193, 209.

Bhatnagar, A. S. (1983). *The Anterior Pituitary Gland.* New York: Raven Press.

Björklund, A., Segal, M. & Steneri, U. (1979). Functional reinnervation of rat hippocampus by locus coeruleus implants. *Brain Res.*, **170**, 409.

Blinkov, S. M. & Glezer, I. I. (1968). *The Human Brain in Figures and Tables.* New York: Plenum Press.

Blinzinger, W. & Kreutzberg, G. W. (1968). Displacement of synaptic terminals from regenerating motoneurons by microglial cells. *Z. Zellforsch.*, **85**, 145.

Blomquist, A. G. & Lorenzini, C. A. (1965). Projection of dorsal roots and sensory nerves to cortical sensory motor regions of squirrel monkey. *J. Neurophysiol.*, **28**, 1195.

Blum, J. S., Chow, K. L. & Pribram, K. H. (1950). A behavioral analysis of the organisation of the parieto-temporo-preoccipital cortex. *J. comp. Neurol.*, **93**, 53.

Boeke, J. (1935). *Handbuch der Neurologie*, vol. 1. Berlin: Springer.

Boulder Committee (1970). Embryonic vertebrate central nervous system: revised terminology. *Anat. Rec.*, **166**, 257.

Booth, J. *et al.* (1950). See Glees (1961a), p. 119.

Botelho, St Y (1965). Proprioceptive, vestibular and cerebellar mechanisms in the control of movement. *Amer. Physiol. Ther. Assoc.*, **45**, 7.

Brandt, P. W. (1962). A consideration of the extraneous coats of the plasma membrane. *Circulation*, **26**, 1075.

Breig, A. (1953). *Integration linearer kutaner Schmerzreize.* Stuttgart: G. Thieme.

Breipohl, W. (1986). Thermoreceptors. In *Biology of the Integument, Vol. 2 Vertebrates*. Berlin: Springer.

Bremer, F. (1935). Cerveau isolé et physiologie du sommeil. *C.R. Soc. Biol.*, **118**, 1235.

Bremer, F. (1954). The neurophysiological problem of sleep. In: *Brain Mechanisms and Consciousness*. Oxford: Blackwell.

Brightmann, M. W. (1965a). The distribution within the brain of ferritin injected into the cerebrospinal fluid compartments. I Ependymal distribution. *J. Cell. Biol.*, **26**, 99.

Brightmann, M. W. (1965b). The distribution within the brain of ferritin injected into the cerebrospinal fluid compartments II. Parenchymal distribution. *Amer. J. Anat.*, **117**, 193.

Brightmann, M. W. & Reese, T. S. (1969). Junctions between intimately apposed cell membranes in the vertebrate brain. *J. Cell Biol.*, **40**, 648.

Brindley, G. S. (1960). *Physiology of the Retina and Visual Pathway.* London: Edward Arnold.

Brisson, A. & Unwin, P. N. T. (1985). Quaternary structure of the acetylcholine receptor. *Nature*, **315**, 474.

Brizzee, K. R. & Jacobs, L. A. (1959). The glia / neuron index in the submolecular layers of the motor cortex in the cat. *Anat. Rec.*, **134**, 97.

Brizzee, K. R., Vogt, J. & Khartehko, X. (1964). Postnatal changes in glia/neuron index with a comparison of methods of cell enumeration in white rats. *Prog. Brain Res.*, **4**, 136.

Brodal, A. (1948). *Neurological Anatomy in Relation to Clinical Medicine.* Oxford: Clarendon Press.

Brodal, A. (1957). *Reticular Formation of the Brain Stem: Anatomical Aspects and Functional Correlations.* Edinburgh: Oliver & Boyd.

Brodal, A. & Fänge, R. (1963). *The Biology of Myxine.* Oslo: Oslo University Press.

Brodmann, K. (1909). *Vergleichende Lokalisationslehre der Grosshirnrinde Barth.* Leipzig.

Brown, A. G. (1981). *Organisation in the Spinal Cord, the Anatomy and Physiology of Identified Neurons.* Berlin: Springer.

Brownson, R. H. (1960). The effect of X-irradation on the perineuronal satellite cells in the cortex of aging brains. *J. Neuropath. exp. Neurol.*, **19**, 407.

Brysch, I., Creutzfeldt, O. D., Hayes, N. L. & Schlinge, K. H. (1984). The 2nd intralaminar thalamocortical projection system. *Anat. Embryo.*, **169**, 111.

Bürgi, S. (1957). Das Tectum Opticum. Seine Verbindungen bei der Katze und seine Bedeutung beim Menschen. *Deut. Z. Nervenhk.*, **176**, 701.

Burn, J. H. (1967). Release of noradrenaline from the sympathetic postganglionic fibre. *Brit. med. J.*, **5546**, 197.

Bushe, K. A. & Glees, P. (1968). *Chirurgi des Gehirns und des Ruchenmarks im Kindes und Jugendalter.* Stuttgart: Hippokrates.

Butler, J. A. V. (1954). *Inside the Living Cell*, p. 58. London: Allen & Unwin.

Cammermeyer, J. (1970). The life history of the microglia cell: a light microscopic study. *Neurosci. Res.*, **3**, 44.

Campbell, G. & Lieberman, A. R. (1979). Presynaptic dendrites in the olivary pretectal nucleus of the albino rat. *J. Anat.*, **129**, 863.

Campos-Ortega, J. A., Glees, P. & Neuhoff, V. (1968).

Ultrastructural analysis of individual layers in the lateral geniculate body of the monkey. *Z. Zellforsch.*, **87**, 82.

Carlton, M. & Welt, C. (1980). Somatic-sensory cortex (SM1) of the pro-simian primates, *Galago crassicaudatus*. Organisation of mechanoreceptor input from the hand in relation to cytoarchitecture. *J. comp. Neurol.*, **189**, 249.

Carpenter, R. H. S. (1984). *Neurophysiology*. London: Edward Arnold.

Choi, J. K. (1963). The fine structure of the urinary bladder of the toad, *Bufo marinus*. *J. Cell Biol.*, **16**, 53.

Chomsky, N. (1969). *The Acquisition of Syntax in Children from Five to Ten*. Cambridge (Mass.): MIT Press.

Chow, K. L. & Nissen, H. W. (1955). Interocular transfer of learning in visually naive and experienced infant chimpanzees. *J. comp. Physiol. Psychol.*, **48**, 229.

Chusid, J. G. & McDonald, J. J. (1967). *Correlative Neuroanatomy and Functional Neurology*. Los Altos (Calif.): Lange Medical Publications.

Clark Howell, F. (1966). *Early Man*. London: Time-Life International.

Conrad, K. & Ule, G. (1951). Ein Fall von Korsakow Psychose mit anatomischen Befunden und klinischen Betrachtungen. *Deut. Z. Nervenk.*, **165**, 430.

Continillo, F. A. & Glees, P. (1985). Comparative studies into the distribution and transportation of osmiophilic waste products. *Arch. Biol., Bruxelles*, **96**, 337.

Cooper, J. R., Bloom, F. E. & Roth, R. H. (1978). *The Biochemical Basis of Neuropharmacology*. Oxford: Oxford University Press.

Cote, R. H., Biernbaum, M. S., Nicol, G. D. & Bownds, M. D. (1984). Light-induced decreases in cGMP concentration precede changes in membrane permeability in frog rod photoreceptors. *J. Biol. Chem.*, **259**, 9635.

Creutzfeldt, O. D. (1983). *Cortex cerebri: Leistung, strukturelle und funtionelle Organisation der Hirnrinde*. Berlin: Springer.

Creutzfeldt, O. & Jung, R. (1961). Neuronal discharge in cat's motor cortex during sleep and arousal. In *The Nature of Sleep*, pp. 131–70. London: Ciba.

Creutzfeldt, O. & Struck, G. (1962). Neurophysiologie und Morphologie der chronisch isolierten Cortexinsel der Katze: Hirnpotentiale und Neuronentatigkeit einer isolierten Nervenzellpopulation ohne afferente Fasern. *Arch. Psychiat. Z. ges. Neurol.*, **203**, 708.

Critchley, M. (1953). The Parietal Lobes. Excerpts from review in *Neurology*, vol. 4. New York: Harper.

Dallenbach, K. M. (1927). Dr Fernberger on the range of attention experiment. *Amer. J. Psychol.*, **39**, 479.

Darwin, C. R. (1836). *Zoology of the Voyage of the 'Beagle'*.

Darwin, C. R. (1859). *On the Origin of Species by Means of Natural Selection, or the Preservation of Favoured Races in the Struggle for Life*. London: John Murray.

Davson, H. (1967). *Physiology of the Cerebrospinal Fluid*. Edinburgh: Churchill Livingstone.

Dawnay, N. A. H. & Glees, P. (1986). Somatotopic analysis of fibre and terminal distribution in the primate corticospinal pathway. *Devl. Brain Res.*, **26**, 115.

Day, M. H. (1967). *Guide to Fossil Man* (A Handbook of Human Paleontology). London: Cassell.

De Beer, J. (1964). *Bildatlas der Evolution*. New York: Thomas Nelson.

Deiters, O. (1865). *Untersuchungen uber Gehirn und Ruchenmark des Menschen und der Saugetiere*. Braunschweig.

Dekaban, A. (1959). *Neurology of Infancy*. Baltimore: Williams & Wilkins.

Delgado, J. M. R. (1963). Effect of brain stimulation on task-free situations. *Electroenceph.*, suppl. 24.

De Robertis, E. (1964). *Histophysiology of Synapses and Neurosecretion*. Oxford: Pergamon.

De Robertis, E., Nowinsky, W. W. & Saez, F. A. (1960). *General Cytology*, 3rd edn. London: Saunders.

Desmedt, J. E. (1971). Somatosensory cerebral evoked potentials in man. In: *Handbook of Electro-encephalography and Clinical Neurophysiology*, vol. 9, pp. 55–82, ed. A. S. Rémond. Amsterdam: Elsevier.

de Vries, H. (1949). Struktur und Lage der Tektorialmembran in der Schnecke untersucht mit neueren Hilfsmitteln. *Acta otolaryng., Stockholm*, **7**, 334.

Diamond, I. T. & Hall, W. C. (1969). Evolution of neocortex. *Science*, **164**, 251.

Diamond, M. C., Law, F., Rhodes, H., Linder, B., Rosenzweig, M. K., Krech, D. & Bennett, E. L. (1966). Increases in cortical depths and glia numbers in rats subjected to enriched environment. *J. comp. Neurol.*, **128**, 117.

Dogiel, A. S. (1893a). Zur Frage uber den feineren Bau des sympathischen Nervensystems bei Saugetieren. *Arch. mikrask. Anat.*, **46**, 305.

Dogiel, A. S. (1893b). *Der Bau der Spinalganglien des Menschen und der Säugetiere*. Jena: Gustav Fischer.

Donaldson, H. H. (1885). On the temperature sense. *Mind*, **10**, 399.

Dowdall, M. J. (1981). Nerve terminal sacs from *Torpedo* electron organ: a new preparation for the study of presynaptic cholinergic mechanisms at the molecular level. In *Cholinergic Mechanisms and Psychopharmacology*, p. 359, ed. D. J. Jenden. New York: Plenum.

Downer, J. L. de C (1959). Changes in visually guided behaviour following midsagittal divisions of optic chiasm and corpus callosum in monkey (*Macaca mulatta*). *Brain*, **82**, 251.

Droogleever Fortyn, J. (1960). *The Contributions of Cortex, Telencephalon, Diencephalon and Midbrain to the State of Sleeps and Wakefulness* (11th International Meeting of Neuro-biologists, Amsterdam 1959). Amsterdam: Elsevier.

Duke-Elder, W. St (1958). *System of Ophthalmology*. London: Henry Kimpton.

Duval, M. (1872). *Structure et usages de la rétine*. Paris.

Ebbecke, V. (1951). *Johannes Müller, der gross rheinische Physiologe, mit einem Neudruck von Johannes Müllers Schrift: Über die phantastischen Gesichserscheinungen*. Hannover: Schmorl u. von Seefeld Nachf.

Eccles, J. C. (1953). *The Neurophysiological Basis of Mind*. Oxford: Clarendon Press.

Eccles, J. C. (1968). The development of the cerebellum of vertebrates in relation to the control of movement. *Naturwiss.*, **56**, 525.

Economo, C. von (1929). Schlafttheorie. *Ergebn. Physiol.*, **28**, 312.

Edinger, L. (1904). *Vorlesungen uber den Bau der nervosen Zentralorgane des Menschen und der Tiere.* Leipzig: Vogel.

Edinger, T. (1950). Die Palaeoneurologie am Beginn einer neuen Phase. *Experientia.*, **6**, 250.

Edinger, T. (1955). Hearing and smell in cetacean history. *Mschr. Psychiat. Neurol.*, **129**, 37.

Ehrenberg, C. G. (1834). Beobachtungen einer unbekannten aufbauenden Structur des Seelenorgans bei Menschen und thieren. *Abh. Konigl. Akad. Wiss. Berlin*, 665.

Elliot Smith, G. (1919). The significance of the cerebral cortex (Croonian lectures). *Brit. med. J.*, **758**.

Engström, H. & Wersäll, J. (1958). The ultrastructural organization of the organ of Corti and of the vestibular sensory epithelia. *Exp. Cell Res.*, **5**, 460.

Erlanger, J. & Gasser, N. S. (1937). *Electrical Signs of Nervous Activity.* Philadelphia: University of Pennsylvania Press.

Erlanger, J., Gasser, N. S. & Bishop, G. H. (1924). The compound nature of the action current of nerve as disclosed by the cathode ray oscillograph, *Amer. J. Psychol.*, **70**, 624.

Fawcett, D. W. (1969). *Die Zelle: Ein Atlas der Ultrastrukture.* Munich & Schwarzenberg.

Feldberg, W. & Sherwood, S. L. (1954). Injections of drug into the lateral ventricles of the cat. *J. Physiol.*, **123**, 148.

Feremutsch, K. (1955). Das Grosshirn einer Mikrocephalia vera. *Wschr. Psychiat. Neurol.*, **129**, 58.

Feremutsch, K. & Grunthal, E. (1952). *Beitrage zur Entwicklungsgeschichte und normalen Anatomie des Gehirns.* Basel: Karger.

Ferrier, D. (1876). *The Function of the Brain.* London: Smith, Elder & Co.

Flechsig, P. E. (1876). *Die Leitungsbahnen im Gehirn und Ruchenmark des Menschen.* Leipzig: Engelmann.

Flechsig, P. E. (1927). *Meine myelogenetische Hirnlehft.* Berlin: Springer.

Fleischhauer, K. (1960a). Fluorescenzmikroskopische Untersuchungen an der Faserglia. *Z. Zellforsch.*, **51**, 467.

Fleischhauer, K. (1960b). Neuroglia, Ergebnisse und Probleme. *Deut. Med. Wschr.*, **85**, 2035.

Fleischhauer, K. (1963). The hippocampus as the site of origin of the seizure discharge produced by tubocurarine acting from the cerebral ventricles. *J. Physiol., Lond.*, **168**, 435.

Fontana, F. (1782). *Treatise on the Venom of the Viper, etc. To which are annexed observations on the primitive structure of the animal body*, etc., 2 vols. London.

Forel, A. H. (1887). Einige hirnanatomische Betrachtungen und Ergebnisse. *Arch. Psychiat. Nervenkr.*, **18**, 162.

Friede, R. L. (1954). Der quantitative Anteil der Glia an der Cortexentwicklung. *Acta Anat.*, **20**, 290.

Fritsch, G. & Hitzig, E. (1870). Uber die elektrische Erregbarkeit des Grosshirns. *Arch. Anat. Physiol.*, p. 332.

Fulton, J. F. (1949). *Physiology of the Nervous System.* Oxford: Oxford University Press.

Fulton, J. F. & Jacobsen, C. F. (1935). The functions of the frontal lobes: a comparative study in monkeys, chimpanzees and man. *Abstr. 2nd Int. Neurol. Cong.* London.

Galambos, R. (1962). *Nerve and Muscles. An Introduction to Biophysics.* London: Doubleday.

Galambos, R. & Morgan, C. T. (1958). *The Neural Basis of Learning.* Handbook of Physiology & Neurophysiology III. Baltimore: Williams & Wilkins.

Gardner, B. T. & Gardener, R. A. (1971). Two way communication with an infant chimpanzee. In *Behaviour of Non-human Primates*, vol. 4, ed. A. M. Schrier & F. Stollnitz. New York: Academic Press.

Gasser, H. S. & Erlanger, J. (1927). The role played by the sizes of the constituent fibers of a nerve trunk in determining the form of action of its action potential wave. *Amer. J. Physiol.*, **80**, 522.

Gastaut, H. (1954). The brain stem and cerebral electrogenesis in relation to consciousness. In *Brain Mechanisms and Consciousness.* Oxford: Blackwell.

Gaze, R. M. (1958). The representation of the retina on the optic lobe of the frog. *Quart. U. exp. Physiol.*, **43**, 209.

Gellerstedt, N. (1933). Zur Kenntnis der Hirnveränderungen bei der normalen Altersinvolution. *Upsala Lak. Förh.*, **38**.

Gerlach, J. von (1872a). Über die Struktur der grauen Substanz des menschlichen Grosshirns. Vorläufige Mittelung. *Zentbl. med. Wiss.*, **10**, 273.

Gerlach, J. von (1872b). Von dem Rüchermark. In Stricker, Handbuch der Lert von der Geweben, vol. 2, pp. 665. London (English translation).

Gilles, F. H., Leviton, A. & Dooling, E. C. (1983). *The Developing Human Brain. Growth and Epidemiologic Neuropathology.* Boston: John Wright.

Gilliatt, R. W. & Pratt, R. T. C. (1952). Disorders of perception and performance in a case of right-sided cerebral thrombosis. *J. Neurol. Neurosurg. Psychiat.*, **15**, 264.

Glees, P. (1940). Termination of optic fibres in the lateral geniculate body. *Nature*, **146**, 747.

Glees, P. (1942). Observations on the structure of the connective tissue sheaths of cutaneous nerves. *J. Anat.*, **77**, 2.

Glees, P. (1944). The contribution of the medial fillet and strio-hypothalamic fibres to the dorsal supra-optic decussation, with a note on the termination of the lateral fillet. *J. Anat.*, **78**, 113.

Glees, P. (1952a). Leistungsfahigkeit von Menschen mit nur einer Hirnhalfte. *Umschau*, **14**, 42.

Glees, P. (1952b). Ludwig Edinger (1855–1918). *J. Neurophysiol.*, **15**, 251.

Glees, P. (1955). *Neuroglia, Morphology and Function.* Oxford: Blackwell.

Glees, P. (1957). *Morphologie und Physiologie des Nervensystems.* Stuttgart: Georg Thieme.

Glees, P. (1958a). The biology of the neuroglia: a summary. In *Biology of Neuroglia*, Ch. 15, ed. W. F. Windle. Springfield (Ill.): Thomas.

Glees, P. (1958b). Die Endigungsweise der ipsilateralen und kontralateralen Sehfasern im Corpus geniculatum laterale des Affen. *Verh. Anat. Ges., Jena*, p. 57.

Glees, P. (1961a). *Experimental Neurology*. Oxford: Clarendon Press.

Glees, P. (1961b). Terminal degeneration and trans-synaptic atrophy in the lateral geniculate body of the monkey. In *The Visual System: Neurophysiology and Psychophysics*, ed. R. Jung & H. Kornhuber. Berlin: Springer.

Glees, P. (1961c). Unser Gehirn nur zur Hälfte benutzt? *Die Welt*, 275/61.

Glees, P. (1962). Das Gehirn. In *Lehrbuch der Physiologie des Menschen*, 2 vols. Munich: Urban & Schwarzenberg.

Glees, P. (1964). Meilensteine in der geschichtlichen Entwicklung der Grosshirnhistologie. In *Med. in Gesch. und Kultur, Boerhaave bis Berger*, pp. 211–24, ed. R. Herrlinger & K. E. Rothschuh. Stuttgart: Gustav Fischer.

Glees, P. (1967). Ist unser Zentralnervensystem links und rechts gleichwertig? *Triangle*, **8**, no. 3.

Glees, P. (1971). *Das Menschliche Gehirn*. Stuttgart: Hippokrates.

Glees, P. (1978). *Il Cervello Umano*. Milan: Feltrinelli.

Glees, P. (1980). Functional reorganization following hemispherectomy in man after small experimental lesions in primates. In *Recovery of Function. Theoretical Considerations for Brain Injury Rehabilitation*, ed. P. Bach-y-Rita. Bern: Hans Huber.

Glees, P. (1982). Evolutional, developmental and clinical aspects of brain stem organisation. In *Tumors of the Central Nervous System in Infancy and Childhood*, eds. D. Voth, P. Gutjahr & C. Langmaid. Berlin: Springer.

Glees, P. (1985). Removal of osmophilic waste material from neurons. In Proceedings of the International Workshop on Age Pigments. Biological Markers in Aging and Environmental Stress? *Arch. Biol. (Brussels)*, **96**, 350.

Glees, P. & Bailey, R. A. (1951). Schichtung und Fasergrösse des Tractus spino-thalamicus des Menschen. *Mschr. Psychiat. Neurol.*, **122**, 129.

Glees, P. & Cole, J. (1954). Comparison of anterior parietal lesions (areas 3, 1 and 2) with posterior parietal lesions (areas 5 and 7) in trained monkeys. International Neurological Congress, Lisbon, 1953.

Glees, P., Cole, J., Whitty, C. W. M. & Cairns, H. (1950). The effects of lesions in the cingular gyrus and adjacent areas in monkeys. *J. Neurol., Lond.*, **13**, 178.

Glees, P. & Griffiths, H. B. (1952). Bilateral destruction of the hippocampus in a case of dementia. *Mschr. Psychiat. Neurol.*, **123**, 193.

Glees, P. & Hasan, M. (1976a). *Lipofuscin in Neuronal Ageing and Diseases*. Stuttgart: Georg Thieme.

Glees, P. & Hasan, M. (1976b). Morphologische und physiologische Grundlagen des zentralen vegetativen Nervensystems. In *Klinische Pathologie des vegetativen Nervensystems*, vol. 1, ed. A. Sturm & W. Birkmayer. Stuttgart: Gustav Fischer.

Glees, P., Hasan, M. & Tischner, K. (1966a). Trans-synaptic neuronal atrophy in the lateral geniculate body of the monkey. *J. Physiol.*, **188**, 17.

Glees, P., Hasan, M. & Tischner, K. (1966b). Ultrastructural features of transneuronal atrophy in monkey geniculate neurones. *Acta Neuropath.*, **7**, 361.

Glees, P. & James, F. E. (1957). Cerebellar abnormality as a possible factor in amentia in a case of microcephaly. *Psychiat. Neurol.*, **134**, 362.

Glees, P. & Le Gros Clark, W. E. (1941). The termination of optic fibres in the lateral geniculate body of the monkey. *J. Anat.*, **75**, 295.

Glees, P. & Meller, K. (1968). *Morphology of Neuroglia*, vol. 1, ed. G. H. Bourne. London: Academic Press.

Glees, P. & Neuhoff, V. (1967). Preparing the lateral geniculate body for various methods assessing trans-synaptic neuronal atrophy. *J. Physiol.*, **191**, 96.

Glees, P. & Spoerri, P. E. (1978). Surface processes of olfactory receptors. *Cell Tissue Res.*, **188**, 49.

Glees, P. & White, W. G. (1958). Resettlement of a case of hemispherectomy for the treatment of infantile hemiplegia. *Trans. Ass. Industr. Med. Officers*, **7**, 127.

Glees, P. & Zander, E. (1950). Der Tractus tegmento-olivaris des Menschen. *Mschr. Psychiat. Neurol.*, **120**, 22.

Godschalk, M., Lemon, R. N., Niss, H. G. & Kuypers, H. G. J. M. (1981). Behaviour of neurons in monkey periarcuate and precontrol cortex before and during visually guided arm and hand movements. *Exp. Brain Res.*, **214**, 113.

Goldscheider, A. (1886). Histologische Untersuchungen über die Endigungsweise der Hautsinnesnerven beim Menschen. *Arch. Anat.*, 191.

Golgi, C. (1886). *Sulla fina anatomia degli organi centrali del sistema nervoso*. Milan.

Golgi, C. (1894). *Untersuchungen uber den feineren Bau des zentralen und peripheren Nervensystems*. Jena: Gustav Fischer.

Goody, W. & Reinhold, M. (1952). Some aspects of human orientation in space. *Brain.*, **75**, 472.

Goody, W. & Reinhold, M. (1953). Some aspects of human orientation in space. *Brain.*, **76**, 337.

Gorski, R. & Wahle, R. (1966). *Brain and Behaviour*, vol. 3. Berkeley: University of California Press.

Graft, A. S. de (1967). *Anatomical Aspects of the Cetacean Brain Stem*, ed. H. J. Prakke & H. M. G. Prakke. Assen: Van Gorcum.

Gray, E. G. (1959). Electron microscopy of synaptic contacts on dendritic spines of the cerebral cortex. *Nature*, **183**, 1592.

Gray, E. G. & Guillery, R. (1966). Synaptic morphology in the normal and degenerating nervous systems. *Int. Rev. Cytol.*, **19**, 173.

Gregory, R. S. (1966). *Eye and Brain: the Psychology of Seeing*. London: World University Library.

Grinvald, A., Anglioter, L., Freeman, D. A., Hiebesheim, R. & Maules, A. (1984). *Nature*, **308**, 848.

Grundfest, H., Shane, A. M. & Freygang, W. (1953). The effect of sodium and potassium on the impedance change accompanying the spike in the squid giant axon. *J. gen. Physiol.*, **37**, 25.

Grünthal, E. (1948). Für Frage der Entstehimg der Mensdenhinus. *Mschr. Psychiat. Neurol.*, **115**, 129.

Guth, L. (1957). The effects of glossopharyngeal nerve transection on the circumvallate papilla of the rat. *Anat. Rec.*, **128**, 715.

Guth, L. (1958). Taste buds on the cat's circumvallate papilla after re-innervation by glossopharyngeal, vagus and hypoglossal nerves. *Anat. Rec.*, **10**, 25.

Guttmann, L. (1953). *Principles of Reconditioning Severely Injured Men*, with particular reference to the management of paraplegia (Symposium on Stress). Washington: Walter Reed.

Haeckel, E. (1874). *Anthropagenie oder Entwicklungsgeschichte des Menschen*. Leipzig: Englemann.

Hallervorden, J. (1957). Das normale und pathologische Altern des Gehirns. *Nervenarzt*, **28**(10), 433.

Hamberger, A., Hansson, H.-A. & Sjöstrand, J. (1971). Surface structure of isolated neurons. Detachment of nerve terminals during axon regeneration. *J. Cell Biol.*, **47**, 319.

Hamlyn, L. H. (1962). The fine structure of the mossy fibre ending in the hippocampus of the rabbit. *J. Anat.*, **96**, part 1.

Hamlyn, L. H. (1963). An electron microscope study of pyramidal neurons in the Ammon's horn of the rabbit. *J. Anat.*, **97**, 189.

Hannover, A. (1840). Die Chromsaure ein vorzugliches Mittel bei mikroskopischen Untersuchungen. *Müller's Physiol.*, 549.

Hansson, H.-A. & Norström, A. (1971). Glial reactions induced by colchicine-treatment of the hypothalamic-neurohypophysial system. *Z. Zellforsch.*, **13**, 294–310.

Hardisty, M. W. (1979). *Biology of the Cytostomes*. London: Chapman & Hall.

Harlow, H. F. (1944). Studies in discrimination learning by monkeys. I The learning of discrimination serves and the reversal of discrimination serves. II Discrimination learning without primary reinforcement. *J. gen. Psychol.*, **30**, 3.

Harlow, H. F., Davis, R. T., Settlage, P. H. & Meyer, D. R. (1952). Analysis of frontal and posterior association syndromes in brain-damaged monkeys. *J. comp. Psychol.*, **45**, 419.

Haug, H. (1967). Uber die exakte Festelling der Anzahl Nervenzellen pro Volumeneinheit des Cortex cerebri. *Acta Anat.*, **67**, 53.

Haug, H. (1970). Der makroskopische Aufbau des Gross-hirns. In *Ergebnisse der Anatomie und Entwicklungs-geschichte*, vol. 43, issue 4. Berlin: Springer.

Haymaker, W. (1969). Effects of ionizing radiation on nervous tissue. In *Structure and Function of the Nervous Tissue III*, ed. G. H. Bourne, pp. 441–518. New York: Academic Press.

Hecht, S., Schaler, S. & Pirenne, M. H. (1942). Energy, quanta and vision. *J. gen. Physiol.*, **25**, 819.

Held, H. (1906). Zur weiteren Kenntnis der Nervendenfusse und zur Struktur der Sehzellen. *Abh. Kgl. sachs Gesellsch. Wissensch., math.-phys. Kl.*, **29**, 143.

Helmholtz, H. (1842). De fabrica systematis nervosi evertebratorum, Berlin (Inaugural dissertation).

Hensel, H. & Zotterman, Y. (1951). The response of mechanoreceptors to thermal stimulation, *J. Physiol., Lond.*, **115**, 16.

Hermann, L. (1883). *Handbuch der Physiologie, F.C.W.* Leipzig: Vogel.

Hess, R. (1964). The EEG in sleep. *Electroenceph. Clin. Neurophysiol.*, **16**, 44–5.

Hess, W. R. (1947). *Vegetative Funktionen und Zwischenhirn*. Basel: Schwabe.

Hess, W. R. (1954). *Das Zwischengehirn Syndrome, Lokalisation Funktion*, 2nd edn. Basel: Schwabe.

Hess, W. R. (1964). Der Schlaf als Phänomen des integralen Organismus. *Praxis*, **41**, 1355.

Hess, W. R. (1965). Sleep as a phenomenon of the integral organism. In *Sleep Mechanisms*, ed. K. Akert, C. Ball & J. P. Schade, pp. 3–8. Amsterdam: Elsevier.

Hill, A. V. (1932). *Chemical Wave Transmission in Nerve*. Cambridge: Cambridge University Press.

Hill, D. K. (1950). The effect of stimulation on the opacity of a crustacean nerve trunk and its relation to fibre diameter. *J. Physiol., Lond.*, **111**, 283.

Hillebrand, H. (1966). Quantitative Untersuchungen über postnatale Entwicklung der Glia im Corpus callosum der Katze. *Z. Zellforsch.*, **79**, 459.

Hodgkin, A. L. (1951). The ionic basis of electrical activity in nerve and muscle. *Biol. Rev.*, **26**, 339.

Hodgkin, A. L. (1958). Ionic movements and electrical activity in giant nerve fibres. *Proc. Roy. Soc. Med.*,: B148, 1.

Hodgkin, A. L. (1964). *The Conduction of the Nervous Impulse*. Liverpool: Liverpool University Press.

Hodgkin, A. L. & Huxley, A. F. (1939). Action potentials rewarded from inside a nerve fibre. *Nature*, **144**, 710.

Hodgkin, A. L. & Huxley, A. F. (1945). Resting and action potentials in single nerve fibres. *J. Physiol., Lond.*, **104**, 176.

Hodgkin, A. L. & Keynes, R. D. (1954). Movements of cations during recovery in nerve. *Soc. Exp. Biol. Sympos.*, **8**, 423.

Horsley, V. (1909). The function of the so-called motor area of the brain. *Brit. med. J.*, **2**, 125.

Hubel, D. H. (1960). Single unit activity in lateral geniculate body and optic tract of unrestrained cats. *J. Physiol., Lond.*, **91**.

Hubel, D. H. & Wiesel, T. N. (1959). Receptive field of single neurones in the cat's striate artex. *J. Physiol., Lond.*, **148**, 574.

Hubel, D. H. & Wiesel, T. N. (1977). Functional architecture of macaque monkey visual cortex. *Proc. Roy. Soc.*, **B198**, 1.

Hubel, D. H. & Wiesel, T. N. (1979). Brain mechanism of vision. *Sci. Amer.*, **24**, 150.

Huisman, A. M., Kuypers, H. G. J. M. & Verburgh, C. A. (1981). Quantitative differences in collateralization of the descending spinal pathways from red nucleus and other brain stem cell groups in rat as demonstrated with the multiple fluorescent retrograde tracer technique. *Brain Res.*, **209**, 271.

Huxley, J. & Kettlewell, H. B. D. (1965). *Charles Darwin and his World*. London: Thames & Hudson.

Huxley, J. S. (1964). Evolution – The Modern Synthesis. New York: Wiley.

Hyden, H. (1960). The neuron. In *The Cell*, vol. 4, p. 215, eds. J. Brachet & A. E. Mirsky. New York: Academic Press.

Irvine, W. (1955). *Apes, Angels and Victorians. A joint biography of Darwin and Huxley.* London: Weidenfeldt & Nicolson.

Jacobsohn, L. (1906). Über die Kerne des menschlichen Hirnstammes. Phys.-math. Klasse, Anhang Abh. 1 Königl. Akad. Wiss.

Jacobsohn, L. (1909). Über die Kerne des menschlichen Hirnstammes. Aus dem Anhang zu den Abhandlungen der koeningl. preuss. Akademie der Wissenschaften.

Jasper, H. H., Proctor, L. D., Knighton, R. S., Noshay, W. C. & Costello, R. T. (eds.) (1958). Reticular Formation of the Brain. Henry Ford Hospital Internal Symposium. Boston: Little & Brown.

Jeffrey, G., Cowey, A. & Kuypers, H. G. J. M. (1981). Bifurcating retinal ganglion cell axons in the rat, demonstrated by retrograde double labelling. *Exp. Brain Res.*, **44**, 34.

Jenkins, W. L. (1938). A critical examination of Nafe's theory of thermal sensitivity. *Amer. J. Psychol.*, **51**, 424.

Jones, D. G. (1975). *Synapses and Synaptosomes: Morphological Aspects.* London: Chapman & Hall.

Joppich, G. & Schulte, F. J. (1968). *Neurologie des Neugeborenen.* Berlin: Springer.

Joseph, J. (1954). Nuclear population change in degenerating posterior column of rabbits spinal cord. *Anat.*, **21**, 356–65.

Jouvet, M. & Jouvet, D. (1966). A study of the neurophysiological mechanisms of dreaming. *Electroenceph. Clin. Neurophysiol.*, **15**, 133–57. In *Sleep, Wakefulness, Dreaming and Memory* (Neurosciences Research Program), eds. W. Nauta, W. Koella & C. Guarton. Brooklin, vol. 4, no. 1 (Mass.).

Jung, R. (1949). Über die Beteiligung des Thalamus, der Stammganglien und des Ammonhorns am Elektro-krampf. *Arch. Psychiat. Z. Neurol.*, **184**, 63.

Jung, R. (1953). Neuronal discharge. Third International Electroencephalogram Congress.

Kandel, E. R. (1983). Neurobiology and molecular biology: the second encounter. *Cold Spring Harbor Symp. Quant. Biol.*, **48**, 891.

Kandel, E. R. & Schwartz, J. H. (eds.) (1982a). *Principles of Neuroscience.* New York: Elsevier.

Kandel, E. R. & Schwartz, J. H. (1982b). Molecular biology of learning: modulation of transmitter release. *Science.*, **218**, 433.

Karchin, A., Wässle, H. & Schnitzer, J. (1986). Immunocytochemical studies on astroglia of the cat retina under normal and pathological conditions. *J. comp. Neurol.*, (in press).

Karlson, P. & Lüscher, M. (1959). 'Pheromones': a new term for a class of biological active substances. *Nature*, **183**, 55–6.

Kastorf, F. (1920). Über die Verschmelzung der Wärmeempfindung bei rhythmisch erfolgenden Reizen. *Z. Biol.*, **71**, 1.

Katz, B. (1952). *Different Forms of Signalling Employed in the Nervous System.* Inaugural lecture delivered at University College, London. London: Lewis.

Kazemi, H. & Johnson, D. C. (1986). Regulation of cerebrospinal fluid acid–base balance. *Physiological Reviews*, **66**, 953.

Kershman, J. (1938). The medulloblast and medulloblastoma. *Arch. Neurol. Psychiat.*, **40**, 937.

Kershman, J. (1939). Genesis of microglia in the human brain. *Arch. Neurol. Psychiat.*, **41**, 24.

Kety, S. S. (1955). Blood flow and metabolism of the human brain in health and disease. In *Neurobiochemistry: The Chemical Dynamics of Brain and Nerve*, eds. Elliott, Page & Quastel. Springfield (Ill.): Thomas.

Keverne, E. B. (1983). Pheromonal influences on the endocrine regulation of reproduction. *Trends in Neurosci.*, **6**, 381.

Kirsche, E. W. (1964). Regenerative Vorgange im Telencephalon von Ambystoma mexicanum. *J. Hirnforsch.*, **6**, no. 6.

Klüver, H. (ed.) (1942). *Visual Mechanism.* Lancaster (Penn.): Cattele Press.

Klüver, H. (1957). *Behaviour Mechanisms in Monkeys.* Chicago: Chicago University Press.

Klüver, H. (1965). Neurobiology of normal and abnormal perception. In *Psychopathology of Perception.* New York: Grune & Stratton.

Koehler, O. (1951). Der Vogelgesang als Vorstufe von Musik und Sprache. *J. Ornithol.*, **93**, part 1.

Koestler, A. (1967). *The Ghost in the Machine.* London: Hutchinson.

Köhler, W. (1925). *The Mentality of Apes.* New York: Harcourt Brace.

Kölliker, R. A. (1853). *Manual of Human Histology.* London.

Kölliker, R. A. (1890). Uber den feineren Bau des Ruckenmarks. *Sitzungsb. phys. med. Gesellsch. Wurzburg*, p. 44.

Kölliker, R. A. (1896). *Handbuch der Gewebelehre der Mausden*, vol. 2 Nervensystem. Leipzig: Engelmann.

Kornmüller, A. E. (1935). Die biolekrischen Erscheinungen architektonischer Felder der Grosshirnrinde. *Biol. Rev.*, **10**, 383.

Kornmüller, A. E. (1947). *Die Elemente der nervosen Tatigkeit.* Stuttgart: Georg Thieme.

Kornmüller, A. E. (1950). Erregbarkeitssteuende Elemente und Systeme des Nervensystems; Grundriss ihrer Morphologie, Physiologie und Klinik. *Fortschr. Neurol. Psychiat.*, **18**, 438.

Kreutzberg, G. W. (1966). Autoradiographische Untersuchung uber die Beteiligung von Gliazellen an der axonalen Reaktion im Facialiskern der Ratte. *Acta Neuropath.*, **7**, 149.

Kreutzberg, G. W. (1969). Neuronal dynamics and axonal flow, IV. Blockage of intraaxonal enzyme transport by colchicine. *Proc. Nat. Acad. Sci. USA*, **62**(3), 722.

Kreutzberg, G. W. & Barron, K. D. (1978). 5-Nucleotidase of microglial cells in facial nucleus during axonal reaction. *J. Neurocytol.*, **7**, 601.

Kreutzberg, G. W., Barron, K. D. & Schubert, P. (1978).

Cytochemical localisation of 5-nucleotidase in glial plasma membranes. *Brain Res.*, **158**, 247.

Kuffler, S. W. (1952). Neurons in the retina: organisation, inhibition and excitation problems. *Cold Spring Harb. Symp. quant. Biol.*, **17**, 281.

Kurth, G. (1965). *Die (Eu) Homininen. Ein Jeweilsbild nach dem Kenntnisstand von 1964. Menschl. Abstammungslehre, Fortschritte der Anthropogenie.* Stuttgart: Gustav Fischer.

Kuypers, H. G. J. M. (1981). Anatomy of the descending pathways. In *Handbook of Physiology – The Nervous System II*, eds. D. B. D. U. A. F. Adolf & C. J. Wilter. Baltimore: Williams & Wilkins.

Kuypers, H. G. J. M., Schwarcbart, M., Resvold, A. & Hishkin, M. (1965). Occipito-temporal corticocortical connections in the rhesus monkey. *Exp. Neurol.*, **2**, 245.

Lamb, T. D. (1986). Transduction in vertebrate photoreception: the roles of cGMP and calcium. *Trends in Neurosci.*, **9**, 224.

Langman, J., Guerrant, R. L. & Freeman, B. G. (1966). Behaviour of neuro-epithelial cells during closure of the neural tube. *J. Comp. Neurol.*, **127**, 399.

Lassek, A. M. (1940). The human pyramidal tract II. A numerical investigation of the Betz cells of the motor area. *Arch. Neurol. Psychiat., Chicago.*, **44**, 718.

Lassek, A. M. (1941a). The pyramidal tract of the monkey. A Betz cell and pyramidal enumeration. *J. comp. Neurol.*, **74**, 193.

Lassek, A. M. (1941b). The human pyramidal tract III. Magnitude of the large cells of the motor area. *Arch. Neurol. Psychiat., Chicago.*, **45**, 964.

Lassek, A. M. (1942a). The pyramidal tract. The effect of pre- and post-central cortical lesions in the fibre components of the pyramids in monkeys. *J. Nerv. Ment. Dis.*, **95**, 721.

Lassek, A. M. (1942b). The pyramidal tract. A study of retrograde degeneration in the monkey. *Arch. neurol. Psychiat., Chicago*, **48**, 561.

Lassek, A. M. (1943). The pyramidal tract. A study of the large motor cells of area 4 and the fibre components of the pyramid in the spider monkey (*Atelus ater*). *J. comp. Neurol.*, **79**, 407.

Lassek, A. M. (1957). *The Human Brain from Primitive to Modern.* Springfield (Ill.): Thomas.

Lassen, N. A., Ingvar, D. H. & Skinhoj, E. (1978). Brain function and blood flow. *Sci. Amer.*, **239**, 50.

Lawson, C. A. (1958). *Language, Thought and the Human Mind.* Ann Arbor (Mich.): University of Michigan Press.

Ledermüller, M. F. (1758). *Versuch zu einer gründlichen Vertheidigung der Samenthierchen, nebst einer Beschreibung der Leeuwenhoekischen Mikroskopen und einem Entwurf zu einer vollständigen Geschichte des Sonnenmikroskopes*, etc. Nürnberg.

Leeuwenhoek, A. (1674–1694). More observations from Mr Leeuwenhoek. *Phil. Trans. Roy. Soc.*, **9**, 178.

Le Gros-Clark, W. E. (1958). *History of Primates.* London: British Museum Publications.

Lemon, R. N. & Muir, R. B. (1983). Responses of hand and forearm muscles to pyramidal tract stimulation during voluntary hand movement in the monkey (*Macaca nemestrina*). *J. Physiol.*, **338**, 31.

Lemon, R. N., Muir, R. B. & Mantel, G. (1983). Control of hand and finger movement in the macaque monkey. *J. Anat.*, **137**, 410.

Lenneberg, E. N. (1967). *Biological Foundation of Language.* New York: Wiley.

LeVay, S., Hubel, D. H. & Wiesel, T. N. (1975). Pattern of ocular dominance columns in macague visual cortex revealed by a reduced silver stain. *J. comp. Neurol.*, **159**, 559.

Levi-Montalcini, R. (1966). The nerve growth factor. In *Molecular Basis of Some Aspects of Mental Activity*, ed. O. Walaas, Proceedings of a NATO Advanced Study Institute held at Drammen, Norway, 2–14 Aug. 1965, vol. 1. London: Academic Press.

Liddell, E. G. T. (1960). *The Discovery of Reflexes.* Oxford: Clarendon Press.

Loewi, O. (1921). Uber humorale Ubertragbarkeit der Herznervirkung. *Pflügers Arch.*, **189**, 239.

Lorenz, K. (1963). *Das sogenannte Bose. Zur Naturgeschichte der Aggression.* Vienna: Borotha-Schoeler.

Lorenz, K. (1965). Uber tierisches und menschliches Verhalten. *Aus dem Werdegang der Verhaltenslehre*, Munich: Piper. (English translation (1966)): *Evolution and Modification of Behavior.* Chicago: The University of Chicago Press.

MacLean, P. D. (1949). Psychosomatic disease and the visceral brain. *Psychosom. Med.*, **11**, 339.

MacLean, P. D. (1954). The limbic system and its hippocampal formation: studies in animals and their possible application to man. *J. Neurosurg.*, **2**, 29.

McFie, J., Piercy, M. F. & Zangwill, O. L. (1950). Visual–spatial agnosia associated with lesions of the right cerebral hemisphere. *Brain*, **73**, 167.

Macphail, E. M. (1982). *Brain and Intelligence in Vertebrates.* Oxford: Clarendon Press.

Magoun, H. W. (1958). *The Waking Brain.* Springfield (Ill.): Thomas.

Mahl, G. F., Rothenberg, A., Delgado, J., Hamlin, H. (1964). Psychological response in the human to intracerebral electrical stimulation. *Psychosom. Med.*, **26**, 4.

Marriott, F. H. C., Morris, V. B. & Pirenne, M.H. (1959). The minimum flux of energy detectable by the human eye. *J. Physiol., Lond.*, **145**, 369.

Martin, J. B., Reichlin, S. & Brown, G. M. (1977). *Clinical Neuroendocrinology.* Philadelphia: F. A. Davis.

Maxwell, D. S. & Kruger, L. (1965). The fine structure of astrocytes in the cerebral cortex and their response to focal injury produced by heavy ionizing particles. *J. Cell Biol.*, **25**, 141.

Meller, K. (1968). *Histo- und Cytogenese der sich entwickelnden Retina. Eine elektronenmikroskopische Studie.* Stuttgart: Gustav Fischer.

Meller, K. & Glees, P. (1969). *Neurobiology of Cerebellar Evolution and Development.* (First International Symposium), American Medical Association.

Milhorat, T. H. (1972). *Hydrocephalus and the Cerebrospinal*

Fluid. Baltimore: Williams & Wilkins.

Minkowski, M. (1913). Experimentelle Untersuchungen über die Beziehungen der Grosshirnrinde und der Netzhaut zu den primären optischen Zentren, besonders zum Corpus geniculatum externum. *Arb. hirnanat. Inst., Zürich.*, **7**, 255.

Mollon, J. D. (1982). Colour vision and colour blindness. In *The Senses*, eds. H. B. Barlow & J. D. Mollon, Cambridge: Cambridge University Press.

Moniz, E. & Lima, A. (1936). Premiers essais de psychochirurgie, technique et résultats. *Lisboa med.*, **13**, 152.

Morgan, C. T. (1961). *Introduction to Psychology*, 2nd edn. London: McGraw-Hill.

Moruzzi, G. & Magoun, H. (1949). Brain stem reticular formation and activation of the EEG. *Electroenceph. clin. Neurophysiol.*, **1**, 455.

Moss, T. H. & Lewkowicz, S. J. (1983). The axon reaction in motor and sensory neurones of mice studied by a monoclonal antibody marker of neurofilament protein. *J. Neurol. Sci.*, **60**, 267.

Mountcastle, V. B. (1967). Modality and topographic properties of single neurons of cat's somatic sensory cortex. *J. Neurophysiol.*, **20**, 408.

Mugnaini, E. & Walberg, F. (1964). Ultrastructure of neuroglia. *Ergeb. Anat. Entwicklungsgesch.*, **37**, 197.

Muir, R. B. & Lemon, R. N. (1983a). Antidromic excitation of motorneurons by intramuscular electrical stimulation. *J. Neurosci. M.*, **8**, 73.

Muir, R. B. & Lemon, R. N. (1983b). Corticospinal neurons with a special role in precision grip. *Brain Res.*, **261**, 312.

Müller, J. (1834). Bestatigung des Bell'schen Lehrsatzes, dass die doppelten Wurzeln der Ruchenmarksnerven verschiedene Funktionen haben, durch neue und entscheidende Experimente. In *Handbuch der Physiologic des Menschen für Vorlesungen*, vol. 1. Koblenz.

Muralt, V. von (1958). *Neue Ergebnisse der Nervenphysiologie*. Berlin: Springer.

Myers, R. E. (1956a). Localization of function within the corpus callosum-visual gnostic transfer. *Anat. Rec.*, **124**, 339.

Myers, R. E. (1956b). Function of corpus callosum in interocular transfer. *Brain*, **79**, 358.

Myers, R. E. (1959). Localization of function in the corpus callosum. *AMA Arch. Neurol. Psychiat.*, **1**, 74.

Myers, R. E. & Sperry, R. W. (1958). Interhemispheric communication through the corpus callosum. *AMA Arch. Neurol. Psychiat.*, **80**, 298.

Nafe, J. P. (1934). The pressure, pain and temperature senses. In *Handbook of General Experimental Psychology*, ed. C. Murchison. Worcester (Mass.): Clark University Press.

Nafe, J. P. (1938). Dr W. L. Jenkins on the vascular theory of warmth and cold. *Amer. J. Physiol.*, **51**, 763.

Netter, F. H. (1953). *Ciba Collection of Medical Illustrations, Vol. 1 The Nervous System*. Ciba Pharmaceuticals Products Inc.

Newport, G. (1834). On the nervous system of the *Sphinx ligustin*. Linn. during the latter stages of its pupa and its imago state and on the means by which its development is affected. *Phil. Trans. Roy. Soc.*, 389–423.

Nisbett, A. (1976). *Konrad Lorenz*. Cambridge: Heffers.

Nissl, Fr. (1894). Uber die Sogenannte. Granula der Nervenzellen. *Neurolog. Zentbl.*, **13**, 676, 781, 810.

Nissl, Fr. (1903). *Die Neuronenlehre und ihre Anhänger*. Jena: Gustav Fischer.

Oertel, O. & Glees, P. (1949). *Leitfaden der Topographischen Anatomie*. Basel: Karger.

Oksche, A. (1964). *The Fine Structure of the Neurosecretory System of Birds in Relation to its Functional Aspects*. Excerpta Medica International Congress Series, no. 83. Amsterdam: Elsevier.

Oksche, A. & Vaupel von Harnack, M. (1965). Vergleichende elektronenmikroskopische Studien am Pinealorgan. In *Structure and Function of the Epiphysis Cerebri*, (Progress in Brain Research, vol. 10). Amsterdam: Elsevier.

Olds, J. & Molner, B. (1954). Positive reinforcement produced by electrical stimulation of septal area and other regions of the brain. *J. Comp. Physiol. Psychol.*, **47**, 419.

Oppenheimer, D. R., Palmer, E. & Weddell, G. (1958). Nerve endings in the conjunctiva. *J. Anat., Lond.*, **92**, 321.

Orbach, H. S., Cohen, L. R. & Grinvald, A. (1985). Optical mapping of electrical activity in rat somato-sensory and visual cortex. *J. Neurosci.*, **5**, 1886.

Orthner, H. (1957). Pathologische Anatomie der vom Hypothalamus ausgelosten Bewusstseinsstorungen. First International Congress of Neurology. *Acta med. Belg.*

Oswald, J. (1962). Sleeping and waking. In *Physiology and Psychology*. Amsterdam: Elsevier.

Oswald, J., Taylor, A. & Triesman, M. (1960). Discriminative responses to stimulation during human sleep. *Brain.*, **83**, 440.

Pallis, C. (1984a). Children in a persistent vegetative state. *Brit. med. J.*, **289**, 1307.

Pallis, C. (1984b). *Brainstem Death: The Evolution of a Concept. Kidney Transplantation*, 2nd edn. New York: Grune & Stratton.

Papez, J. W. (1937). A proposed mechanism of emotions. *Arch. Neurol. Psychiat., Chicago*, **38**, 725.

Papez, J. W. (1958). The visceral brain, its components and connections. In *Reticular Formation of the Brain*, ed. H. H. Jasper, L. D. Proctor, R. S. Knighton, W. C. Noshay & R. T. Costello. Boston: Little, Brown & Co.

Parkenberg, H. (1966). The number of nerve cells in the cerebal cortex of man. *J. comp. Neurol.*, **1**, 128.

Parkinson, J. (1817). *Essay on the Shaking Palsy*. London.

Patten, B. M. (1947). *Human Embryology*. London: Churchill.

Pavlov, I. P. (1927). Conditioned reflexes: An investigation of the activity of the cerebral cortex. *Trans. G.U.*

Peiper, A. (1961). *Die Eigenart der kindlichen hirntatigkeit*, VEB, 3rd edn. Leipzig: Georg Thieme.

Pendleton, C. R. (1928). The cold receptor. *Amer. J. Psychol.*, **40**, 353.

Penfield, W. (1928). Neuroglia and microglia (the metallic). In *McLung's Handbook of Microscopical Techniques*. New York: Hoeber.

Penfield, W. & Boldrey, E. (1937). Somatic motor and sensory representation in the cerebral cortex of Man, as studied by electrical stimulation. *Brain*, **60**(4), 389.

Penfield, W. & Rasmussen, T. (1950). *The Cerebral Cortex of Man*. New York: Macmillan.

Peters, A., Palay, S. L. & Webster, H. de F. (1970). *The Fine Structure of the Nervous System*. New York: Harper & Row.

Pfeifer, R. A. (1930). *Grundlegende Untersuchungen fur die Angioarchitektonik des menschlichen Gehirns*. Berlin: Springer.

Phillips, C. G. (1955). The dimensions of a cortical motor point. *J. Physiol., Lond.*, **129**, 20.

Piaget, J. (1955). *Language and Thought of the Child*. New York: Meridian.

Pirenne, M. H. (1948). Chemistry of visual processes. *Nature*, **161**, 725.

Pirenne, M. H. (1953). Absolute visual thresholds. *J. Physiol., Lond.*, **123**, 409.

Pirenne, M. H. (1956). Physiological mechanisms of vision and the quantum nature of light. *Biol. Rev.*, **31**, 194.

Platzer, W. (1956a). Die Arteria carotis interna im Bereiche des Keilbeines bei Primaten. Über den sogenannten 'Carotis-Siphon'. *Morphol. Jb.*, **97**, 220–48.

Platzer, W. (1956b). Der Carotissiphon und seine anatomische Grundlage. *Röntgenfortschritte*, **84**(2), 200–6.

Ploog, D. (1953). Physiologie und Pathologie des Schafes. *Fortschr. Neurol. Psychiat.*, **21**, 15–56.

Ploog, D. (1961). Untersuchungen am Totenkopfaffen: Die cerebrale Lokalisation der männlichen Genitalfunktion und die Bedeutung dieser Funktion für das soziale Verhalten. *Klin. Wochensch.*, **39**, 12.

Ploog, D. (1964). Verhaltensforschung und Psychiatrie, estratto da Psychiatrie der Gegenwart. In Grundlagenforschung der Psychiatrie, parte B. Berlin: Springer.

Ploog, D., Fichter, M., Doerr, P. & Pkirke, K. M. (1981). Anorexia nervosa – Neurobiologie, Psychosomatik und Verhaltenstherapie. *Internist*, **22**, 7.

Ploog, D. & MacLean, P. D. (1963). On functions of the mamillary bodies in squirrel monkey. *Exp. Neurol.*, **7**, 115. 115.

Polyak, S. (1957). *The Vertebrate Visual System*. Chicago: Chicago University Press.

Porter, K. R. & Bonneville, A. M. (1965). *Einführung in die Feinstruktur von Zellen und Geweben*. Berlin: Springer.

Portmann, A. (1965). *Einführung in die vergleichende Morphologie der Wirbeltiere*. Basel: Schwabe.

Purkinje, J. E. (Purkyně) (1948). *Opera Selecta Cura Societatis Spolek Českých Lékařň*. Prague.

Purves, M. J. (1972). *The Physiology of the Cerebral Circulation*. Cambridge: Cambridge University Press.

Raischle, M. E., Grubb, R. L., Mokhtar, H. G., Eichling, J. O. & Ter-Pogossian, M. M. (1976). Correlation between regional cerebral blood flow and oxidative metabolism. *Arch. neurol.*, **33**, 523.

Ramón y Cajal, S. (1900). *Studien uber die Hirnrinde des Menschen*. Leipzig.

Ramón y Cajal, S. (1928). *Degeneration and Regeneration of the Nervous System*. Oxford: Oxford University Press.

Ramón y Cajal, S. (1935). Die Neuronenlehre. In *Handbook of Neurology*, vol. 1, p. 887. Berlin: Springer.

Ramón y Cajal, S. (1952). Histologie du Systeme Nerveux, de l'Homme et des Vertebrates. Instituto Ramon Y Cajal, Madrid.

Ramón y Cajal, S. (1955). *Studies on the Cerebral Cortex (Limbic Structures)*. London: Lloyds-Luke.

Ranson, S. W. (1911). Non-medullated nerve-fibres in the spinal nerves. *Amer. J. Anat.*, **12**, 67.

Remark, R. (1843). Uber den Inhalt der Nervenprimitiv-rohren. *Arch. Anat. Physiol.*, 197.

Rennels, M. L. & Nelson, E. (1975). Capillary innervation in the mammalian central nervous system. An electron-microscopic demonstration. *Amer. J. Anat.*, **144**, 233.

Retzius, G. (1884). *Das Gehörorgan der Wirbeltiere*. Königliche Buchdruckerei, Stockholm: P. A. Norstedt & Söhne.

Robinson, D. L. & Petersen, S. E. (1985). The neurobiology of attention. In *Mind and Brain*, eds. J. E. LeDoux & W. Hirst, p. 142. Cambridge: Cambridge University Press.

Roessmann, U. & Friede, R. L. (1968). Entry of labelled monocyte cells in the central nervous system. *Acta Neuropathol.*, **10**, 359.

Rose, J. E., Galambos, R. & Hughes, J. R. (1959). Micro-electrode studies of the cochlear nuclei of the cat. *Bull. Johns Hopk. Hosp.*, **104**, 211–51.

Sacks, O. (1982). *Awakenings*. London: Duckworth.

Scheiner, C. (1619). *Oculus seu fundamentum opticum, in quo radius visualis eruitur*. Muhldorf.

Schlesinger, B. (1962). Higher cerebral functions and their clinical disorders. In *The Organic Basis of Psychology and Psychiatry*. New York: Grune & Stratton.

Schwalbe, G. (1881). *Lehrbuch der Neurologie*. Erlangen.

Schwann, T. (1838). *Mikroskopische Untersuchungen über die Ubereinstimmung in der Struktur und dem Wachsthum der Thiere und Pflanzen*. Berlin.

The Biosphere (1970). (Collection of *Scientific American* articles). San Francisco: W. H. Freeman.

Seitelberger, F. (1960). Aufgaben der Hirnforschung in der heutigen Neurologie. *Klin. Wochenschr.*, **72**, 93.

Sherrington, C. S. (1906). *The Integrative Action of the Nervous System*. New York: Charles Scribener's Sons.

Sholl, D. A. (1956). *The Organization of the Cerebral Cortex*. London: Methuen.

Silverstone, T. & Turner, P. (1982). *Drug Treatment in Psychiatry*, 3rd edn. London: Routledge & Kegan Paul.

Skinner, B. F. (1938). *The Behaviour of Organisms: an Experimental Analysis*. New York: Appleton Century.

Spatz, H. (1964). Vergangenheit und Zukunft des Menschenhirns. In *Jahrbuch 1964 der Akademie der Wissenschaften und der Literatur*. Wiesbaden: Franz Steiner.

Sperry, R. W. (1955). On the neural basis of the conditioned response. *Brit. J. Anim. Behav.*, **3**, 41.

Sperry, R. (1964). *Problems Outstanding in the Evolution of Brain Function*. New York: The American Museum of Natural History.

Sperry, R. W. (1966). Brain bisection and mechanisms of consciousness. In *Brain and Conscious Experience*, ed. J. C. Eccles, pp. 298–313. Berlin: Springer.

Sperry, R. W., Stamm, J. S. & Miner, N. (1956). Relearning tests for interocular transfer following division of optic chiasma and corpus callosum in cats. *J. comp. Physiol. Psychol.*, **49**, 529.

Spoerri, P. E. & Glees, P. (1977). Subsurface cisterns in the Cynomonolgus retina. *Cell. Tiss. Res.*, **182**, 33.

Stämpfli, R. (1954). Saltatory conduction in nerves. *Physiol. Rev.*, **34**, 101.

Stephan, H. (1967). Zur Entwicklungshöhe der Primaten nach Merkmalen des Gehirns. In *Neue Ergebnisse der Primatologie*. Stuttgart: Gustav Fischer.

Stephan, H. & Andy, Q. J. (1964). Quantitative comparisons of brain structures from insectivores to primates. *Progr. Brain Res.*, **3**.

Steven, D. H. (1981). *Anatomy of the Domestic Animals: III The Cerebral Circulation*. University of Cambridge, Subdepartment of Veterinary Anatomy Publications.

Stilling, B. (1859). *Neue Untersuchungen über den Bau des Rückenmarks*. Kassel.

Stirling, W. (1876). On the reflex functions of the spinal cord. *Edinb. med. J.*, **21**(ii), 914, 1092.

Stöhr Jr., P. (1928a). Das periphere Nervensystem. *Mollendorffs Handb. mikr. Anat. Menschen*, **4**, 202.

Stöhr, P. (1928b). *Mikroskopische Anatomie des Vegetativen Nervensystems*. Berlin: Springer.

Stöhr, P. (1951). *Lehrbuch der Histologie und Mikroskopischen Anatomie der Menschen*. Berlin: Springer.

Strugnold, H. & Karbe, M. (1925). Die Topographie des Kältesinnes auf Cornea und Conjunction. *Z. Biol.*, **83**, 189.

Stryer, L. (1986). Cyclic GMP cascade of vision. *Ann. Rev. Neurosci.*, **9**, 87–119.

Sunderland, S. (1968). *Nerves and Nerve Injuries*. London: Livingstone.

Szenágothai, J. & Rajkovits, K. (1959). Über den Ursprung der Kletterfasern des Kleinhirns. *Z. Anat. Entw. Gesch.*, **121**, 130–41.

Taggert, P. & Gibbons, D. (1967). Motor-car and the heart rate. *Brit. med. J.*, **1**, 411.

Talbot, S. A. & Marshall, W. H. (1941). Physiological studies on neural mechanisms of visual localization and discrimination. *Ass. Res. Ophthal. 12th Annual Meeting*, p. 63.

Tasaki, I. (1948). The excitatory and recovery process in the nerve fibre as modified by temperature changes. *Biochem. Biophys. Acta*, **3**, 498.

Tasaki, I. (1952). Properties of myelinated fibres in frog sciatic nerve and in the spinal cord as examined with microelectrodes. *Jap. J. Physiol.*, **3**, 73.

Tasaki, I. & Freygang, W. H., Jr (1955). The parallelism between the action current and membrane resistance at a node of Ranvier. *J. gen. Physiol.*, **39**, 211.

Tasaki, I. & Takeuchi, T. (1941). Der am Ranvierschen Knoten entstehende Aktionsstrom und seine Bedeutung für die Erregungsleitung. *Pflügers Arch. ges. Physiol.*, **244**, 696.

Teuber, H. L., Battersby, W. S. & Bender, M. B. (1960). *Visual Field Defects after Penetrating Missile Wounds of the Brain*. Cambridge (Mass.): for the Commonwealth Fund by Cambridge–Harvard University Press.

Thenius, R. & Hofer, H. (1960). *Stammesgeschichte der Säugetiere, Abschn. 3, Palaoneurolgie*. Berlin: Springer.

Thomas, T. N. & Redburn, D. A. (1979). 5-Hydroxy-tryptamine-neurotransmitter of bovine retina. *Exp. Eye Res.*, **28**, 55–61.

Thorpe, W. H. (1956). *Learning and Instinct in Animals*. London: Methuen.

Thuiller, G., Rumpf, P. & Thuiller, J. (1959). Préparation et étude pharmacologique préliminaire des esters diméthylaminoéthyliques de divers acides agissant comme régulateurs de croissance des végétaux. *C.R. hebdo. seances Acad. Sci.*, **249**, 2081.

Tinbergen, N. (1951). *The Study of Instinct*. Oxford: Clarendon Press.

Tobias, P. V. (1969). Brain-size, grey matter and race – fact or fiction?, *Amer. J. Phys. Anthrop.*, **32**, 3.

Toole, J. F. & Patel, A. N. (1967). *Cerebrovascular Disorders*. New York: McGraw-Hill.

Truex, R. C. (1959). *Human Neuroanatomy*. Baltimore: Williams & Wilkins.

Uchizono, K. (1975). *Excitation and Inhibition: Synaptic Morphology*. Tokyo: Igaku Shoin.

Ule, G. (1950). Korsakow-Psychose nach doppelseitiger Ammonshornzerstörung mit transneuronaler Degeneration der Corpora mammillaria. *Deut. Z. Nervenhk.*, **156**, 446.

Valentin, G. (1836). Uber den Verlauf aund die letzten Enden der Nerven. *Nova Acta Akad. nat. cur.*, **18**, 51.

Vaughn, J. E., Lowary Hinds, P. & Shoff, R. P. (1970). Electronmicroscopic studies of Wallerian degeneration in rat optic nerves. I. The multipotential glia. *J. comp. Neurol.*, **140**, 175.

Vaughn, J. E. & Pease, D. C. (1970). Electronmicroscopic studies of Wallerian degeneration in rat optic nerves. II. Astrocytes, oligodendrocytes and advential cells. *J. comp. Neurol.*, **140**, 207.

Vogel, W. (1962). See Glees (1964), Fig. 5.

Vogt, O. & Vogt, C. (1906). Der Wert der myelogenetischen Felder der Grosshirnrinde (Cortex Palii). *Anat. Anz., Jena.*, **29**, 273.

Vogt, O. & Vogt, C. (1919). Die psychologische Bedeutung der architektonischen Rindenreizung. *J. Psychol.*, **25**, suppl. 1, 127.

Voth, D. & Glees, P. (1985). *Cerebral Vascular Spasm*. Berlin: Walter de Gruyter.

Wagner, H.-J., Pilgrim, Ch. & Brandl, J. (1974). Penetration and removal of horseradish peroxidase injected into the cerebrospinal fluid. Role of cerebral perivascular spaces, endothelium and microglia. *J. Acta neuropath.* (Berlin), **27**, 299–315.

Wald, G. (1968). The molecular basis of visual excitation. *Nature*, **219**, 800.

Waldeyer-Hartz, H. W. G. von (1891). Über einige neuere Forschungen im Gebiete der Anatomie des Central-nervensystems. *Deut. med. Wschr.*, **17**, 1231, 1244, 1267, 1287, 1331, 1352.

Walter, W. Grey (1953). *The Living Brain*. New York: W. W. Norton.

Wässle, H. (1982). Morphological types and central projections of ganglion cells in the cat retina. In *Progress in Retinal Research*, ed. N. Osborne & G. Chader. Oxford: Pergamon Press.

Wässle, H. (1984). Retinale Ganglienzellen und ihre Projektion in die visuellen Gehirnzentren. In *Pathophysiologie des Sehens*, ed. V. Herzan. Stuttgart: Ferdinand Enke.

Weddell, G. (1941). The pattern of cutaneous innervation in relation to cutaneous sensibility. *J. Anat., Lond.*, **75**, 346.

Weddell, G., Palmer, E. & Pallie, W. (1955). Nerve endings in mammalian skin. *Biol. Rev.*, **30**, 159.

Wehmeyer, H. & Casers, H. (1958). Bioelektrische Registrierung der Schlaf-Wach-Periodik beim Tier. *Pflügers Arch. ges. Physiol.*, **267**(3), 298.

Weigert, C. (1885). Uber Schnittserien von Celloidinpraparten des Centralnervensystems zum Zwecke der Marscheidenfärbung. *Z. Wissen. med.*, **2**, 49, 495.

Weigert, C. (1891). Zur Markscheidenfarbung. *Deut. med. Wschr.*, 42.

Weigert, C. (1895). Bertrage zue Kenntnis der normalen menschlichen Neuroglia. In *Festschrift 5o jahr. Jub. Arztl. Verein zu Frankfurt a.M.* Frankfurt.

Weil-Malherbe, H. (1952). Der Energiestoffwechsel des Nervengewebes und sein Zusammenhang mit der Funktion. In *Die Chemie und der Stoffwechsel des Neuvengewebes*. 3rd Colloquium Ges. phyiol. Chemie. Berlin: Springer.

Wendell-Smith, C. P., Blunt, M. J., Baldwin, F. & Paisley, P. B. (1965). Neurone-satellite cell relationship. *Nature.*, **205**, 781.

Willis, T. (1664). Quoted in Purves (1972).

Wilson, S. A. (1913–1914). An experimental research into the anatomy and physiology of the corpus striatum. *Brain*, **36**, 427.

Wolff, J. R. (1965). Elektronenmikroskopische Untersuchungen über Struktur und Gestalt von Astrozyten fortsätzen. *Z. Zellforsch.*, **66**, 811.

Wolff, J. R. (1970). Der Astrocyt als Verbindungsglied zwischen Kapillare und Nervenzellen. *Triangle*, **9**, 153.

Wolstenholme, G. E. W. & O'Connor, M. (1961). Nature of sleep. In *Ciba Foundation Symposium*. Edinburgh: Churchill Livingstone.

Wüstenfeldt, E. (1957). Experimentelle Untersuchungen zum Problem der Schallanalyse im Innenohr. *Z. mikrosk.- anat. Forsch.*, **63**, 327.

Yamada, E. (1955). The fine structure of the gall bladder epithelium of the mouse. *J. biophys. biochem. Cytol.*, **1**, 445.

Young, R. W. (1978). Receptor structure and renewal. *Vision Res.*, **18**, 573.

Zimmermann, E., Karsh, D. & Humbertson, A., Jr (1972). Initiating factors in perineuronal cell hyperplasia associated with chromatolytic neurons. *Z. Zellforsch.*, **114**, 73.

INDEX